GLUCOSE HOMEOSTASIS AND INSULIN RESISTANCE

Leszek Szablewski

Department of General Biology and Parasitology, Center of Biostructure, Medical University of Warsaw. 5 Chalubinskiego Str., 02-004 Warsaw, Poland.
E-mail: leszek.szablewski@wum.edu.pl

CONTENTS

FOREWORD

Insulin resistance is generally taken to mean as a reduced ability of insulin to stimulate glucose transport and utilization. It is a major problem associated with type 2 diabetes mellitus (non-insulin-dependent diabetes mellitus) and is increasing rapidly worldwide. As least one-in-ten people today are destined, on current trends, to develop diabetes at some point during their lifetime. The total number of individuals with diabetes worldwide is scheduled to double in a generation. It is not however well known that insulin resistance also increases the risk of cardiovascular disease.

The progress in molecular biology, genetics, epidemiology and in clinical applications notwithstanding, much more needs to be done. It will be of great importance to identify the molecular mechanisms of insulin resistance and establish most effective combinatorial therapies.

The book entitled "Glucose homeostasis and insulin resistance" edited by dr. Leszek Szablewski provides a broad overview of the molecular, biochemical, and clinical aspects of glucose metabolism and insulin resistance. The chapters will make the reader acquainted with a variety of topics ranging from glucose metabolism and glucose transporters, the hormonal regulation of glucose homeostasis, to insulin resistance and characterization of novel pharmacological approaches on emerging targets for the treatment of diabetes. The non-pharmacological modes of therapy, physical exercise, diet, and weight loss are also included.

Prof. Jacek Malejczyk
Chair and Department of Histology and Embryology,
Center of Biostructure,
Medical University of Warsaw,
Poland

PREFACE

The World Health Organization has defined type 2 diabetes mellitus, a progressive worldwide epidemic. The number of people diagnosed with type 2 diabetes is increasing at an alarming rate in the western societies. The statistics are alarming; 30 million people were diagnosed with diabetes world-wide in 1985. By 1995, the number had risen to 135 million. It has been estimated that by 2010, 220 million people worldwide will be affected by the disease, and at the current rate, there will be some 300 million by the year 2025 as predicted by the WHO. The prevalence of all forms of diabetes is estimated to be 2 – 3% of the world's population, with the number of diabetic patients increasing by 4 – 5% per annum. Moreover, many people with diabetes remain undiagnosed.

The recent and dramatic increase in the prevalence of diabetes can be attributed to several factors. Diabetes has shadowed the spread of the so-called "modern western lifestyle". The westernized high caloric diet (including sucrose, fructose and high saturated fats) has a strong influence on the disturbance of the normal glucose and lipid metabolism leading to the progression of obesity. On the other hand, obesity is strongly associated with type 2 diabetes. It is notable that obesity is present in approximately 80 – 90% of diabetic patients. Obesity also exacerbates the metabolic abnormalities linked to type 2 diabetes, particularly hyperglycemia, hyperlipidemia and hypertension. Diabetes is currently the fifth leading cause of death in the United States. Approximately 95% of all patients with diabetes have type 2 disease.

Type 2 diabetes is the clinical manifestation of long-term metabolic abnormalities involving multiple organs and hormonal pathways that impair the body's ability to maintain glucose homeostasis. This type of diabetes is characterized by impaired insulin secretion from pancreatic β-cells and increased insulin resistance in peripheral tissues resulting in hyperglycemia. Type 2 diabetes mellitus results when insulin secretion by the endocrine pancreas fails to compense for insulin resistance in peripheral tissues. Once type 2 diabetes mellitus has been diagnosed, β-cell function is reduced by up to 50%. Prolonged elevation of blood glucose concentrations causes a number of complications like blindness, renal failure, cardiac and peripheral vascular disease, neuropathy, foot ulcers, and limb amputation. Vascular complications represent the leading cause of mortality and morbidity in diabetic patients. Approximately, 65% of deaths among diabetic patients are due to cardiovascular and cerebrovascular diseases, including myocardial ischemia and stroke.

Leszek Szablewski
Department of General Biology and Parasitology,
Center of Biostructure,
Medical University of Warsaw

CHAPTER 1

Glucose and Lipid Metabolism

A. Glucose Metabolism

Abstract: Glucose is an essential metabolic substrate of all mammalian cells. D-glucose is the major carbohydrate presented to the cell for energy production and many other anabolic requirements. Under normal physiological conditions, it is the sole source energy for the brain. Glucose is obtained directly from the diet. Dietary carbohydrates from which humans gain energy enter the body in different forms, such as monosaccharides, disaccharides, and polysaccharides and more so, also by the synthesis of other substrates in organs such as the liver. Glucose and other monosaccharides are transported across the intestinal wall to the hepatic portal vein and then to liver cells and other tissues. There they are converted to fatty acids, amino acids and glycogen (the liver stores excess glucose as glycogen and little glucose is normally converted to fat), or are oxidized by the various catabolic pathways of cells. In the first rate-determining step of metabolism, glucose is transported across the plasma membrane by the facilitative glucose transporters. Hexokinase then phosphorylates glucose to glucoso-6-phosphate. The product generally enters the glycolytic pathway, generating NADH, ATP, and pyruvate, or the pentose phosphate pathway. In the presence of sufficient oxygen, pyruvate can be fed into mitochondria and fully oxidized to produce more ATP. When oxygen is limited, pyruvate is disposed in the form of lactate and glycolysis becomes the main source for ATP production. Pentose phosphate pathway plays an important role in the synthesis of pentose sugars for DNA and RNA, as well as generation of NADPH for the synthesis of lipids.

GENERAL INFORMATION ON GLUCOSE METABOLISM

Carbohydrate metabolism denotes the various biochemical processes responsible for the formation, breakdown and interconversion of carbohydrates in living organisms. Most mammalian cells depend on a continuous supply of a precursor of glycoproteins, triglycerides and glycogen. Glucose is also an important source of energy being derived by generating ATP (adenosine triphosphate). The major source of dietary carbohydrate for humans is starch from consumed plants. This is supplemented with a small amount of glycogen from animal tissue, and disaccharides such as sucrose from products containing refined sugar and lactose in milk. Digestion in the gut converts carbohydrate (not all, as for example cellulose) to monosaccharides, such as glucose, fructose or galactose. Fructose and galactose are transported to the liver. In this organ, the mentioned monosaccharides are converted to glucose.

Monosaccharides enter metabolism through phosphorylation; they react with ATP and a kinase to yield phosphorylates derivatives. Glucose can be phosphorylated by either hexokinase or glucokinase. The former is involved in the cell's metabolism. Glucokinase is implicated in the either energy storage or in glucose-signaling system. Fructose metabolism is initiated through fructokinase (Fig. **1**) while galactokinase (Fig. **2**) is the first enzyme involved in galactose metabolism.

In the body carbohydrates, and especially glucose, undergo one of the few metabolic fates: 1). It is catabolised to produce high energy product, adenosine triphosphate (ATP). This process occurs in all peripheral tissues, particularly the brain, muscle and kidney. The first step of this process is glycolysis which is the process of oxidation metabolism of glucose molecules to obtain ATP and pyruvate. Pyruvate from glycolysis enters the Krebs cycle in aerobic organisms. 2) Glucose is stored as glycogen in liver and muscle. This process is called glycogenesis which prevents excessive osmotic pressure buildup inside the cell. 3) Glycogenolysis – the breakdown of glycogen into glucose, which provides a glucose supply for glucose-dependent tissues. 4) Gluconeogenesis the *de novo* synthesis of glucose molecules from simple organic compounds. An example in humans is the conversion of a few amino acids in cellular protein to glucose. 5) It is converted to fatty acids and in adipose tissue, the fatty acids are stored as triglycerides (Fig. **3**). The other metabolic pathways of carbohydrates are: the pentose phosphate pathway, which acts in the conversion of hexoses into pentoses and in NADPH (Nicotinamide adenine dinucleotide phosphate) regeneration and carbon fixation (or photosynthesis), in which CO_2 is reduced to carbohydrate – only in plants, algae and bacteria.

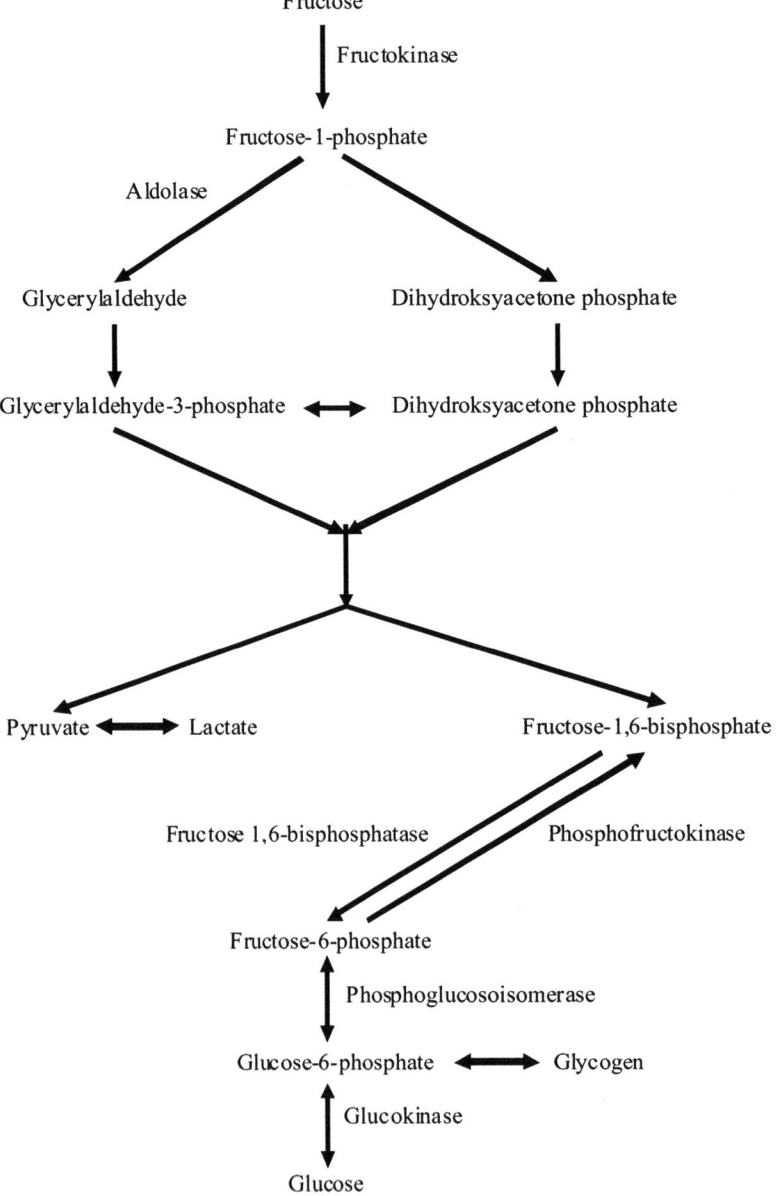

Figure 1: Utilization of fructose in the liver [1].

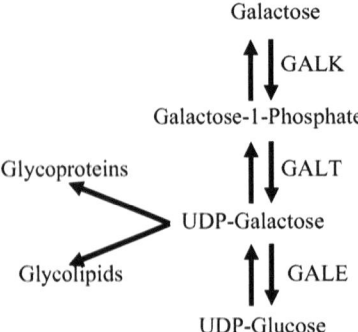

Figure 2: Utilization of galactose in the liver [2]. (GALK – Galactokinase, GALT – Galactose-1-phosphate uridiltransferase, GALE – Uridine diphosphate galactose-4-epimerase, UDP-Galactose – Uridine diphosphate galactose, UDP-glucose – Uridine diphosphate glucose.

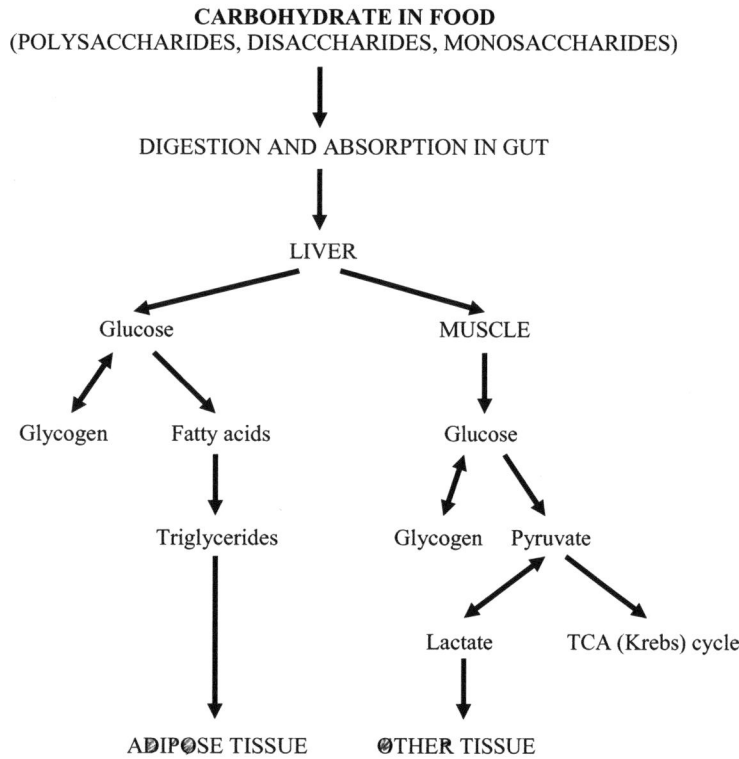

Figure 3: Carbohydrate metabolism in body [3].

GLUCOSE AS A SOURCE OF CELLULAR ENERGY

Glucose is rapidly metabolized to produce ATP, a high energy end product. Because of the cell's high metabolic demand for ATP, glucose is oxidized through a large series of reactions that extract the greatest amount of possible energy from it. The first pathway which begins the complete oxidation of glucose is called glycolysis which takes place in the cytoplasm of the cell.

Glycolysis

Oxidation of glucose to pyruvate is called glycolysis. It was first described by Embden-Meyerhof and Parnas. Hence it is also called as Embden-Meyerhof pathway. Glycolysis occurs virtually in all tissues. Erythrocytes and nervous tissues derive energy mainly from glycolysis. This pathway is unique in the sense that it can proceed in both aerobic (presence of O_2) and anaerobic (absence O_2) conditions.

Glycolysis is the pathway which cleaves the six carbon glucose molecule ($C_6H_{12}O_6$) into two molecules of the three carbon compound pyruvate ($C_3H_3O_3^-$). During the first four steps, glucose undergoes several energy-absorbing steps to facilitate the splitting of glucose into two molecules of glycerylaldehyde-3-phosphate. The following sequences of glycolysis are known collectively as the pay-off phase, where energy is harvested. The end result of glycolysis is two molecules of ATP and two molecules of NADH (Fig. **4**).

One oxidation reaction occurs in the latter part of the pathway. As an electron acceptor, NAD (Nicotinamide adenine dinucleotide) is used. This cofactor is present only in limited amounts and once reduced to NADH, as in this reaction, it must be re-oxidized to NAD to permit continuation of the pathway. This process occurs by the one of the two methods: aerobic metabolism of glucose or anaerobic glycolysis.

Oxidative Decarboxylation

During aerobic metabolism of glucose, pyruvate is transported inside mitochondria. In the mitochondria, pyruvate is oxidized and during this reaction, NAD is uses as an electron and proton acceptor. This process is called oxidative decarboxylation (also known as pyruvate decarboxylation, transition reaction or link reaction) and pyruvate is converted to acetyl coenzyme-A (abbreviated as "acetyl-CoA") (Fig. **5**). Pyruvate dehydrogenase catalyzes the conversion of pyruvate into acetyl-CoA through oxidative decarboxylation. The carboxyl group of pyruvate leaves the molecule as CO_2 and the remaining two carbons become acetyl-CoA.

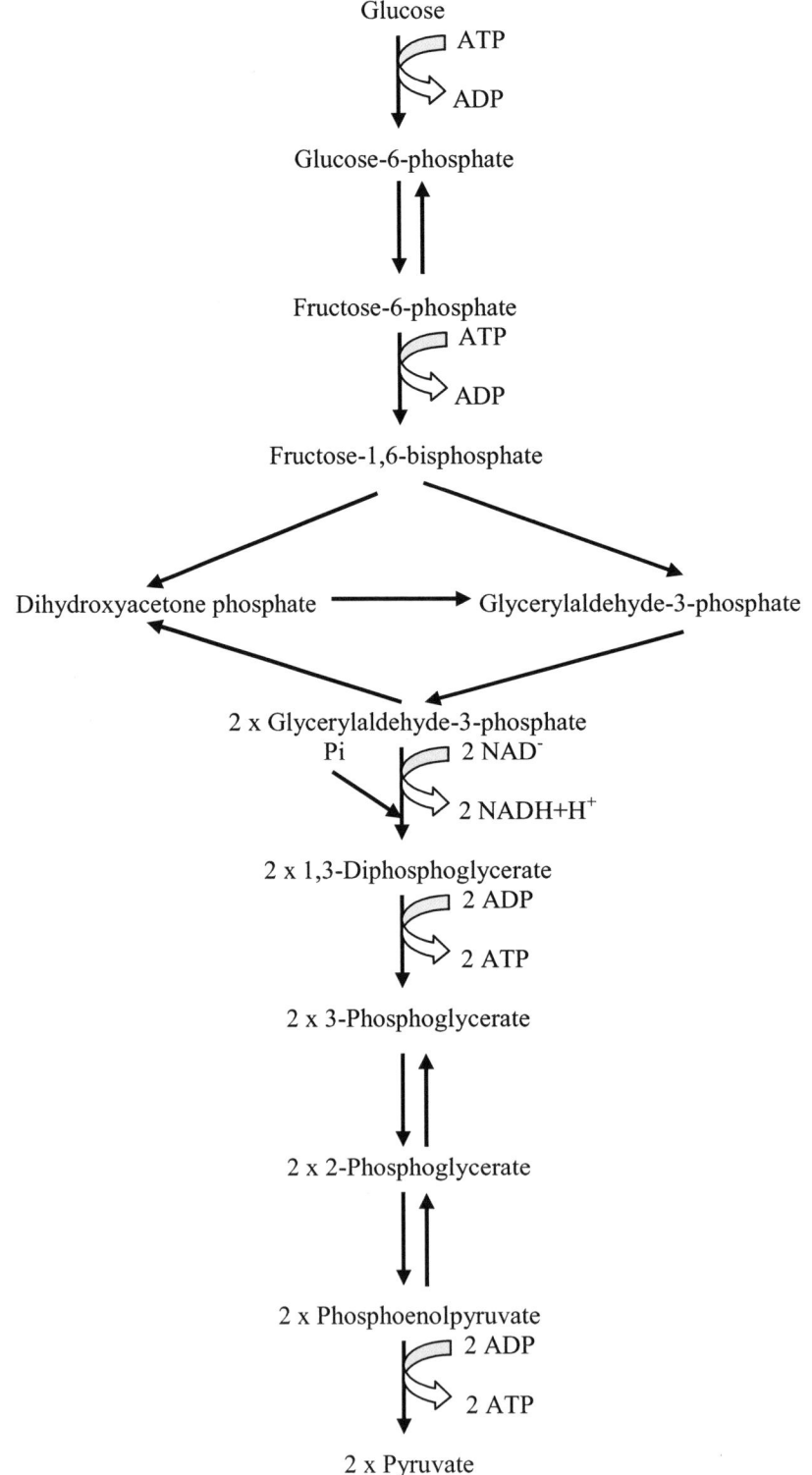

Figure 4: The diagram an outline of glycolysis [3].

$$\text{1) Pyruvate} + \text{TPP} \xrightarrow{\text{E1}} \text{hydroxyethyl-TPP} + CO_2$$

$$\text{2) Hydroxyethyl-TPP} + \text{lipoamide} \xrightarrow{\text{E1}} \text{S-acetyldihydrolipoamide} + \text{TPP}$$

$$\text{3) S-acetyldihydrolipoamide} + \text{CoA-SH} \xrightarrow{\text{E2}} \text{dihydrolipoamide} + \text{acetyl-CoA}$$

$$\text{4) Dihydrolipoamide} + \text{FAD} \xrightarrow{\text{E3}} \text{lipoamide} + FADH_2$$

$$\text{5) } FADH_2 + NAD^+ \xrightarrow{\text{E3}} \text{FAD} + \text{NADH} + H^+$$

Figure 5: Oxidative decarboxylation [4]. The process is catalyzed by three enzymes: pyruvate dehydrogenase (E1), dihydrolipoamide transacetylase (E2), dihydrolipoamide dehydrogenase (E3) and five coenzymes (includes NAD^+ and coenzyme A which appear in the overall reaction, as well as thiamine pyrophosphate, lipoic acid, and flavin adenine dinucleotide – attached to E1, E2, and E3, respectively). TPP – coenzyme thiamine pyrophosphate, FAD – flavin adenine dinucleotide [4, modified].

The overall equation can be summarized as:

$$\text{2 Pyruvate} + \text{2 } NAD^+ + \text{2 CoA-SH} \rightarrow \text{2 Acetyl-CoA} + \text{2 } CO_2 + \text{2 NADH} + H^+$$

This reaction occurs twice since each glucose (6 carbons) produce 2 pyruvates (3 carbons each). Consequently, these processes produce 2 NADH + H^+

Krebs Cycle

Further series of reactions is collectively called "Krebs Cycle", also known as the "Citric Acid Cycle" or the "Tricarboxylic Acid Cycle" (Fig. **6**). Through a series of reactions, acetyl-CoA is oxidized ultimately to CO_2. The Krebs cycle is one of the most important reaction sequences in biochemistry. Not only is this series of reactions responsible for most of the energy needs in complex organisms, the molecules that are produced in these reactions can be used as building blocks for a large number of important processes, including the synthesis of fatty acids, steroids, cholesterol, amino acids for building proteins, and the purines and pyrimidines used in the synthesis of DNA.

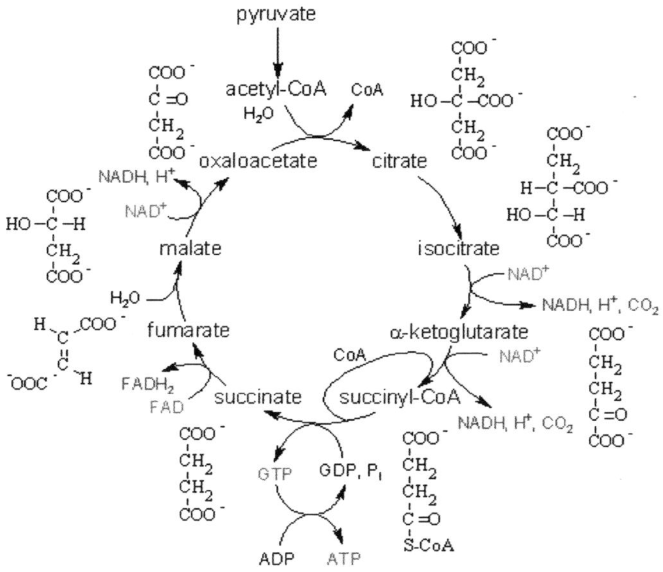

Figure 6: Overview of Krebs cycle [3, 4]

Fuel for the Krebs cycle comes from lipids (fats), carbohydrates, and proteins (amino acids), which produce the molecule acetyl-CoA. Acetyl coenzyme-A reacts in the first step of the eight sequences of reactions that comprise the Krebs cycle, all of which occur inside mitochondria (mitochondrial matrix) of eukaryotic cells. While the Krebs cycle does produce CO_2, this cycle does not produce significant chemical energy in the form of ATP directly. This reaction sequence does not require any oxygen. Instead, this cycle produces NADH + H^+ and $FADH_2$, which feed into the respiratory cycle, also located inside the mitochondria (inner mitochondrial membrane). It is the electron transport chain that is responsible for the production of large quantities of ATP and consumption of oxygen. In addition, the electron transport chain converts NADH + H^+ and $FADH_2$ into reactants that the Krebs cycle requires to function. Thus, if oxygen is not present, the electron transport chain cannot function, which halts the Krebs cycle. For this reason, the Krebs cycle is considered an anaerobic pathway for energy production.

If carbohydrates are the fuel for Krebs cycle, this cycle occurs twice since each glucose produces 2 pyruvates and then in the process of oxidative decarboxylation two molecules of acetyl-CoA.

Electron Transport Chain

Mitochondria is the site of oxidative phosphorylation, a series of reactions that utilize the energy from NADH + H^+ and $FADH_2$ electron carriers to produce more ATP. Embedded in the inner membrane of the mitochondria are the series of proteins that use the stored energy from NADH + H^+ and $FADH_2$ to pump protons into the membrane space. This results in an electrical and chemical gradient of protons. The enzyme ATP synthase (ATPase) uses the proton gradient to drive the reaction of producing ATP from ADP and inorganic phosphate (Fig. **7**).

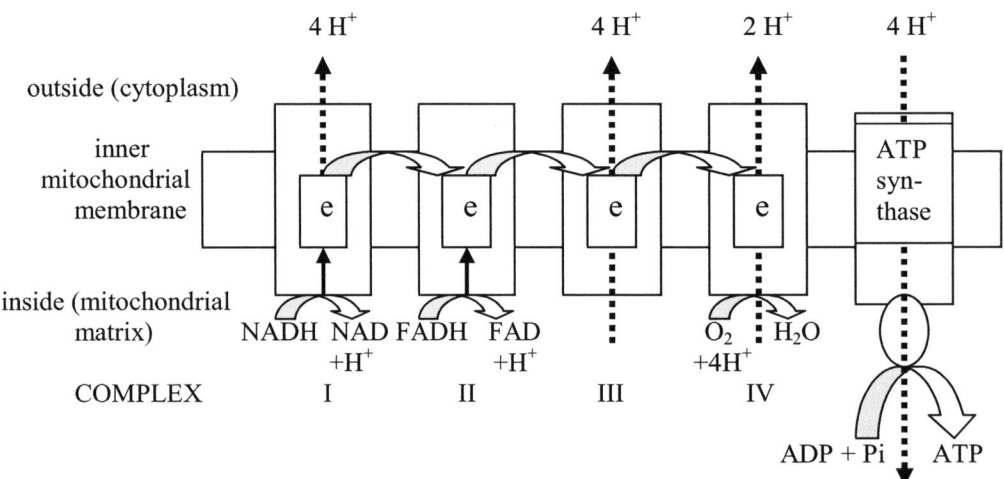

Figure 7: Electron transport chain and proton gradient formation in the mitochondria [3, 4, modified].

The electron transport chain consists of a series of proteins (called cytochromes) that are embedded in the inner mitochondria membrane and an enzyme ATP synthase (ATPase). There are four complexes, namely, I, II, III, IV. Ubiquinone (within the membrane) carries the electrons between complexes I and III, and cytochrome *c* (in the membrane space) carries the electrons between complexes III and IV.

Reduced NAD (as NADH + H^+) enter the chain at complex I, releasing hydrogen atoms which split into protons (H^+) and electrons (e^-). Reduced FAD (as $FADH_2$) does the same but enters the chain at complex II.

The electrons are successively passed down the chain of cytochromes from I to IV, each time releasing some their energy. This energy is then used by complexes I, III, and IV to pump protons actively across the membrane into the intermembrane space (complex II isn't a proton pump).

In complex IV, the electrons are combined with protons and oxygen to form water, the final end-product. The oxygen acts as the final electron acceptor and without oxygen, soothe reaction does not proceed and therefore only anaerobic respiration is possible.

The energy from the electrons is now stored in the form of a proton gradient across the inner mitochondrial membrane and the reservoir of proton ions creates a chemiosmotic gradient across the membrane. Thus, the protons move back into the matrix down this chemiosmotic gradient, but can only do so through the ATP synthase. The enzyme ATPase is of mushroom shape, with the "stalk" (F0 subunit) embedded in the membrane and the "head" (F1 subunit) goes through a series of conformational changes, which cause ADP (adenosine diphosphate) and Pi (inorganic phosphate) to be bound together to form ATP. The end result of electron transport chain is three molecules of ATP, if a donor of protons and electrons is NADH + H$^+$, and one molecule of H_2O. In the case of FADH$_2$ the end result of electron transport chain is two molecules of ATP and one molecule of H_2O (Fig. **8**).

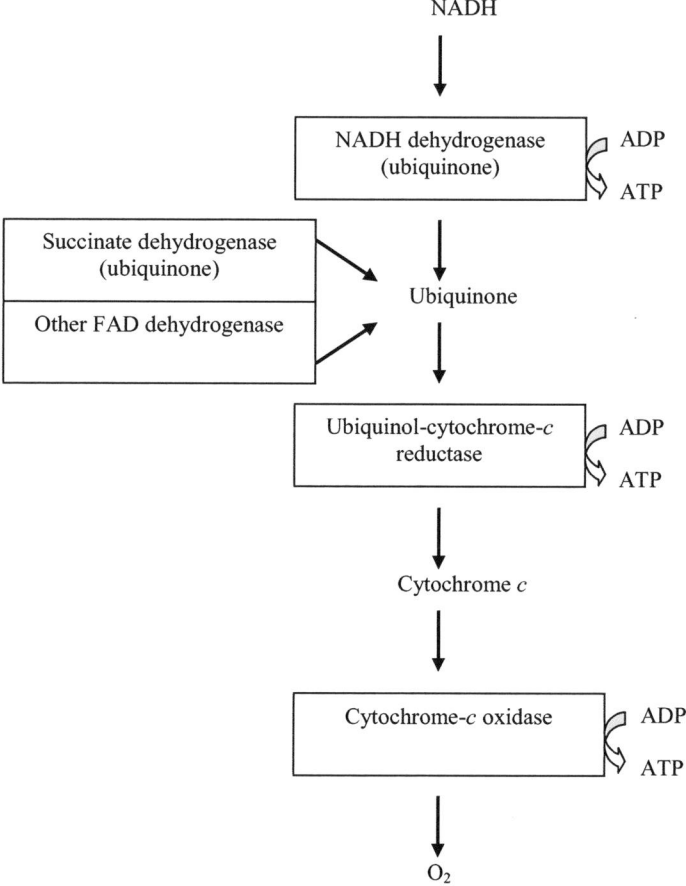

Figure 8: Synthesis of ATP during electron transport chain [3, 4, modified].

The Metabolism of Lactate

The anaerobic glycolysis occurs in the absence of oxygen (anaerobically). This single reaction is ideally suited to utilization in heavily exercising muscle where oxygen supply is often insufficient to meet the demands of aerobic metabolism. During anaerobic glycolysis, earlier obtained pyruvate is reduced to a compound called lactate (or, as in the case of yeast, the first step is a decarboxylation of pyruvate and then, acetylaldehyde is reduced to an ethanol). The reduction of pyruvate to lactate is coupled to the oxidation of NADH + H$^+$ to NAD. Glycolysis and reduction of pyruvate to lactate are coupled to the net production of two molecules of ATP from one molecule of glucose. The formation of lactate as an end product from glucose extracts only a relatively small amount of the bond energy (about 5%) contained in glucose. Accumulation of lactate also causes a reduction in intracellular pH. Therefore lactate is removed to other tissues and dealt with by one of the two mechanisms:

1) Lactate is converted back to pyruvate. The pyruvate then proceeds to be further oxidized by a second mechanism, the aerobic metabolism of glucose finally producing a large amount of ATP.

2) Conversion of lactate to glucose in the process of gluconeogenesis.

Conversion of Lactate to Pyruvate

The conversion of lactate to pyruvate is enzymatically catalyzed by lactate dehydrogenase. In this reaction, lactate becomes oxidized (loses two electrons) and is converted to pyruvate. NAD^+ gains two electrons (is reduced) and is converted to $NADH + H^+$. The coupling of oxidation-reduction reactions is often depicted in the following manner:

lactate $\xrightarrow{\hspace{3cm}}$ dehydrogenase

lactate + NAD $\xleftarrow{\hspace{3cm}}$ pyruvate + NADH + H^+

GLUCONEOGENESIS

Gluconeogenesis is a metabolic pathway that results in the generation of glucose from non-carbohydrate carbon substrates such as lactate, glycerol, and glucogenic amino acids. All must be converted to oxaloacetate. There is no pathway in animals for net conversion of acetyl-CoA to oxaloacetate (occurs in plants, glyoxylate cycle).

One common substrate is lactic acid, formed in the skeletal muscle in the absence of oxygen. Lactate may also come from red blood cells, which obtain energy solely from glycolysis. Erythrocytes have no membrane-bound organelles for aerobic respiration (mitochondria). All citric acid cycle intermediates, through conversion to oxaloacetate, amino acids other than lysine or leucine, and glycerol can also function as substrates for gluconeogenesis. Transamination or deamination of amino acids facilitates entering of their carbon skeleton into the cycle directly (as pyruvate or oxaloacetate), or indirect via the citric acid cycle.

Lactate is the predominate source of carbon atoms for glucose synthesis by gluconeogenesis. During anaerobic glycolysis in skeletal muscle, pyruvate is reduced to lactate by lactate dehydrogenase (LDH). This reaction serves two critical functions during anaerobic glycolysis. Firstly, for lactate formation, the LDH reaction requires NADH + H^+ and yields NAD^+ which is then available for use by the glyceraldehyde-3-phosphate dehydrogenase reaction of glycolysis. These two reactions are, therefore, intimately coupled during anaerobic glycolysis. Secondly, the lactic acid produced by the lactate dehydrogenase reaction is released to the blood stream and transported into liver. Here it is converted to glucose. The glucose is then returned to the blood for use by muscle as an energy source and to replenish glycogen stores. This cycle is termed the Cori cycle (Fig. **9**).

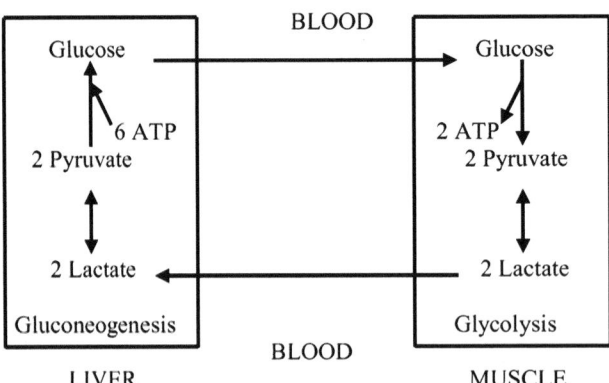

Figure 9: The Cori cycle.

The Cori cycle involves the utilization of lactate, produced by glycolysis in non-heaptic tissues (such as muscle and erythrocytes), as a carbon source for hepatic gluconeogenesis. In this way the liver can convert the anaerobic byproduct of glycolysis, lactate, back into more glucose for reuse by non-hepatic tissues. The gluconeogenesis of the cycle (on its own) is a net consumer energy, costing the body 4 moles of ATP more than are produced during glycolysis. Therefore, the cycle cannot be sustained indefinitely.

The process of gluconeogenesis uses some of the reactions of glycolysis (in reverse direction) and some reactions unique to this pathway to re-synthesize glucose (Fig. **10**).

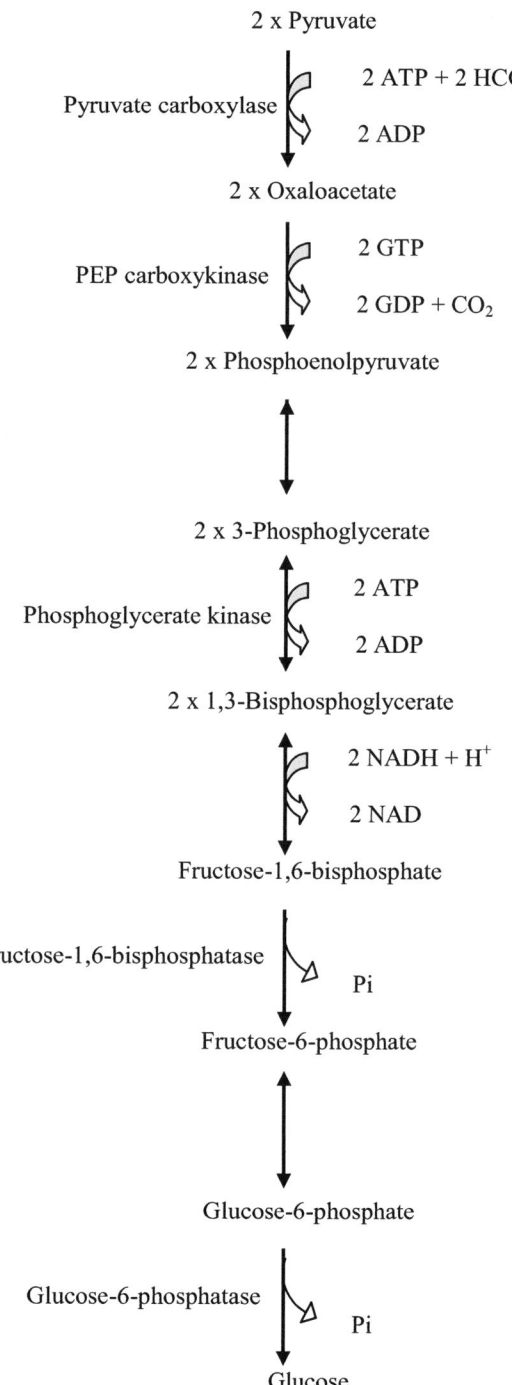

Figure 10: The process of gluconeogenesis [3, 5].

This pathway requires an energy input (as ATP), but has the role of maintaining a circulating glucose concentration in the blood stream even in the absence of dietary supply. Gluconeogenesis maintains the glucose supply to fast twitch muscle fibers.

Two enzymes specific for gluconeogenesis, phosphoenolpyruvate carbokinase and fructose-1,6-bisphosphatase, are opposed by the glycolytic enzymes pyruvate kinase and 6-phosphofructo-1-kinase. The enzyme glucose-6-phosphatase catalyzes the terminal step in both the gluconeogenic and glycogenolytic pathways and is opposed by the glycolytic enzyme glucokinase.

Fatty acids cannot be converted into glucose in animals with the exception of odd-chain fatty acids, which yield propionyl-CoA, a precursor for succinyl-CoA. Glycerol, which is a part of all triacylglycerols, can also be used in gluconeogenesis.

In organisms in which glycerol is derived from glucose (e.g., humans and other mammals), glycerol is sometimes not considered a true gluconeogenic substrate, as it cannot be used to generate new glucose.

GLYCOGENESIS

Glycogenesis is the process of glycogen synthesis in which glucose molecules are added to chains of glycogen for storage in liver and muscle. This process acts during rest periods following the Cori cycle, in the liver, and also activated by insulin in response to high glucose levels, for example after a carbohydrate containing meal.

For the synthesis of a molecule of glycogen, the starting point is the protein glycogenin, self-glucosylating enzyme that can create short chains of glucose attached to itself. Once the chains contain more than 10 glucose residues, they act as a primer for proglycogen synthase to elongate them. Once molecules of proglycogen are established in a cell, further synthesis is controlled by the enzyme, glycogen synthase. This enzyme elongates existing glucose chains by transferring a new glucose residue onto the free reducing end of the chain. The reaction is depicted in the following manner:

$$\text{UDP-glucose} + \text{glycogen (glucose)}_n \rightarrow \text{glycogen (glucose)}_{n+1} + \text{UDP}$$

The newly-attached glucose is derived from uridine diphosphate glucose (UDP-glucose), which is made by UDP-glucose pyrophosphorylase:

$$\text{UDP-glucose pyrophosphorylase}$$

$$\text{Glucose 1-phosphate} + \text{UTP} \longrightarrow \text{UDP-glucose} + \text{PP}_i$$

where UTP is a uridine triphosphate. By itself, this is a readily reversible reaction; however, the subsequent hydrolysis of pyrophosphate to two inorganic phosphates (PP_i) will readily occur, and this will drive the reaction over the product side.

Glycerol is a precursor for the synthesis of triacylglycerols and phospholipids in the liver and adipose tissue. When the body uses stored fat as a source of energy, glycerol and fatty acids are released into the bloodstream. The glycerol component can be converted to glucose by the liver and provides energy for cellular metabolism. Before glycogen can enter the pathway of glycolysis or gluconeogenesis (depending on physiological conditions), it must be converted to their intermediate glyceraldehyde 3-phosphate.

The enzyme glycerol kinase is present only in the liver. In adipose tissue, glycerol 3-phosphate is obtained from dihydroxyacetone phosphate (DHAP) with the enzyme glycerol-3-phosphate dehydrogenase.

GLYCOGENOLYSIS

When the blood sugar levels fall, glycogen stored in the tissue, especially glycogen of muscle and liver may be broken down. This process of breakdown of glycogen is called glycogenolysis (Fig. **11**).

Glycogenolysis (also known as "Glycogenlysis") is the catabolism of glycogen by removal of a glucose monomer through cleavage with inorganic phosphate to produce glucose-1-phosphate. This derivative of glucose is then converted to glucose-6-phosphate, an intermediate in glycolysis.

Glycogenolysis occurs in the muscle and liver, where glycogen is stored by low blood glucose concentrations. Liver cells can consume glucose 6-phosphate in glycolysis, or remove the phosphate group using the enzyme glucose 6-phosphatase and release the free glucose into the bloodstream for uptake by other cells. Since muscle cells lack glucose 6-phosphatase, they cannot convert glucose-6-phosphate into glucose, and therefore use the glucose-6-phosphate for their own energy demands. However, since the glucose residues present as the branching points of the glycogen molecule are removed as free glucose (rather than as glucose-6-phosphate), even muscle cells are able to release a small amount of glucose into the bloodstream.

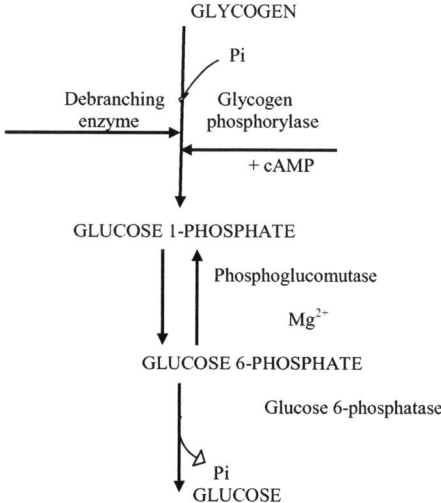

Figure 11: The process of glycogenolysis [3, 5].

Glycogenolysis requires three enzymes:

1) Glycogen phosphorylase (breaks down glucose polymer at α-1-4 linkages, yielding glucose-1-phosphate and a shorter glycogen molecule),

2) Debranching enzyme transferase / α-1,6-Glucosidase (bifunctional enzyme) (transfers α-1-6-linked glucose to end the of glycogen chain for glycogen phosphorylase, and removes the glucose present at the branching point as free glucose),

3) Phosphoglucomutase (converts glucose-1-phosphate to glucose-6-phosphate).

The comparison of different glucose metabolic pathways is seen in Fig. **12**.

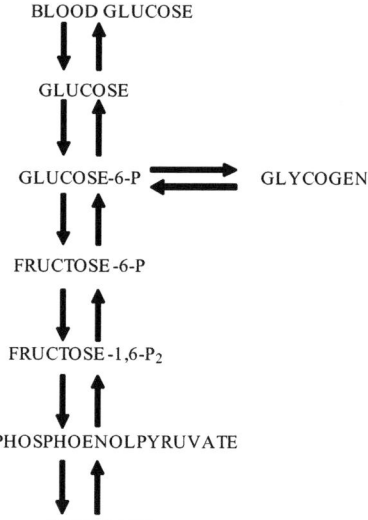

Figure 12: Substrate cycles in the glycolytic/gluconeogenic and glycogenic/glycogenolytic pathways that are involved in the regulation of glucose production by the liver [6].

PENTOSE PHOSPHATE PATHWAY

The pentose phosphate pathway (also called phosphogluconate pathway, or hexose monophosphate shunt [HMP shunt]) is primarily a cytoplasmic anabolic pathway that converts the 6 carbons of glucose to 5 carbons (pentose) sugars and reducing equivalents. However, this pathway does oxidize glucose and under certain conditions can completely oxidize glucose to CO_2 and H_2O. The primary functions of this pathway are:

1)   1) To generate reducing equivalents, in the form of $NADPH + H^+$, for reductive biosynthesis reactions within cells.

2)   2) To provide the cell with ribose-5-phosphate for the synthesis of the nucleotides and nucleic acids.

3)   3) Although not a significant function of the pentose phosphate pathway, it can operate to metabolize dietary pentose sugars derived from the digestion of nucleic acids as well as rearrange the carbon skeleton of dietary carbohydrates into glycolytic/gluconeogenic intermediates.

There are two distinct phases in the pathway [4, 5, and 7]. The first is the oxidative phase, in which $NADPH + H^+$ is generated, and the second is the non-oxidative synthesis of 5 carbon sugars (Fig. **13**). The pathway is one of the three main routes the body creates reducing molecules to prevent oxidative stress, accounting for approximately 10% of $NADPH + H^+$ production in humans.

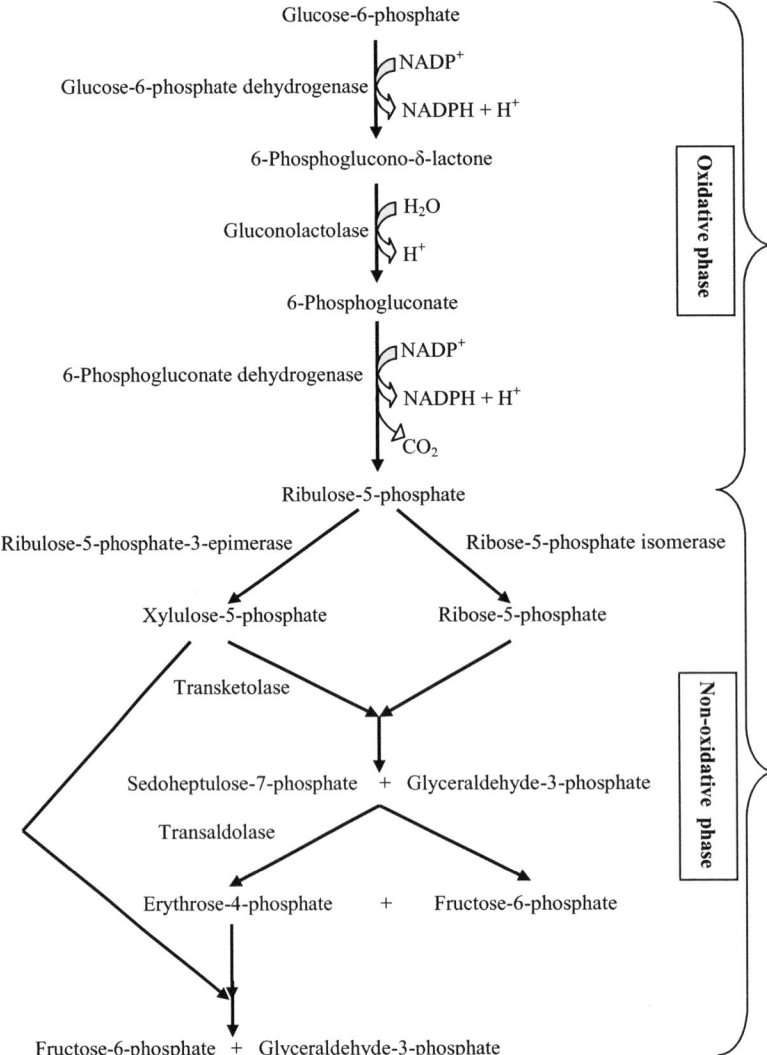

Figure 13: Pentose phosphate pathway [5, 7].

This pathway is an alternative to glycolysis. While it does involve oxidation of glucose, its primary role is anabolic rather than catabolic. For most organisms, it takes place in the cytosol. In plants, most of the functions take place in plastids.

The biosynthesis of fatty acids and steroid utilizes large amounts of NADPH + H$^+$. As a consequence, hepatocytes, adipocytes, cells of the adrenal cortex, lactating mammary gland have high levels of the pentose phosphate pathway enzymes. In fact 30% of the oxidation of glucose in the liver occurs via the pentose phosphate pathway. Erythrocytes utilize the reactions of the pentose phosphate pathway to generate large amounts of NADPH + H$^+$ used in the reduction of glutathione to the sulfhydryl form. Also the conversion of ribonucleotides to deoxyribonucleotides requires NADPH + H$^+$. Rapidly proliferating cells need large amounts of NADPH + H$^+$.

In summary, the pentose phosphate pathway primarily generates NADPH + H$^+$, ribose-5-phosphate, fructose-5-phosphate, and glyceraldehyde-3-phosphate. Glyceraldehyde-3-phosphate can be shunted to glycolysis and oxidized to pyruvate. Alternatively, glyceraldehyde-3-phosphate can be utilized by the gluconeogenic enzymes to generate more 6 carbon sugars (fructose-6-phosphate or glucose-6-phosphate).

Oxidative Phase

In this phase, two molecules of NADP$^+$ are reduced to NADPH + H$^+$, utilizing the energy from the conversion of glucose-6-phosphate into ribose-5-phosphate. The first step in this series of reactions is the dehydrogenation of glucose-6-phosphate into 6-phosphoglucono-δ-lactone. In this process, NADPH + H$^+$ is generated. The second step is the oxidative decarboxylation of 6-phosphoglucono-δ-lactone to ribulose-5-phosphate. This reaction generates another molecule of NADPH + H$^+$. The final step is the isomerization of ribulose-5-phosphate into ribose-5-phosphate.

The entire set of reactions can be summarized as follows:

1)   Glucose-6-phosphate + NADP$^+$ → 6-phosphoglucono-δ-lactone + NADPH + H$^+$

2)   2) 6-phosphoglucono-δ-lactone + H$_2$O → 6-phosphogluconate + H$^+$

3)   6-phosphogluconate + NADP$^+$ → ribulose-5-phosphate + NADPH + H$^+$

The overall reaction for this process is:

Glucose-6-phosphate + 2 NADP$^+$ + H$_2$O → ribose-5-phosphate + 2 NADPH + 2 H$^+$ + CO$_2$.

Non-Oxidative Phase

The non-oxidative reactions of the pentose phosphate pathway primarily generate ribose-5-phosphate. The pentose phosphate pathway also converts dietary 5 carbon sugars into both 6 (fructose-6-phosphate) and 3 (glycerylaldehyde-3-phosphate) carbon sugars which can then be utilized by the pathway of glycolysis. The primary enzymes involved in the non-oxidative steps of pentose phosphate pathway are transaldolase and transketolase.

The entire set of reactions can be summarized as follows:

1)   Ribulose-5-phosphate → ribose-5-phosphate

2)   Ribulose-5-phosphate → xylulose-5-phosphate

3)   3) Xylulose-5-phosphate + ribose-5-phosphate → glyceraldehyde-3-phosphate + sedoheptulose-7-phosphate

4)   4) Sedoheptulose-7-phosphate + glyceraldehyde-3-phosphate → erythrose-4- phosphate + fructose-6-phosphate

5)   5) Xylulose-5-phosphate + erythrose-4-phosphate → glyceraldehyde-3-phosphate + fructose-6-phosphate

B. Lipid Metabolism

TRIGLYCERIDE

Triglyceride (more properly known as triacylglycerol, TAG or triacylglyceride) is a glyceride in which the glycerol is esterified with three fatty acids. Triglycerides are formed from a single molecule of glycerol, combined with three fatty acids on each of the OH groups. Ester bonds form between each fatty acid and the glycerol molecule. The fatty acids present in triglycerides are predominantly saturated. The chemical formula is:

$$RCOO\text{-}CH_2CH(\text{-}OOCR')CH_2\text{-}OOCR''$$

where R, R', and R'' are longer alkyl chains. The three fatty acids RCOOH, R'COOH and R''COOH can be all different, all the same, or only two the same. (Fig. **14**).

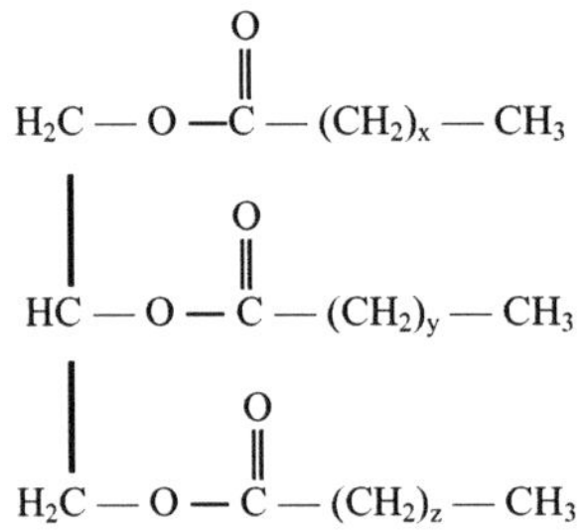

Figure 14: The general chemical formula of fat triglyceride.

Chain lengths of the fatty acids in naturally occurring triglycerides can be of varying lengths, but 16, 18, and 20 carbons are the most common. Natural fatty acids found in animals (include humans) are typically composed only of even number of carbon atoms due to the way they are biosynthesized from acetyl-CoA. Most natural fats contain a complex mixture of individual triglycerides.

Triglycerides, which are the main storage form of fat in the body, serve as building blocks for cells and used to create energy. They are made in the liver from proteins and carbohydrates, and also come from the fats in food. The major building block for the synthesis of triglycerides in cells other than adipocytes, is glycerol. Adipocytes lack glycerol kinase, therefore dihydroxyacetone phosphate, produced during glycolysis, is the precursor for triglyceride synthesis in adipose tissue (Figs. **15, 16**). This means that adipocytes must have glucose to oxidize in order to store fatty acids in the form of triglycerides. Fatty acids are stored for future as triglycerides in all cells, but primarily in adipocytes of adipose tissue.

LIPOGENESIS

Lipogenesis is the process by which simple sugars such as glucose are converted to fatty acids. Fatty acids are subsequently esterified with glycerol to form triglycerides that are packed in very low-density lipoprotein (VLDL) and secreted from the liver. Lipogenesis encompasses the process of fatty acid synthesis and subsequent triglyceride synthesis.

Like many metabolic pathways, the processes of fatty acid biosynthesis and fatty acid degradation (oxidation) are mediated by separate sets of enzymes, so that biosynthesis and oxidation do not run simultaneously. Also, while β-oxidation occurs in mitochondria, fatty acid synthesis occurs in the cytoplasm. The other major difference is the use of nucleotide co-factors. Oxidation of fats involves the reduction of FAD and NAD. Synthesis of fats involves the oxidation of $NADPH + H^+$.

Lipogenesis starts with acetyl-CoA and builds up by the addition of two carbon units. The overall equation for fatty acid synthesis is [3 – 5, and 8]:

Acetyl-CoA + 7 malonyl-CoA + 14 NADPH + 14 H^+ → palmitic acid + 7 CO_2 + 14 NADP + 8 CoA-SH + 6 H_2O

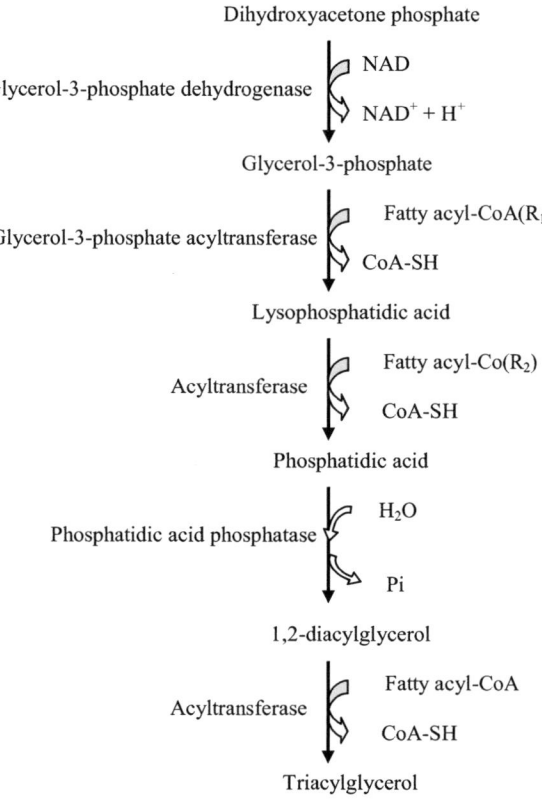

Figure 15: Triglyceride synthesis [8].

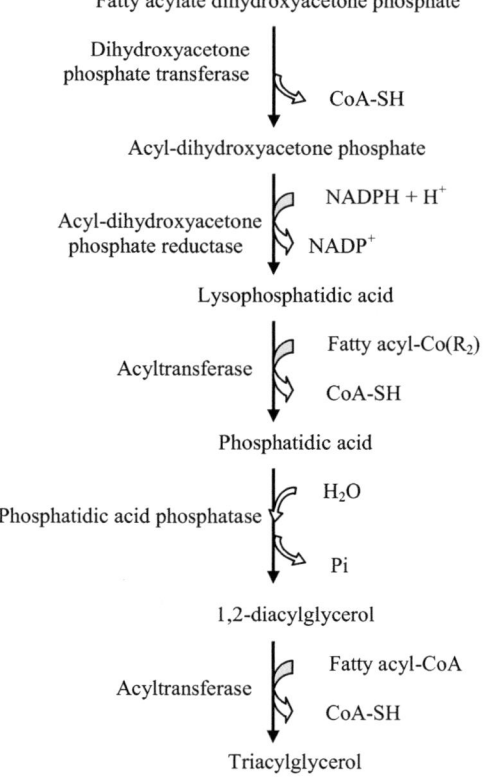

Figure 16: The second reaction pathway of triglyceride synthesis utilizes the peroxisomal enzyme dihydroxyacetone phosphate acyltransferase [8].

The process requires large amounts of NADPH + H^+, which are derived from the pentose phosphate pathway, and the sole product obtained is palmitic aid. Longer fatty acids can be synthesized from this palmitate in the endoplasmic reticulum, and unsaturations are also added here. Many of the enzymes for the fatty acid synthesis are organized into a multienzyme complex called fatty acid synthase.

Fatty acid synthesis begins in the mitochondria, where any free acetate is activated in the presence of ATP and CoA-SH to form acetyl-CoA. Acetyl-CoA is generated in the mitochondria primarily from two sources: the pyruvate dehydrogenase reaction and fatty acid oxidation. Acetyl-CoA is then transported to the cytoplasm.

In the cytoplasm, acetyl-CoA is carboxylated by acetyl-CoA carboxylase to form malonyl-CoA:

$$\text{Acetyl-CoA} + \text{ATP} + \text{HCO}_3^- \rightarrow \text{malonyl-CoA} + \text{ADP} + \text{Pi} + H^+$$

This process requires ATP, CO_2 and biotin, as a cofactor. The synthesis of malonyl-CoA is the first committed step of fatty acid synthesis, and the enzyme that catalyzes this reaction, is the major site of regulation of fatty acid synthesis. To continue fatty acid synthesis, acetyl-CoA and malonyl-CoA must bind to a specific peptide – acyl carrier protein (ACP). The extensions phase of the fatty acid synthesis begins with the formation of acetyl-S-ACP and malonyl-S-ACP by acetyl-CoA-ACP transacylase and malonyl-CoA-ACP transacylase respectively:

$$\text{Acetyl-CoA} + \text{ACP} \rightarrow \text{acetyl-S-ACP} + \text{CoA}$$

$$\text{Malonyl-CoA} + \text{ACP} \rightarrow \text{malonyl-S-ACP} + \text{CoA}$$

All of these reactions of fatty acid synthesis are carried out by the multiple enzymatic activities of fatty acid synthase. The fat synthesis involves 4 enzymatic activities: β-keto-ACP synthase, β-keto-ACP reductase, 3-OH acyl-ACP dehydratase and enoyl-CoA reductase. The reduction reactions require NADPH + H^+ oxidation to NADP.

The synthesis of fatty acids with an odd number of carbon atoms begins with a specific enzyme acetyl transacylase with the formation of propionyl-ACP from propionyl-CoA. The four reactions of the chain extension in the fatty acid synthesis are condensation, reduction, dehydration and reduction:

The first cycle is completed when crotonyl-ACP is reduced and butyryl-ACP is formed. In the second round, butyryl-ACP condenses with malonyl-ACP. Then the reactions are followed as in the first round 2 carbon atoms are then added in each round. This goes on until palmitate (C16) has been formed. There are 6 rounds during this process. Palmitate is taken away by ACP and there palmitate and ACP arise. The chain extension stops after the formation palmitate.

Palmitate is the primary fatty acid synthesized by fatty acid synthase. It can then undergo separate elongation and/or unsaturation to yield other fatty acid molecules. A further chain extension and the insertion of double bonds is catalyzed by other enzyme systems in endoplasmic reticulum. The process of elongation involves condensation of acyl-CoA groups with malonyl-CoA. The obtained product, two carbons longer, undergoes reduction, dehydration and reduction yielding saturated fatty acids.

Saturated fatty acids have no double bond between carbons. Unsaturated fatty acids have at least one double bond. Each double bond produces a "bend" in the molecule (Fig. **17**).

Desaturation involves 4 broad specificity fatty acyl-CoA desaturases. These enzymes introduce unsaturation at C4, C5, C6 or C9. The electrons from the oxidized fatty acids during desaturation are transferred to cytochrome b5 and then NADH-cytochrome b5 reductase. These electrons are un-coupled from mitochondrial oxidative phosphorylation and, therefore, do not yield ATP [8].

LIPOLYSIS

Lipolysis is the chemical decomposition and release of fat from adipose tissue. During this process, free fatty acids are released into the bloodstream and circulate throughout the body. This process predominates over lipogenesis when additional energy is required. The triglycerides within the adipocyte are acted upon by a multi-enzyme complex called hormone sensitive lipase (HSL), which hydrolyzes the triglyceride into free fatty acids and glycerol. These lipases act consecutively on triglycerides, diglycerides, and monoglycerides. Triglyceride lipase regulates the rate of lipolysis, because its activity is low.

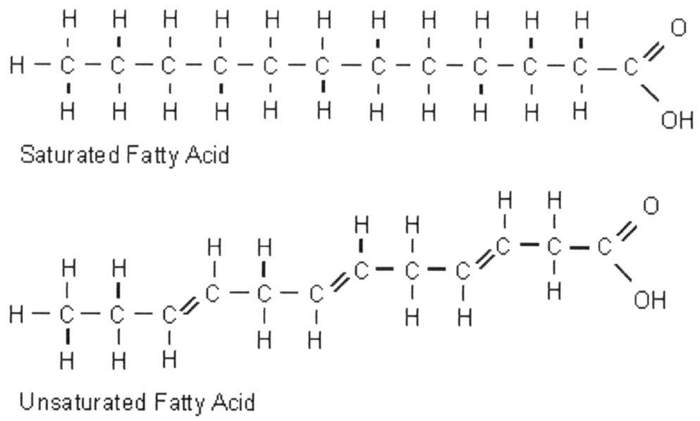

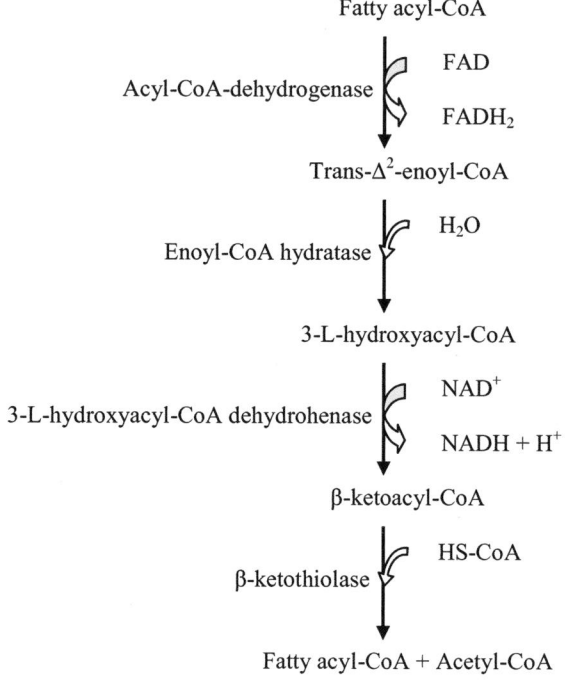

Saturated Fatty Acid

Unsaturated Fatty Acid

Figure 17: The molecule of saturated and unsaturated fatty acid [3, 4].

Triglycerides undergo hydrolysis by lipases and are broken down into glycerol and fatty acids. Once released into the blood, the free fatty acids bind to serum albumin for transport to tissues. The glycerol also enters the bloodstream and is absorbed by the liver or kidney. Here it is converted to glycerol-3-phosphate by the enzyme glycerol kinase. Hepatic glycerol-3-phosphate is mostly converted into dihydroxyacetonephosphate and then glycerylaldehyde-3-phosphate to rejoin the glycolysis or gluconeogenesis pathway.

B-OXIDATION OF FATTY ACIDS

The process of β-oxidation is named after the carbon number atom in the β-position of the fatty acyl-CoA which becomes the most oxidized during the cyclic redox reactions that remove the fatty acyl chain. The beta carbon becomes the new carboxyl end of the shortened (n-2) fatty acyl-CoA (Fig. **18**).

Fatty acyl-CoA

Acyl-CoA-dehydrogenase   FAD
                                FADH$_2$

Trans-Δ^2-enoyl-CoA

Enoyl-CoA hydratase   H$_2$O

3-L-hydroxyacyl-CoA

3-L-hydroxyacyl-CoA dehydrohenase   NAD$^+$
                                          NADH + H$^+$

β-ketoacyl-CoA

β-ketothiolase   HS-CoA

Fatty acyl-CoA + Acetyl-CoA

Figure 18: Pathway of β-oxidation [3, 4, 8]

The acyl-CoA dehydrogenase is specific for the length of the acyl chain being oxidized. Three types of the dehydrogenase exist in mitochondria: type I (EC 1.3.99.12; long chain) which oxidizes C12 – C18 fatty acids, type II (EC 1.3.99.3) which oxidizes C4 – C14 fatty acids, and type III (EC 1.3.99.2; butyryl dehydrogenase) which oxidizes C4 and C6 acyl-CoA substrates.

The oxidation of fatty acids occurs in 5 distinct steps:

1) The first step is the activation of the fatty acid, wherein it is converted to an acyl-CoA.

2) The second step is an enzymatic dehydrogenation of the CoA thioester, which produces a double bond in the α, β position.

3) In step 3, a specific hydrase adds a molecule of water across the newly formed double bond.

4) Step 4 involves oxidation of the β-hydroxyl group to a ketone.

5) In step 5, the enzyme β-ketothiolase splits off acetyl-CoA, thus producing a fatty acyl-CoA with two less carbon

The energy yield per cycle is 5 mols of ATP for each round; 2 mols per $FADH_2$ (goes into complex II) and 3 mols per $NADH + H^+$ (goes into complex I).

The fatty acids that occur in nature can be saturated or unsaturated, and can have an even or odd number of carbons. There are enzymatic pathways available to handle every type of fatty acid.

- Saturated fatty acids with an even number of carbons are oxidized to acetyl-CoA only.

- Fatty acids with an odd number of carbons produce acetyl-CoA and one molecule of propionyl-CoA, which then can enter the Krebs cycle.

- Unsaturated fatty acids require special handling. β-oxidation of unsaturated fatty acids poses a problem since the location of a cis bond prevents the formation of a trans-Δ^2 bond. These situations are handled by an additional two enzymes:

- if the acyl-CoA contains a cis-Δ^3 bond, then cis-Δ^3-Enol-CoA isomerase will convert the bond to a trans-Δ^2 bond, which is a regular substrate;

- if the acyl-CoA contains a cis- Δ^4 double bond, then dehydrogenation yields a 2,4-dienoyl intermediate, which is not a substrate for enoyl-CoA hydratase. However, the enzyme 2,4-Dienoyl-CoA reductase reduces the intermediate, using $NADPH + H^+$, into trans-Δ^3-enoyl-CoA. This compound is converted into a suitable intermediate by 3,2-Enoyl-CoA isomerase.

To summarize:

- odd numbered double bands are handled by the isomerase;

- even numbered double bonds by the reductase and the isomerase.

Fatty acids must be activated in the cytoplasm before being oxidized in the mitochondria. Activation is catalyzed by fatty acyl-CoA ligase (also called acyl-CoA synthetase or thiokinase) [8].

$$\text{Fatty acid} + \text{ATP} + \text{CoA} \rightarrow \text{Acyl-CoA} + \text{PPi} + \text{AMP}$$

Oxidation of fatty acids occurs in the mitochondria.

LIPOPROTEINS

Because lipids are insoluble, they are transported around the body as protein complexes called lipoproteins. Lipoproteins are associations of proteins and lipids that undergo changes in their passage through the circulation. These associations involve special proteins, called apolipoproteins or apoproteins. The structure of a lipoprotein typically involves the assembly of the more polar lipids, phospholipid, free cholesterol and protein on the exterior of a sphere where they can interface with the aqueous environment, and neutral lipids such as cholesterol ester and triglyceride, in the centre [9]. The apoproteins can be classified into two main groups: hydrophobic and amphipathic.

The hydrophobic apolipoprotein B (apoB) is essential for initiating the assembly of triglyceride-rich lipoproteins in enterocytes and hepatocytes. Hepatocytes translate the entire gene to produce a very high molecular mass protein B (apoB$_{100}$) and enterocytes edit the mRNA for apoB at 48% of the length to produce apoB$_{48}$ [10]. ApoB remains associated with the particle through its metabolism to low-density lipoprotein. The amphipathic apoproteins may exchange between lipoproteins. They include apoAI, apoAII, apoAIV, apoAV, apoCI, apoCII, apoCIII, and apoE as well as several lesser-known apoproteins [10]. Apoproteins AI – AV are found predominantly on high-density lipoproteins. ApoCII activates lipoprotein lipase and apoCIII inhibits it. ApoE is an important apoprotein for the clearance of remnants of the triglyceride-rich lipoproteins [10].

Lipoproteins were originally classified as α-, β-, and pre-β-lipoproteins according to their migration during electrophoresis. These represent high-density lipoprotein, low-density lipoprotein and very low-density lipoprotein. Lipoproteins are classified by their buoyant density which inversely reflects their size.

Chylomicron

In the small intestine absorbed dietary acids are converted into triglycerides and are packaged and secreted into the bloodstream as chylomicrons, a lipoprotein particle rich in triglycerides and apoB$_{48}$. Chylomicrons leave the intestine via the lymphatic system and enter the circulation at the left subclavian vein. In the capillaries of adipose tissue and muscle, the fatty acids of chylomicrons are removed from the triacylglycerols by lipoprotein lipase, which is found on the surface of the endothelial cells of the capillaries. The free fatty acids are then absorbed by the tissues and the glycerol backbone of triacylglycerols is returned, via the blood, to the liver and kidneys. Glycerol is converted to the dihydroxyacetone phosphate. Chylomicron remnants are taken up by the liver via the apoE receptor or via the chylomicron remnant receptor, which is a member of the LDL receptor-related protein. Chylomicrons function to deliver dietary triacylglycerols to adipose tissue and muscle and dietary cholesterol to the liver.

The properties of chylomicrons are: density < 0,95 g/ml; size 75 – 1200 nm; apoproteins B$_{48}$, CII, CIII, AIV; protein 1 – 2% of mass; triglyceride 85 – 90% of mass; phospholipids 8% of mass; cholesteryl esters 3% of mass; free cholesterol 1% of mass; free fatty acids 0% of mass.

Very Low-Density Lipoprotein (VLDL)

VLDLs transport endogenous lipid from the liver to the cells. Very low-density lipoproteins are synthesized in the liver, fulfill a lipid transport function. The triacylglycerols, synthesized in liver from both fat and carbohydrate, are packaged into VLDLs and released into the circulation for delivery to the various tissues (primarily adipose tissue and muscle) for storage or production of energy through oxidation. VLDLs are the molecules formed to transport endogenous derived triacylglycerols to extra-hepatic tissues. The triacylglycerols in these particles are hydrolyzed by lipoprotein lipase in the plasma and in the liver, generating small, cholesterol-enriched lipoproteins known as intermediate-density lipoproteins [11]. Smaller VLDLs and intermediate density lipoproteins are referred to as VLDL remnants and are atherogenic lipoproteins [12, 13]. About half of the VLDL remnants are cleared directly by the liver. The remainder are converted to low-density lipoprotein containing only apoB$_{100}$, and end product of VLDL catabolism and the major cholesterol-transporting lipoprotein in the plasma [11].

The properties of VLDL are: density 0,95 – 1,006 g/ml; size 30 – 80 nm; apoproteins B$_{100}$, CII, E, CIII, AI; protein 6 – 12% of mass; triglyceride 55 – 65% of mass; phospholipids 18 – 20% of mass; cholesteryl esters 12 – 15% of mass; free cholesterol 15 – 20% of mass; free fatty acids 1% of mass.

Intermediate-Density Lipoprotein (IDL)

Intermediate-density lipoproteins are transient and form during the conversion of VLDL to low-density lipoprotein. They are not normally detectable in the plasma. Cholesteryl ester from high-density lipoprotein is transferred to IDL by the action of cholesteryl ester transfer protein (CETP). IDL loses most of apolipoprotein except apoB and is converted to low- density lipoprotein by the action of hepatic lipase.

The properties of IDL are: density 1,006 - 1019 g/ml; size 25 – 35 nm; apoproteins B_{100}, E; protein 10 – 20% of mass; triglyceride 15 – 30% of mass; phospholipids 25 – 27% of mass; cholesteryl esters 32 – 35% of mass; free cholesterol 8 – 10% of mass; free fatty acids 1% of mass.

Low-Density Lipoprotein (LDL)

Low-density lipoproteins are formed from VLDL and carry cholesterol to the cells. LDL is taken up by liver and other tissues in an endocytotic process that involves the LDL receptor. During the transformation of VLDL remnants to LDL, a process thought to be dependent in part on hepatic lipase, all apoproteins other than apoB are lost and apoB assumes the correct conformation to bind the LDL receptor. This lipoprotein provides the bulk of the total cholesterol in the plasma of humans and acts as the source of cholesterol for cells which require this substance [9].

The properties of LDL are: density 1,019 – 1,063 g/ml; size 18 – 26 nm; apoproteins B_{100}; protein 20 – 25% of mass; triglyceride 8 – 12% of mass; phospholipids 20 – 28% of mass; cholesteryl esters 37 – 48% of mass; free cholesterol 8 – 10% of mass; free fatty acids 1% of mass.

High-Density Lipoprotein (HDL)

High-density lipoproteins are the most dense lipoproteins and are involved in the transport of cholesterol from the cells back to the liver (reverse cholesterol transport). HDL is formed by the transfer of cholesterol and phospholipids out ApoA-1 to generate pre β-HDL. This process is catalyzed by the ATP-binding cassette (ABC) A1 transporter (ABCA1), which is expressed in the peripheral tissues, intestine and liver. The cholesterol in the nascent pre β-HDL is then esterified by lysolecithin cholesterol acetyltransferase as part of a process that generates mature spherical HDL. Another ABC transporter (ABCG1) is able to load more cholesterol onto mature HDL from peripheral tissues and along with ABCA1 is important in allowing macrophages to efflux artery wall cholesterol, which prevents atherosclerotic vessel disease. HDL cholesterol-esters are taken up by receptor BI in the liver and after hydrolysis the resulting free cholesterol is metabolized to bile acids [14]. HDL can be further subdivide into HDL_2 and HDL_3. HDL_2 and HDL_3 derived from nascent HDL as a result of the acquisition of cholesteryl esters.

The properties of HDL_2 are: density 1,063 – 1,112 g/ml; size 9 – 12 nm; apoproteins AI, AII, AIV, CI, CII, CIII; protein 35 – 45 of mass; triglyceride 5 – 15% of mass; phospholipids 32 – 43 of mass; cholesteryl esters 20 – 30 % of mass; free cholesterol 5 – 10% of mass; free fatty acids 0% of mass.

The properties of HDL_3 are: density 1,112 – 1,210 g/ml; size 3 – 5 nm; apoproteins AI, AII; protein 50 – 60% of mass; triglyceride 3 – 5 % of mass; phospholipids 32 – 43% of mass; cholesteryl esters 20 – 30 % of mass; free cholesterol 5 – 10 % of mass; free fatty acids 0% of mass.

REFERENCES

[1]   Elliott SS, Keim NL, Stern JS, Teff K, Havel PJ. Fructose, weight gain, and the insulin resistance syndrome. Am J Clin Nutr 2002;76(5):911-922
[2]   Elsea SH, Lucas RE. The mousetrap: What we can learn when the mouse model does not mimic the human disease. ILAR J 2002;43(2):66-79
[3]   Nelson DL, Cox MM. Lehninger Principles of Biochemistry. WH Freeman & Co, 2004
[4]   Murray RK, Granner DK, Harper HA, Mayes PA, Rodwell VW. Harper's illustrated biochemistry. McGraw-Hill Professional Ed, 2003 (26th ed.)
[5]   Horton R, Moran LA, Scrimgeour G, Perry M, Rawn D. Principles of Biochemistry. Pearson Prentics Hall, 2006 (4th ed.).
[6]   Nordlie RC, Foster JD, Lange AJ. Regulation of glucose production by the liver. Annu Rev Nutr 1999;19:379-406
[7]   King MW. The Medical Biochemistry Page. Pentose Phosphate Pathway. 2009. Available from: http://themedicalbiochemistrypage.org/pentose-phosphate-pathway
[8]   King MW. The Medical Biochemistry Page. Lipid Synthesis. 2009. Available from: http://themedicalbiochemistrypage.org/lipid-synthesis

[9]   Marais D. Lipoprotein metabolism and its derangements. CME 2003;21,7:384-390

[10]   Marais AD. Normal and abnormal lipid and lipoprotein metabolism. CME 2009;27,3:118-122

[11]   Mahley RW, Ji Z-S. Remnant lipoprotein metabolism: key pathways involving cell-surface heparan sulfate proteoglycans and apolipoprotein E. J Lipid Res 1999;40:1-16

[12]   Mahley RW. Atherogenic lipoproteins and coronary artery disease: concepts derived from recent advances in cellular and molecular biology. Circulation 1985;72:943-948

[13]   Mahley RW, Weisgraber KH, Innerarity TL, Rall SC Jr. Genetic defects in lipoprotein metabolism. Elevation of atherogenic lipoproteins caused by impaired catabolism. J Am Med Assoc 1991;265:78-83

[14]   Tall AR. Plasma high density lipoproteins. J Clin Invest 1990;86:379-384

CHAPTER 2

Glucose Transporters

Abstract: Glucose is obtained directly from the diet, principally following the hydrolysis of ingested disaccharides and polysaccharides, and by the synthesis from other substrates in organs such as the liver. Glucose derived from the diet is transferred from the lumen of the small intestine, and both dietary glucose and glucose synthesized within the body have to be transported from the circulation into target cells. These processes involve the transfer of glucose across plasma membranes. Because for its hydrophilicity, glucose cannot penetrate the lipid bilayer, and specific carrier proteins are required to its diffusion. These transporters comprise two structurally and functionally distinct groups, whose members have been identified over the past two decades, namely: the Na^+-dependent glucose co-transporters (SGLT, members of a larger family of Na^+-dependent transporters, gene name *SLC5A*) and the facilitative Na^+-independent sugar transporters (GLUT family, gene name *SLC2A*). The number of known glucose transporters has expanded considerably over the past few years. These various transporters exhibit different substrate specificities, kinetic properties and tissue expression profiles. The number of distinct genes products, together with the presence of several different transporters in certain tissues and cell, indicates that glucose delivery into cells is a process of considerable complexity.

TRANSPORT ACROSS CELL MEMBRANES

Cell membranes act as barriers to most, but not all, molecules. Cell membranes are differentially (or semi-) permeable barriers separating the inner environment. Molecules and ions move spontaneously down their concentration gradient (i.e. from a region of higher to a region of lower concentration) by diffusion. Molecules and ions can be moved against their concentration, but this process, called active transport, requires the expenditure of energy (usually from ATP). Lipid bilayers are impermeable to most essential molecules and ions.

The lipid bilayer is permeable to water molecules and a few other small, uncharged, molecules like oxygen and carbon dioxide. These diffuse freely in and out of the cell. On the other hand, lipid bilayers are not permeable to cations (such as K^+, Na^+, Ca^{2+}), anions (such as Cl^- and HCO_3^-), small hydrophilic molecules like glucose and macromolecules like proteins and RNA. Therefore transport systems for these substances are required.

Transport of Small Molecules

Passive Transport

Diffusion

This involves movement of solutes, with the direction being by relative concentrations. Diffusion of different substances does not interfere with each other (no competition). Substances can cross membranes by diffusion. They can dissolve in the lipids of the membrane (hydrophobic). Diffusion is the mechanism of movement of inorganic ions. Diffusion of water down its concentration is called osmosis. Osmosis is a special term used for the diffusion of water through cell membranes. Although water is a polar molecule, it is able to pass through the lipid bilayer of the plasma membrane. Transmembrane proteins that form hydrophilic channels accelerate the process, but even without these, water is still able to get through.

Carrier-Mediated Transport

Transporters are two general classes: channels and carriers. Channels are usually simple peptides or small proteins of which the outside surface is hydrophobic and the inside hydrophilic, e.g. gramicidin. Gated channels are more complex, they have gates that open in response to a chemical, mechanical or electrical stimulus.

-   Uniporter – is an integral membrane protein that is involved in facilitated diffusion. It can be either a channel or a carrier protein. Uniport carriers mediate transport of a single solution and transport it only with the solute gradient (uniporters may not utilize energy).

The transmembrane channels, uniporter channels that permit facilitated diffusion can be opened or closed. They are said to be "gated".

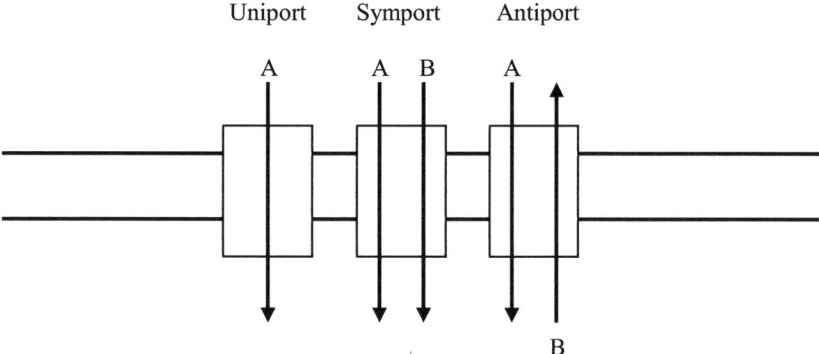

Figure 1: Classes of carrier proteins.

There are different ways in which the opening of uniporter channels may be regulated (types of gated ion channels):

a)   Voltage-regulated (Voltage-gated) ion channels. In so called "excitable" cells like neurons and muscle cells, some channels open or close in response to change in the charge (measured in volts) across the plasma membrane. For example, as an impulse passes down a neuron, the reduction in the voltage opens sodium channels in the adjacent portion of the membrane. This allows the influx of Na^+ into the neuron and thus the continuation of the nerve impulse.

b)   Stress-regulated (Mechanically-gated) ion channels. They are regulated by physical pressure on the transporter. For example – in the ear, sound waves cause the stress-regulated channels in the ear to open, sending an impulse to the vestibulocochlear nerve.

c)   Ligand-regulated (Ligand-gated) by the binding of a ligand to either the intracellular (intracellular ligand) or extracellular (extracellular ligand) side of the cell. In both cases, the ligand is not the substance that is transported when the channel opens.

As examples of external ligand which bind to a site on the extracellular side of the channels are: acetylcholine (the binding of neurotransmitter acetylcholine at certain synapses opens channels that admit Na^+ ions to initiate a nerve impulse or muscle contraction) and gamma amino butyric acid, GABA, (binding of gamma amino butyric acid in the central nervous system admits Cl^- ions into the cell and inhibits the creation of a nerve impulse).

Internal ligands bind to a site on the intracellular side of the channel. Examples: "second messengers", like cyclic AMP (cAMP) and cyclic GMP (cGMP), regulate channels involved in the initiation of impulses in neurons in response to odors and light respectively. The other example of internal ligand is ATP, which is needed to open the channel that allows Cl^- and HCO_3^- ions out of the cell.

-   Symporter – is an integral membrane protein that is involved in the movement of two or more molecules or ions across the plasma membrane in the same direction, and is therefore a type of cotransporter. Typically, the ion(s) move down the electrochemical gradient, allowing other molecule(s). Examples of symporter – SGLT1 in the intestinal epithelium transports Na^+ ions and glucose across luminal membrane of the epithelial cells so that it can be absorbed into the bloodstream. The same, $Na^+/K^+/2Cl^-$ symporter in the loop of Henle in the renal tubules of the kidney transports 4 molecules of 3 different types.

-   Antiporter – is an integral membrane protein that is involved in the transport of two species of ion or other solutes, which are pumped in opposite directions across a membrane. One of these species is allowed to flow from high to low concentration which yields the energy to drive the transport of the other solute from a low concentration region to a high one. A substrate binds and is transported across the membrane. Then another substrate binds and is transported in the other direction. Only exchange is catalyzed, not net transport, because the carrier protein cannot undergo the conformational transition in the absence of bound substrate. An example is the adenine nucleotide translocase, which catalyzes exchange of ADP for ATP across the inner mitochondrial membrane. The other example is the sodium-calcium exchanger (antiporter), which allows three Na^+ ions into the cell to transport one Ca^{2+} ion out.

Facilitated Diffusion of Molecules

Facilitated diffusion is a process of diffusion, a form of passive transport facilitated by transport proteins. Polar molecules and charged ions are dissolved in water but they can not diffuse freely across cell membranes, due to the hydrophobic nature of the phospholipids that make up the lipid bilayers. Facilitated diffusion is a spontaneous passage of molecules or ions across a biological membrane passing through specific transmembrane transport proteins. Proteins act as carriers or pores permit flux of substances that cannot diffuse directly through the membrane. These transmembrane proteins form a water-filled channel through which the polar molecules or ions can pass down its concentration gradient. Larger proteins are transported by transmembrane carrier proteins. Facilitated diffusion occurs across cell membrane only.

In facilitated diffusion, particle on one side of the membrane binds to carrier protein site. Channel reconfigures, exposing the carrier protein site to the solution on the other side of the membrane and then particle dissociates from the carrier protein and diffuses into the solution on the other side. It may move several particles simultaneously in the same direction (symport) or in opposite direction (antiport). Facilitated diffusion channels are generally selective. Examples include the bacterial lactose permease or GLUT – glucose transporter found in plasma membrane of all human cells.

Active Transport

Active transport is the pumping of molecules or ions through a membrane against their concentration gradient. It requires a transmembrane protein (usually a complex of them) called a transporter and energy. The source of this energy is ATP. The energy of ATP may be used directly or indirectly.

Primary Active Transport

Primary active transport, also called direct active transport, directly uses energy to transport molecules across a membrane. Some transporters bind ATP directly and use the energy of its hydrolysis to drive active transport. Most of the enzymes that perform this type of transport are transmembrane ATPases. A primary ATPase universal to all cellular life is the sodium-potassium pump, which helps maintain the cell potential. A Na^+/K^+ATPase is present in nearly every cell in the body. It pumps 3 Na^+ ions out in exchange of 2 K^+ ions pumped in (cost = 1 ATP). The parietal cells of stomach use H^+/K^+ATPase to secrete gastric juice. A Ca^{2+}ATPase is located in the plasma membrane of all eukaryotic cells. It uses the energy provided by one molecule of ATP to pump one Ca^{2+} ion out of the cell.

Secondary Active Transport

Secondary active transport, also called indirect active transport, uses the energy already stored in the gradient of a directly-pumped ion. In secondary active transport, one species of solute moves along its electrochemical gradient, allowing a different species of move against its own electrochemical gradient. This movement is in contrast to primary active transport, in which all solutes are moved against their concentration gradients, fueled by ATP.

The two main forms of this are antiport (also called counter-transport) and symport (also called co-transport).

Antiport pumps. In antiport pumps, the driving ion diffuses through the pump in one direction providing the energy for the active transport of some other molecule or ion in the opposite direction. As an example Ca^{2+} ions are pumped out of the cells by sodium-driven antiport pumps.

Symport pumps. In this type of indirect transport, the driving ion (Na^+) and the pumped molecule pass through the membrane pump in the same direction. Examples are: 1) Na^+/glucose transporter. This membrane protein allows sodium ions and glucose to enter the cell together. The sodium ions flow down their concentration gradient while the glucose molecules are pumped up theirs. Later, the sodium ion is pumped back out of the cell by the Na^+/K^+ATPase. 2) The Na^+/iodide transporter. This symporter pumps iodide ions into the cells of the thyroid gland and also into the cells of the mammary gland.

Transport of Large Molecules (Vesicular Transport)

Membranes transport larger molecules that are difficult to permeate the membrane by engulfing the substance and forming internal vesicles. Uptake of the substance by such a mechanism is called endocytosis; the secretion is called exocytosis.

Endocytosis

Endocytosis is the process of formation of vesicles containing fluid or solid material which occurs mainly in animal cells. The substances involved for all cells are fluids and nutrients; whereas for specialized cells, debris and pathogens. The substance to be transported binds to the cell membrane receptors, resulting in invagination of cell membrane invaginates, forming vesicle containing the transported substance culminating vesicle in the migration of the intracellularly. The two main categories are pinocytosis and phagocytosis.

- Pinocytosis is a nonspecific uptake of extracellular solution. Whatever is present in the solution is taken up by the cell.

- Phagocytosis. In phagocytosis the cell forms pseudopodia that engulf macromolecules. The pseudopodia fuse, and the membrane pinches off, forming an internal vesicle. Phagocytes are macrophages that line blood channels of liver (spleen) and eat up aging erythrocytes. Monocytes penetrate the inflamed tissue and remove the invading bacteria.

Exocytosis

Exocytosis is the process of secretion of protein hormones, serum proteins, and extracellular matrix. Exocytosis involves the fusion of vesicles containing fluids and/or solids with the cell membrane. In exocytosis the vesicle migrates to the cell membrane and attaches to it. The vesicle membrane fuses with the cell membrane and vesicle contents are released into the interstitial fluid.

THE TRANSFER OF GLUCOSE ACROSS PLASMA MEMBRANES

Carbohydrate, and glucose in particular, are an important source of energy for most living organism. The first and limiting step in glucose metabolism is the transport across plasma membrane. Because the lipid bilayers that make up cell membranes are impermeable to carbohydrates, carbohydrate-transport systems are required. In eukaryotes, each organism expresses a multitude of sugar uptake systems that are all controlled at different levels in complex ways. The movement of monosaccharides across plasma membranes is controlled by proteins encoded from two structurally and functionally distinct gene families, namely the facilitative glucose transporters (gene symbol *SLC2A*, protein symbol GLUT) and Na^+-dependent glucose transporters (gene symbol *SLC5A*, protein symbol SGLT).

Na^+-Dependent Glucose Cotransporters (SGLT)

The involvement of Na^+ in glucose absorption was first proposed by Riklis and Quastel [1]. The original Na^+/glucose cotransport hypothesis was presented by Crane [2]. This group showed that active glucose absorption by hamster small intestine required sodium ions in the bathing medium. Crane further developed the model of a mobile carrier in the brush border membrane with two binding sites, one for glucose and one for Na^+ [3]. He determined that the continuously maintained outward sodium ions gradient accomplished by Na^+/K^+ATPase on the basolateral membrane was the primary asymmetry providing the driving force for active sugar transport. The phenomenon was considered by the "secondary active transport" (indirect active transport), as the hydrolysis of ATP was indirectly coupled to glucose transport via this electrochemical gradient.

Wright and colleagues developed a new method called expression cloning. The method resulted in SGLT 1 being the first eukaryote cotransporter to be cloned. The first of this type glucose transport protein to be cloned was the high-affinity transporter from rabbit intestine [4]. The human analogue was soon followed by homology cloning [5]. Amino acid comparisons of the human SGLT range from 57 – 71% identity [6]. The members of the SGLT family also share considerable homology among the proteins (21 – 70% amino acid identity to SGLT 1) [8, 19]. The sodium/glucose cotransporters are the founding members of a large gene family (*SLC5A*), the SGLTs or sodium/substrate symporters family (SSSF), containing over 450 members [7 – 9]. So far, there are 11 human genes described which are expressed in different tissues. The functions of six are tightly coupled plasma membrane Na^+/substrate cotransporters for solutes such as glucose, myo-inositol and iodide, one is a Na^+/Cl^-/choline cotransporter, and another is a glucose-activated ion channel [8]. The exon organization of eight genes is similar in that each comprises 14 – 15 exons, the choline transporter (CHT) is encoded in eight exons and Na^+-dependent myo-inositol transporter (SMIT) in one exon.

The *SLC5A* genes code for proteins of 659 – 672 residues, with a predicted mass of 73 kDa. Experimental and computational analyses indicate the model contains 14 transmembrane α-helices (TMH) with both the hydrophobic NH_2 terminus and the COOH terminus of TMH 14 facing the extracellular solution [7, 10]. The transporter contains a single glycosylation site. All probably use the consensus N-linked glycosylation site (N^{248}) between TMH 6 and 7 [7]. However SGLT contains a single glycosylation site. Glycosylation is not required for functioning of the protein. Phosphorylation sites are suggested between transmembrane helices 5 and 6 [11] and between transmembrane helices 8 and 9 [12].

The process of intestinal sugar transport has been described by Wright and colleagues [13]. In the first step, on the luminal side of brush border membrane, two Na^+ ions bind to SGLT 1 and produce a conformational change that permits sugar binding. Another conformational change allows the substrate to enter the enterocyte.

The sugar, followed by the Na^+, dissociates from SGLT1. The Na^+/K^+ATPase in the basolateral membrane is responsible for maintaining the Na^+ and K^+ electrochemical gradients across the cell membrane. SGLT 1 can recycle ~ 1000 times/sec. at 37^0C [9, 16, and 17].

SGLT 1

The Na^+/glucose cotransporter 1 (SGLT 1), encoded by gene *SLC5A1*, is an archetype for the *SLC5* family, which is comprised of Na^+-coupled transporters for sugars, myo-inositol, choline, and organic anions [14]. SGLT 1 is comprised of 15 exons (spanning 72 kb); a possible evolutionary origin from a six-membrane-span ancestral precursor via a gene duplication [15]. The single copy gene for the SGLT 1 is located on human chromosome 22q12.3. The open reading frame codes for a 664-amino acid membrane protein with a predicted weight 73 kDa [9]. According to Zhao and Keating [19], the deduced SGLT 1 is a 662-amino acid polypeptide with a molecular weight of 73 kDa and shows no sequence homology to GLUT protein. SGLT 1 membrane protein contains 14 transmembrane α-helical domains with large hydrophilic loop localized between transmembrane α-helices 13 and 14 of the cytoplasm [10, 18].

The COOH-terminal domain containing the five terminal helices (C5, TMH 10-14, residues 407 – 662 and 410 – 662) is involved in sugar binding (sugar affinity), selectivity, and translocation [20, 21]. The results obtained by Panayotova-Heiermann and colleagues showed that helices 10 – 13 form the sugar permeation pathway for SGLT 1, and N-terminal region of SGLT 1 (helices 1 – 9) may be required to couple Na^+ and glucose transport [22, 23]. Sodium ion and sugar have two separate pathways through SGLT 1: Na^+ permeates through the N-terminal half of the protein, and sugar permeates through the COOH-terminal half. Na^+ binding to N-terminal domain then causes a long-range conformational change in the SGLT 1 to permit sugar binding and translocation [7, 21]. Glutamine 457 is a critical residue because the Q457R mutation causes glucose/galactose malabsorption by blocking sugar translocation [16].

SGLT 1 is predominantly expressed in the brush border membrane of mature enterocytes in the human small intestine, trachea and prostate [7, 8, 19, and 24]. The expression of SGLT 1 in human heart is unexpectedly high, approximately 10-fold higher than that observed in kidney tissue [25]. SGLT 1 has also been detected in the luminal membrane of intracerebral capillary endothelial cells [26].

SGLT 1 (high affinity, low capacity) is largely responsible for glucose and galactose transport across the intestinal brush border. It exhibits a high affinity for D-glucose (Km ~ 0,4 mM) and D-galactose [27]. In the kidney, any remaining glucose is recovered by SGLT 1 thus preventing glucose loss in urine [6]. SGLT 1 does not transport fructose, mannose and xylose [11].

SGLT 1 expression has been observed in many tissues in which glucose is believed to be taken up by the facilitative process, such as the mammary gland and liver [28]. Therefore, SGLT 1 may be multifunctional protein, also functioning as other substrates cotransporter. In the absence of sugar, the SGLT family members (SGLT 1, SMIT 1, NIS – Na^+-iodide) transport Na^+. The rate of Na^+ transport ranges from 8 to 34% of the maximum cotransport rate [9]. Loo and colleagues have found that cotransporters behave as water pumps [30]. In *Xenopus laevis* oocytes expressing SGLT 1, the activation of Na^+-glucose cotransport by the addition of sugar triggers the immediate uptake of water. Coupled-water transport is independent of the osmotic gradient and even occurs against it [9]. In the presence of glucose, cotransport of water occurs [29].

SGLT 1 and other cotransporters behave as channels for water and small hydrophilic solutes when expressed in *Xenopus laevis* oocytes [22, 30]. The rate and direction of the osmotic flow of water are directly proportional to the osmotic gradient. The coupling of water transport to active Na^+-glucose cotransport was investigated by Wright and colleagues. Overexpression of human SGLT 1 in *Xenopus laevis* oocytes revealed that activation of the transporter was associated with an increase in volume of the cell. If oocytes expressing SGLT 1 were incubated in sugar-free solution, no change in oocyte volume was observed. The increase in volume could be accounted for a stoichiometry of two Na^+ ions, one glucose molecule, and 249 water molecules [30]. A channel formed by five C-terminal transmembrane helices of SGLT1 is to transport not only water, but also urea [22, 31]. The urea channel is located in the C5 domain of SGLT 1. The significance of the SGLT 1 channel is that aquaporins and urea transporters are absent from the intestinal brush border, and therefore SGLT 1 may play an important role in fluid and urea transport across the intestine [9]. SGLT 1 plays an important role in water transport, either directly as a water cotransporter or indirectly as a water channel. About 1 mol of glucose is absorbed from the intestine each day and in human small intestine, secondary active transport of water through SGLT 1 can account for five liter water absorption per day [9, 29]. Under steady-state conditions, 35% of water transport occurs by Na-glucose-water cotransport, 35% occurs by osmosis through SGLT 1 and 30% occurs by osmosis through plasma membrane [9].

Patients with SGLT 1 mutations are unable to accumulate sugars within enterocytes. SGLT 1-deficient patients only show a mild renal glucosuria. In summary – mutations in SGLT 1 cause diarrhea associate with glucose/galactose malabsorption.

SGLT 1 may also behave as glucose receptor in heart and brain [9].

SGLT 2

There is a little information available about SGLT 2, owing to its low level of expression [7]. SGLT 2 was isolated from a human kidney library. The single copy gene (*SLC5A2*) for SGLT 2 is located on human chromosome 16p11.2 [32, 33], and is comprised of 14 exons (spanning 8 kb) [19]. The *SLC5A2* gene codes for a 672-amino acid protein with a predicted mass of 73 kDa [7, 19]. SGLT 2 has identities of 59% on SGLT 1 [7]. It secondary structure profile is the same as that for SGLT 1. SGLT 2 is a low affinity (Km = 10 mM), high capacity glucose transporter, and it is highly selective for D-glucose. It cannot efficiently transport D-galactose. SGLT 2 has a high affinity for sodium ions under the same sugar concentration (2 mM) [34, 35]. The SGLT 2 stoichiometry is 1 Na^+ : 1 sugar [34, 36].

SGLT 2 is predominantly expressed on the apical membrane of renal convoluted proximal tubules (S1 and S2 segments) [7, 32, and 34]. It is presumed to be mainly responsible for the reabsorption of D-glucose from the glomerular filtrate. SGLT 2 is also found in the brain and liver [9]. According to Wright and colleagues hypothesis, SGLT 2 may also behave as glucose receptors in the heart and brain [9].

Homozygous and heterozygous nonsense mutations of SGLT 2 are associated with autosomal recessive renal glucosuria in human patients [37, 38].

SGLT 3

SGLT 3 (alias SAAT 1) is coded by gene *SLC5A4* localized on human chromosome 22q12.2-q12.3 [8]. The gene *SLC5A4* is located downstream of gene encoded SGLT 1 (within 0,15 mb) and has similar intron-exon organization, suggesting an ancient gene duplication [7].

SGLT 3 has a low affinity for sugars (Km = 2 mM), and is highly selective for D-glucose [19, 39]. The *SLC5A4* gene codes for a 660-amino acid protein [19] that have identities of 70% to SGLT 1 [7]. The Na^+ Hill coefficient for SGLT 3 is ~ 1,5. It suggests low cooperativity between Na^+ binding sites. The results obtained by Diez-Sampedro and colleagues [39] suggest that SGLT 3 has functional characteristics intermediate between SGLT 1 and SGLT 2. SGLT 3 stoichiometry is the same as that for SGLT 1 – 2 Na^+ : 1 sugar. On the other hand, sugar affinity and specificity are similar to SGLT 2 [39].

Surprisingly, human SGLT 3 does not transport sugar. Instead, glucose generates an inward Na^+ current that depolarizes the membrane potential. Therefore, SGLT 3 is not a glucose transporter but a glucose sensor [9, 19, and 40].

SGLT 3 is expressed in the kidney, uterus and testis [8]. It is also expressed in the intestinal autonomic nervous system, skeletal muscle and brain. This may be related to the hypothesis that SGLT 3 is a glucose sensor. The other sites of SGLT 3 expression are cholinergic neurons in the enteric nervous system; cholinergic neurons mediate enteric reflexes after a meal. SGLT 3 is predicted to play a role in determining intestinal motility [9].

SGLT 4, SGLT 5, SGLT 6

Limited functional and structural studies have been carried out with SGLT 4, SGLT 5 and SGLT 6. There are very limited reports on the function of mentioned glucose cotransporters [6, 9].

Gene for SGLT 4 (*SLC5A9*) is localized on human chromosome 1p32 [8]. SGLT 4 is expressed in small intestine, kidney, liver, lung and brain [8]. Results obtained by Tazawa and colleagues suggest that SGLT 4 would have unique physiological functions, i.e. absorption and/or reabsorption of D-mannose and D-fructose, in addition to D-glucose [41].

Genes encoding SGLT 5 and SGLT 6 (*SLC5A10* and *SLC5A11*) are localized on human chromosomes 17p11.2 and 16p12.1, respectively [8]. The first mentioned glucose cotransporter is expressed in the kidney, and the second – in small intestine, brain, kidney, liver, heart and lung [8].

Facilitative Glucose Transporters (GLUT)

The facilitative transporters (GLUT) utilize the diffusion gradient of glucose and other sugars across plasma membranes and exhibit different substrate specificities, kinetic properties and tissue expression profile. The first transporter to be isolated, GLUT 1, was cloned from HepG2 cell line [42].

The GLUTs belong to the major facilitator super family, which is a group of transmembrane proteins that transport a wide range of solutes such as amino acids, sugars, nucleotides, drugs, peptides, organic and inorganic anions, metabolites, neurotransmiters, polyols etc. The major facilitator super family includes thousands of sequenced members and is present in organisms ranging from bacteria to human.

The GLUTs are intrinsic membrane proteins which differ in tissue-specific expression and response to metabolic and hormonal regulation [19, 43, and 44].

In human, 14 members of the mammalian glucose transporter (GLUT) family, encoded by genes *SLC2A* have been identified [45]. There are 12 hydrophobic α-helical segments, suggesting that this family of transporters may have a tertiary structure of 12 transmembrane domains [43, 46]. The transmembrane domain contains a water-filled pathway through which the substrate moves (central aqueous pore or channel through which the substrate crossed the lipid bilayer) [47, 48]. The cytoplasmic domain contains a short N-terminal segment, a large intracellular loop between transmembrane domain 6 and 7 and a large C-terminal segment. The exoplasmic domain contains a large loop bearing a single N-linked oligosaccharide moiety [45, 49, and 50]. Sequence comparison of all 14 family members show that the sequence are more conserved in the putative transmembrane regions and more divergent in the loops between the transmembrane domains and in the C-terminal and N-terminal regions. The most divergent regions are loops 1 and 9 and two terminal regions. The sequences among members of family are 14 – 63% identical and 30 – 7% conservative [19]. For example, human GLUT 1 – GLUT 5 exhibit 39 – 65% sequence identity and 50 – 76% sequence similarity in pairwise comparison [49].

GLUT 1 (or Glut 1 in the case of animals) appears to be the most highly conserved glucose transporter in mammals. Human GLUT 1 exhibits ~ 97 – 98% sequence identity with the analogous rat, mouse, rabbit, and pig proteins. Human GLUT 2, on the other hand, is only ~ 82% identical in sequence to its rat and mouse counterparts [49]. The fact that isoform-specific amino acid sequences are found at the cytoplasmic and exoplasmic domains indicates that they are responsible for tissue-specific regulation of transporter function. The fact that the transmembrane domain primary structure is largely conserved suggests that the glucose channel is basically identical in structure among the members of this family [44]. Sequence alignments of all members also reveal several highly conserved structures: PMY in transmembrane domain 4, QQLSGIN in transmembrane domain 7, GPGPIP/TW in transmembrane domain 10, and VPETKG in the C-terminal tail. Highly conserved amino acids are also in loops: PESPRY/FLL in loop 6 and GRR in loop 8. In addition, there are 18 conserved glycine residues, 11 of them being adjacent to at least one other conserved amino acid [19]. The presence of a common motif suggests that this family may have originated from a common ancestral gene.

Based on the phylogenetic analysis of sequence similarity and characteristic elements, the GLUT family of sugar transporters is divided into three classes [19, 43, 45, and 46].

Class I comprises the thoroughly characterized glucose transporters GLUT 1 – GLUT 4 and GLUT 14 that are distinguishable mainly by their tissue distribution. These members of GLUT family are 48 – 63% identical in human and have been extensively characterized. The larger loop 1 contains glycosylation site (N-45 for human GLUT 1). Residues that appear specific for the class I transporters are a glutamine in α-helical structure 5 (QL motif corresponding with Q161 in GLUT 1 [51] and the STSIF motif in the extracellular loop 7 [52].

Class II includes the fructose-specific transporter GLUT 5 and three related proteins: GLUT 7, GLUT 9, and GLUT 11, which are 36 – 40% identical. The most striking sequence characteristic of class II transporters is the lack of the tryptophan following the conserved GPXXXP motif in helix 10 corresponding with tryptophan 388 in GLUT 1. Glycosylation site is also present in the larger loop 1 [19].

Class III comprises five facilitative glucose transporters: GLUT 6, GLUT 8, GLUT 10, GLUT 12, and HMIT1. This class of transporters is only 19 – 41% identical. Class III GLUTs are characterized by a shorter extracellular loop 1 that lacks a glycosylation site, and by the presence of such site in the larger loop 9 [19]. It is suggested that the class III GLUTs are the "oldest" isotypes, from which class I and class II evolved as an adjustment to the additional requirements of glucose homeostasis in mammals [46].

The detailed information, regarding primary and secondary structure, membrane topology, transport kinetics, and functionally important residues of the GLUT 1 facilitative glucose transporter has been described by Hruz and Mueckler [53].

GLUT 1

The GLUT 1 is known as the erythrocyte, brain or Hep-G2-Type glucose transporter and comprises 3 – 5% of the erythrocyte total membrane protein. The gene for this transporter (*SLC2A1*) maps to chromosome 1p35-p31.3. *SLC2A1* is comprised of 10 exons. The gene is about 33 kb in length and mRNA size is 2,8 kb [54]. The transporter is a highly hydrophobic, heterogeneously glycosylated protein. The deduced protein sequence of GLUT 1 is composed of 492 amino acids with a molecular weight of approximately 54,2 kDa [53]. An extracellular loop of 33 amino acids located between transmembrane segments 1 and 2 is the location of a single site for ASN-linked oligosaccharide addition. On SDS PAGE, GLUT 1 runs as a broad band between 50 – 60 Da, due to N-linked glycosylation at ASN-45.

The original model for GLUT 1 structure [42] predicted the formation of a central aqueous channel formed by the juxtaposition of five of the transmembrane helices (namely 3, 5, 7, 10, and 11) each of which possesses some amphipathic character. The results obtained by Mueckler and Makepeace [62] suggest that transmembrane segment

6 of GLUT 1 contains amino acid side chains essential for transport activity. Helix 6 possesses 6 residues that are sensitive to cysteine substitution with respect to decreased transport activity. Helix 12 has no such residues. This observation suggests that helix 6, unlike helix 12, plays an active role in the transport mechanism [63]. The role of the other sites in GLUT 1 in the process of glucose transport is described by Hruz and Mueckler [53]

Brain GLUT 1 is a multiple-molecular-weight species ranging between 45 – 55 kDa [55 – 57]. The differences in molecular weight are due to differences in N-linked glycosylation. The functional effect of the different glycosylation states is not clear although it is suggested that they are involved in GLUT 1 trafficking [58] and substrate affinity [59]. The larger-molecular-weight glucose transporter protein is present in cerebral cortex and in cerebral microvessels [56]. The lower, 45-kDa GLUT 1 is readily detectable in microvessels-depleted brain membranes (neuronal/glial membranes), and synaptosomes [56, 60]. An intermediate form of GLUT 1 is present in the choroid plexus [61]; however, according to the results obtained by Maher and colleagues [56], in choroid plexus, the lower isoform of GLUT 1 is present.

GLUT 1 appears to be the most ubiquitously distributed of the glucose transporter. It is expressed in many fetal and adult mammalian tissues and cell types. GLUT 1, provides transport in various cells comprising of a barrier between body tissue and blood supply. Thus, endothelial or epithelial-like barrier cells of the brain, eye, peripheral nerve, and placenta all express relatively high level of GLUT 1 [64]. It is expressed also in erythrocytes, granulocytes, agranulocytes, adipocytes, muscle cells, kidney, colon, and fetal tissues [54, 65 – 67]. In the adipocytes and muscle cells, it is present constitutively in the plasma membrane, where it presumably provides low level of glucose required for basal cellular activity [68, 69].

GLUT 1 has high affinity for glucose (Km = 3 – 7 mM) [19]. The other transport substrates of GLUT 1 include galactose, mannose and glucosamine [70, 71].

GLUT 1 is expressed not only in the cell membrane. *In vitro* mitochondrial import of GLUT 1 (Glut 1), immunoblot analysis of mitochondrial proteins, and cellular immunolocalization studies indicated that GLUT 1 (Glut 1), as a 54 kDa protein, localizes to mitochondria in human kidney cells (293 T) and murine fibroblasts (NIH/3T3). The oxidized form of vitamin C, dehydroascorbic acid, enters mitochondria, analogous to the cellular uptake, via facilitative glucose transporter 1 and accumulates mitochondrially as ascorbic acid. It protects mitochondria from oxidative injury [72].

It has been shown that GLUT 1 also plays other functions. Surprisingly, studies using adherent cell lines have shown that GLUT 1 can function as a receptor for human T cell leukemia virus type 1 (HTLV). Infection of CD4[+] T lymphocytes by the human T cell leukemia virus type 1 is mediated by GLUT 1 [73 – 75].

Cancer cells have marked increased rates of glucose metabolism compared with normal cells. Especially, glycolysis has been shown to be increased in cancer cells compared with normal cells [76]. Therefore tumors show increased uptake of glucose compared to normal tissue [77], a response mediated by a number of facilitative glucose transporters located in the cell membrane [78]. The up-regulation of GLUT 1 expression occurs in the transformation process and this increased expression may be a fundamental part of the neoplastic process. However, an alternate interpretation of the data is that increased GLUT 1 protein level in transformed cells may be an indirect effect [79].

As every cell contains the genes for each GLUT family member, the expression of certain GLUT forms was absent in cancer cells which, under normal conditions, would never have been expressed in these tissues [44]. For example, GLUT 1 mRNA was not detected in normal gastric mucosa, and in gastric carcinoma samples, GLUT 1 mRNA was detected in 95% cases [80].

GLUT 1 expression has been shown to be altered also by other tumors, as for example: in human brain tumors [81], renal cell carcinoma [82] breast cancer [83], malignant melanomas [84]. Therefore, it is suggested that GLUT 1 may be a potential marker of prognosis in rectal carcinoma [85].

A large number of studies have been published on the regulation of GLUT 1. Most of these concern the regulation of GLUT 1 in cultured cell lines. More details were described by Mueckler [49].

GLUT 1 deficiency syndrome (De Vivo disease) was first described in 1991 [86]. The disease arises from heritable mutations (all types, including missense mutations, nonsense mutations, insertions, microdeletions and splice-site mutations) in *SLC2A1* gene that impairs monosaccharide uptake, which becomes rate-limiting in tissues where the transporters serve as the main glucose carrier systems [87].

GLUT 2

GLUT 2, the second member of GLUT family, is encoded by *SLC2A2* gene localized on human chromosome 3q26.2-27 and is comprised of 11 exons [19, 46]. The gene is about 31 kb length [19]. The deduced protein sequence of GLUT 2 is composed of 524 amino acids with the molecular weight of 58 kDa [54]. The GLUT 2 amino acid sequences display 81% identity between the human, mouse and rat [19]. GLUT 2 lacks the QLS motif at helix 7 which is thought to confer substrate specificity on the transporter and which may explain the high affinity for glucosamine [70].

GLUT 2 is primarily expressed in hepatocytes and pancreatic β-cells and absorptive epithelial cells of the intestinal mucosa and kidney [88, 89]. In the epithelial cells GLUT 2 is expressed exclusively in the basolateral membrane, where it works in conjunction with the SGLT-cotransporter of the apical membrane to facilitate the absorption and reabsorption of glucose from the intestinal lumen or forming urine into the blood [90, 91]. It was demonstrated that GLUT 2 mRNAs are present in the limited number of brain nuclei, including the nucleus tractus solitarius, the motor nucleus of the vagus, the paravetricular hypothalamic nucleus, the lateral hypothalamic area, the arcuate nucleus and the olfactory bulbs [92]. The kinetic properties allow GLUT 2 to function in the liver where glucose transport must not be rate limiting for influx and efflux.

GLUT 2 is a low affinity transporter for glucose (Km ~ 17 mM), galactose (Km ~ 92 mM), mannose (Km ~ 125 mM), and fructose (Km ~ 76 mM). It is a high affinity transporter for glucosamine (Km ~ 0,8 mM) [70, 93, 94].

GLUT 2 mRNA is detected in 80% of normal gastric mucosal samples. In gastric carcinoma samples, GLUT 2 mRNA is detected in all samples [80]. Overexpression of GLUT 2 has been observed in breast, colorectal, oral, pancreatic tumors, and in the cases of insulinoma. For details see [44].

GLUT 2 has garnered a great deal of attention as a protein that could be involved in pathogenesis of diabetes mellitus. Reductions in β-cell Glut 2 have been observed in several animal models of diabetes [95, 96].

Fanconi-Bickel syndrome is due to heritable mutations in transporter-encoding gene that impair monosaccharide uptake. The syndrome was first described in 1949 [97]. This first patient developed osteopenia, hepatomegaly, and tubular nephropathy, associated with glycosuria, phospaturia, aminoaciduria and proteinuria. A mutation in the GLUT 2 gene was identified by Santer and colleagues [98]. Most patients are homozygous for the disease-related mutations [99].

GLUT 3

There is relatively little information about GLUT 3, especially in humans [49]. The single copy gene (*SLC2A3*) for GLUT 3 is located on human chromosome 12p13.3 [43, 46, and 54]. The gene is comprised of 10 exons (spanning 17 kb) [19]. The open reading frame codes for a 496-amino-acid membrane protein with a predicted weight, 54 kDa [54]. GLUT 3 is highly expressed in the brain [100], especially in neurons [56, 106]. During rat brain development, Glut 3 mRNA was detected only in differentiated neurons. Glut 3 mRNA increased gradually from embryonic day 14, attaining adult levels in most regions by postnatal day 20. The highest levels were found in large projection neurons of the olfactory system, hippocampal formation, neocortex, and deep cerebellar, pontine, and brain stem nuclei. The anatomical distribution of Glut 3 gene expression correlated with developmental and regional patterns of brain glucose utilization. It suggests that, while Glut 1 may have a role in the transfer of glucose across the blood-brain barrier, Glut 3 expression determines brain glucose utilization [101]. However, its expression is restricted to nervous tissue in he mouse, but the GLUT 3 mRNA and GLUT 3 have been detected in other human tissues, including placenta, liver, and kidney [102]. GLUT 3 (Glut 3) is expressed also in fibroblasts [54], mouse embryos [103], sperm [104], human platelets [105], and retinal endothelial cells [107]. In human platelets thrombin stimulate the translocation of GLUT 3 from α-granules to the cell surface [105]. In summary, GLUT 3 mRNA is widely distributed in human tissues [108, 109], in contrast to its distribution in rodent and bovine tissues [110, 111].

GLUT 3 transports glucose with high affinity (Km = 1,4 mM). It also transports galactose (Km = 8,5 mM), mannose, maltose, xylose and dehydroascorbic acid [112, 113].

Unspecific expression of GLUT 3 is observed in tumors. For example, GLUT 3 is expressed in all the melanocytic lesions both benign and malignant [84]. GLUT 3 mRNA was detected in all samples of gastric tumors [80], human brain tumors [81], and in other cases of tumors [44]. In lung, colorectal, ovarian, laryngeal, and breast carcinomas, high levels of GLUT 1 and GLUT 3 in the tumors were significant indicators of decreased survival [114 – 119].

GLUT 4

GLUT 4, classically referred to as the "insulin-responsive" transporter has been widely studied due to its role as the main insulin-sensitive member of this family and thus its role in diabetes. GLUT 4 is a 509 amino acids protein with a molecular weight of approximately 55 kDa. In human, bovine, rat and mouse it is highly conservative with 91 – 96% sequence identity [19, 54]. Gene *SLC2A4* is localized on human chromosome 17p13-43 [54], and is comprised of 11 exons (spanning 6 kb) [19].

GLUT 4 is a member of the facilitative glucose transporter family characterized by preferential expression in muscle and fat tissue, where it is responsible for insulin-stimulated glucose uptake, and for the entry of glucose to muscle during contraction/exercise. GLUT 4 is unique among other members of family in its dynamic cycling within the muscle and adipose cell. Unlike other human GLUT proteins which constitutively reside in the cell membrane, GLUT 4 is stored intracellularly [120], more than 95% of total amount [44]. GLUT 4 is constitutively active for hexose transport, and glucose uptake is regulated by insulin controlling the amount of GLUT 4 in the plasma membrane [121]. In unstimulated cells, GLUT 4 is rapidly removed from the plasma membrane to which it recycles only slowly, leading to a steady-state accumulation in intracellular organelles. It was observed that all of the intracellular GLUT 4 of L6 muscle cells recycles to the plasma membrane within 6 h [126], whereas the existence of such behavior is in dispute in 3T3 L1 adipocytes [127, 128]. In muscle cells, GLUT 4 molecules from the plasma membrane reach the endosomal recycling compartment within 20 min and rapidly exit this compartment 20 min later [126].

In the presence of insulin or another stimulus, such as exercise, the equilibrium of this recycling process is altered to favor the translocation (regulated movement) of GLUT 4 from intracellular storage vesicles to the plasma membrane and, in the case of muscle, to the transverse tubules as well. The net effect is a rise in the maximal velocity of glucose transport into the cell [65, 122]. Activation of the intrinsic activity of the glucose transporters may also contribute to the increased glucose uptake in a post-translocation manner [123]. Within 10 min the level of surface of GLUT 4 increases 2- to 3-fold in skeletal muscle tissue and muscle cells [124] and human adipocytes, but the increase is > 10-fold in rodent adipocytes [125]. Insulin signaling results in changes in GLUT 4 trafficking parameters: GLUT 4 exocytosis is accelerated, whereas GLUT 4 endocytosis is inhibited.

As described above, in unstimulated adipocytes or muscle cells (i.e., the basal state), 5 – 10% of GLUT 4 is located at the cell surface and > 90% is in intracellular compartments. In the muscle fiber, surface GLUT 4 is more abundant in T tubules than in sarcolemma [134]. GLUT 4 is recycled between the plasma membrane and intracellular storage pools. In mature adipocytes and muscle cells, GLUT 4 is a long lived protein ($t_{1/2}$ of about 40 h) so each polypeptide chain is likely to cycle to the plasma membrane many times during its lifetime.

GLUT 4 trafficking in adipocytes differs greatly from that of other recycling proteins in some cells, indicating that GLUT 4 contains specific sequences that control its specialized behavior. For example, the F^5QQI sequence located in the N terminus mediates GLUT 4 internalization through a clathrin adaptin protein complex-2 (AP-2)-dependent pathway in insulin-stimulated adipocytes. The LL^{490} motif is dispensable for both basal and insulin stimulated endocytosis. The $TE^{499}LE^{501}Y$ sequence located in the C terminus is involved in basal retention [135]. N-glycosylation of glucose transporter also plays a role in GLUT 4 translocation [136].

The lipid second messenger, phosphatidic acid is produced by phospholipase D in a variety of intracellular signaling pathways. Phosphatidic acid transduces the signal by altering the localization and/or activity of its target proteins. A number of proteins are known to be regulated by phosphatidic acid in this way. Insulin appears capable of stimulating phospholipase D activity. The putative phosphatidic acid-binding motif, SQWL, is located in the first intracellular loop of GLUT 4, proximal to the third transmembrane helix and suitably placed to mediate interactions with a membrane lipid molecule. The other members of GLUT family, which are not thought to be regulated by phospholipase D, do not contain SQWL motif. Mutation of the SQWL sequence in 3T3-L1 adipocytes reduces GLUT 4 cell surface exposure in response to insulin by affecting fusion of the GLUT 4-containing vesicles with the plasma membrane [137].

It is unclear, whether in the absence of insulin, GLUT 4 storage vesicles represent a separate, distinct class of vesicles. Several so-called non-specialized proteins have been found to co-localize with GLUT 4 in adipocytes. However, many questions regarding the localization and trafficking pathways of GLUT 4 remained unanswered.

The majority of intracellular GLUT 4 is found in small 50-nm vesicles referred to as GSVs (GLUT4 storage vesicles). The formation of vesicles is catalyzed by a budding stage where coat proteins are recruited to the donor membrane via adaptor proteins [141, 142]. GLUT4 storage vesicles may form either from endosomes or from parts of the trans-Golgi network or both. The existence of a specialized GLUT 4 compartment that is exclusively insulin responsive has been postulated, but such organelle has not been fully biochemically characterized.

In the absence of insulin, GLUT 4 is segregated from the compartment containing the recycling receptors. The studies of protein composition of GLUT 4-containing vesicles reveal the presence of synaptobrevins, vesicle associated membrane protein 2 (VAMP2), cellubrevin (VAMP3), secretory carrier membrane proteins (SCAMP), phosphatidylinositol 4-kinae, GTP-binding protein Rab4, and zinc-dependent aminopeptidase (vp165 – for vesicle protein of molecular weight 165 kDa or gp160 – glycoprotein of molecular weight 160 kDa) [138, 139]. These observations suggest the existence of a GLUT 4 specialized compartment that can be regulated by insulin and is characterized by the presence and functional requirement of VAMP2 for final fusion with the plasma membrane [140].

Its expression is highest in the insulin sensitive tissues including brown and white adipose tissue and skeletal and cardiac muscle. The basal and insulin-induced changes in subcellular distribution of Glut 4 are different between fetal/neonatal and adult rat skeletal muscle. Under basal conditions, sarcolemma associated Glut 4 is higher in the newborn when compared to the adult translating into a higher glucose transport. Insulin-induced translocation of Glut 4 to the sarcolemma and insulin-induced transport is lower in the newborn when compared to the adult [133].

GLUT 4 is a high affinity transporter for glucose with a Km of $1 - 4$ mM when expressed in both *Xenopus* oocytes and Chinese hamster ovary cells [129, 130] or $5 - 6$ mM when expressed in the yeast *Saccharomyces cerevisiae* [131]. It can also transport dehydroascorbic acid and glucosamine (Km ~ 3,9 mM) [131].

Resistance to the stimulatory effect of insulin on glucose utilization is a key pathogenic feature of obesity, metabolic syndrome (also known as the syndrome X) or insulin resistance syndrome and characterized by insulin resistance, dyslipidemia, hypertension, and an increased risk of cardiovascular disease), and most forms of type 2 diabetes [132]. The over-expression of GLUT 4 is observed also in human cancers (breast, gastric, lung and pancreatic) [44].

GLUT 5

GLUT 5 belongs to class II of facilitative glucose transporters family. It was cloned by Burant and colleagues in 1992 [143]. The gene *SLC2A5* encoding GLUT 5 is located on human chromosome 1p36.2 [43, 46]. The gene is comprised of 12 exons (spanning 33 kb) [19]. The deduced protein sequence of GLUT 5 is composed of 501 amino acids with a molecular weight of approximately 43 kDa [11, 54]. GLUT 5 exhibits the weakest inter-isoform homology of any of the members of the GLUT family [144]. This is consistent with its identity as a fructose, rather than a glucose, transporter. Among the seven members of glucose transporter family able to transport fructose, GLUT 5 is the sole transporter specific for fructose, with no ability to transport glucose or galactose. It mediates fructose transport with a Km of ~ 6 mM [143, 145]. Buchs and colleagues have found two protein domains of

GLUT 5 to be responsible for fructose uptake (amino-terminus to first intracellular loop, and the sequence between the 5th and 11th transmembrane stretches [146], whereas at least parts of the carboxyl-terminal of GLUTs seem to be required for transport function [147].

It is expressed at high levels in the apical membrane of enterocytes [148]. GLUT 5 mRNA levels increase with age, and are highest in the adult small intestine [154]. In the intestine, a proximal-distal gradient was observed, with GLUT 5 mRNA levels being higher in the proximal small intestine when compared to the distal small intestine [11]. It is also expressed in high levels in the plasma membrane of mature spermatozoa [143]. Modest to significant levels of GLUT 5 mRNA and/or protein have now been demonstrated in kidney, fat, skeletal muscle and brain [54, 56, 144, and 149]. In muscle and fat cells it is not subject to acute insulin regulation as are GLUT 1 and GLUT 4 [49].

GLUT 5 is of tremendous interest because total fructose consumption has increased dramatically, e. g., in the United States, from ~ 20 to ~ 80 g/day in the last 20- 30 years [150, 151]. Fructose is the major sweetener in Western diets and for a while was used in diabetes therapy because it did not result in acute hyperglycemia. Increased fructose consumption, in particular as carbonated beverages, has been attributed to participate in the increased prevalence of obesity and type 2 diabetes.

Despite the importance of dietary fructose in the development of type 2 diabetes, very few studies have investigated the link between disease and GLUT 5 in insulin-sensitive tissues like skeletal muscle and adipocytes. Although GLUT 5 may be affected by diabetes, GLUT 5 is also particularly affected by levels of dietary fructose that may vary markedly among diabetes patients [145]. Patients with type 2 diabetes exhibited dramatic increases in GLUT 5 mRNA and protein abundance in skeletal muscle [152]. These increases were specific, because expression of GLUT 1, GLUT 3, GLUT 4, GLUT 8, GLUT 11, and GLUT 12 did not change with diabetes and could be reversed with drug enhancing insulin action [145]. There is a four-fold increase in GLUT 5 protein in intestinal epithelium from diabetic subjects [153].

A little else is known about GLUT 5 regulation and its physiological significance in fructose induced hypertension in animal models and humans, however the obtained results suggest, that Glut 5 is essential for the absorption of fructose in intestine and generation of fructose-induced hypertension in mice [155].

GLUT 5 mRNA and protein expression are affected by the development of tumors in certain organ systems. Grover-McKay and colleagues determined the *in vitro* invasive potential of three human breast cancer cell lines and showed that GLUT 1 protein levels increased with invasive potential, and, at the some time, GLUT 5 protein levels decreased with invasive potential [156]. Elevated GLUT 5 expression has been described in many human cancers, including: lung, colorectal, and breast carcinoma (reviewed [44]). Overexpression of GLUT 5 has been described also in human leukemia [157]. GLUT 5 is highly overexpressed in 27% of cancerous tissues tested [145].

Paralleling the increasing concern about the role of fructose in various diseases, the number of studies on GLUT 5 has increased dramatically in the five years [145].

GLUT 6

GLUT 6 (formerly designated GLUT 9) belongs to the class III of facilitative glucose transporters family. It has to be noted that the symbol GLUT 6 has previously been used for a pseudogene derived from the GLUT 3 (*SLC2A3P*) [160]. Human GLUT 6 was cloned from leukocytes by PCR and RACE-PCR amplification on the basis of sequence information obtained from murine expressed sequence tags and a human genomic sequence [158]. The gene *SLC2A6*, encoding GLUT 6 protein is localized on human chromosome 9q34 [43, 46]. It is comprised of 10 exons (spanning 8 kb) [19]. GLUT 6 protein is composed of 507 amino acids.

The cDNA of human GLUT 6 expresses a 46-kDa membrane protein [158]. Human GLUT 6 is predominantly expressed in brain, spleen and peripheral leukocytes [158], however, the presence of a GLUT 6 protein in these tissues has not been demonstrated so far [46]. GLUT 6 protein was detected in testis germinal cells [159]. It exhibits glucose transport activity, however, the transporter appears to be a low-affinity facilitator (Km = 5 mM) [46].

The intracellular localization of GLUT 6 is due to single dileucine motif present in N-termini. Mutation of the motif to alanines gave rise to expression of the protein in the plasma membrane. The insulin treatment has been reported not to induce protein translocation to the cell surface [161].

GLUT 7

GLUT 7 is the most recently cloned GLUT member. The human GLUT 7 has been cloned from a human intestinal cDNA library by using a PCR-based strategy [162]. It has been assigned to the class II of the GLUT family on the basis of sequence similarity [163]. The gene (*SLC2A7*) is adjacent to the GLUT 5 gene (*SLC2A5*) on the chromosome 1p36.22 [19, 46]. It is comprised of 12 exons (spanning 23 kb) [19]. The encoded protein is comprised of 524 amino acid residues and shares 68% similarity and 53% identity with GLUT 5, its most closely related isoform [162].

GLUT 7 is primarily expressed in the apical membrane of the small intestine (distal region) and colon, although mRNA has been detected in the testis and prostate as well [151, 163].

GLUT 7 has a high affinity for both glucose ($Km = 0,3$ mM) and fructose. It does not transport galactose, 2-deoxy-D-glucose and xylose [162].

The observation that the distribution of GLUT 7 is limited to the distal region of the small intestine, the ileum, which does not contain high concentrations of glucose and fructose, suggests that GLUT 7 does not play a major role in taking up glucose and fructose from the diet. It may be important toward the end of a meal when luminal concentrations of hexoses in the ileum are low [151, 162].

The unusual substrate specificity and close sequence identity with GLUT 5 suggest that GLUT 7 represents an intermediate between class II GLUTs and the class I member GLUT 2. Comparison between these proteins may provide key information as to the structural determinants for the recognition of fructose as a substrate [162]. Cheeseman introduced the hypothesis that GLUT proteins may have a substrate selectivity filter at the exofacial opening of their translocation pore [163].

GLUT 8

GLUT 8 (formerly designated GLUTX1) was independently cloned by Ibberson and colleagues [164] and by Doege and colleagues [165]. The gene (*SLC2A8*) is located on chromosome 9q33.3, is 11 kb in length and contains 10 exons [19, 43] encoding a protein of 477 amino acids. *In vitro* translated GLUT 8 migrates as a 35-kDa protein [166], however, COS-7 cells transfected with GLUT 8 cDNA expressed a 42-kDa protein [165]. GLUT 8 exhibits significant sequence similarity with the members of the GLUT family (29,4% of amino acids identical with GLUT 1) [165].

GLUT 8 is a high affinity transporter for glucose ($Km \sim 2$ mM) [166].

In human tissues, the GLUT 8 mRNA was predominantly found in testis, but not in testicular carcinoma. Lower amounts of the mRNA were detected is skeletal muscle, heart, small intestine, and brain [165]. GLUT 8 protein was detected in the hippocampus of streptozotocin diabetic rats [167] and mouse blastocyst [168]. Facilitative glucose transporter 8 was detected in the acrosomal region of mature spermatozoa [171] and blood retinal barrier [172]. GLUT 8 was detected also in endometrium and endometrial adenocarcinoma [174].

The GLUT 8 cycles between intracellular vesicles and the plasma membrane. It is primarily located in intracellular compartments under basal conditions. GLUT 8 has been found to be associated with endosomes, lysosomes and membranes of endoplasmic reticulum [166] and the distribution of GLUT 8 is not affected by insulin treatment in adipose cells [169, 170]. In different cells systems, none of the conventional signals tested induced a translocation of GLUT 8 to the plasma membrane. Therefore, GLUT 8 appears to catalyze transport of sugars or sugar derivatives through intracellular membranes [166].

The GLUT 8 mRNA and protein are differentially regulated in the liver, depending on the prenatal and postnatal developmental stage of mice, GLUT 8 mRNA and protein are also differentially regulated in mice liver in response to physiologic and diabetes milieu [173].

GLUT 9

GLUT 9 (earlier designated as GLUTX) sequence was identified independently by two groups [175] and was designated GLUTX [176] and GLUT 9 [177]. The human *SLC2A9* gene is localized on chromosome 4p15.3-p16 and is approximately 214 bp in length [19]. The gene encodes two isoforms through the use of alternative promoters. The *SLC2A9* gene consists of 12 exons coding for a 540-amino acid protein (the major isoform of GLUT 9). An alternative splice variant of GLUT 9 RNA consists of 13 exons and codes for a putative protein of 512 amino acids (GLUT9ΔN isoform). The predicted proteins differ only in their N terminus, suggesting a different subcellular localization and possible physiological role [19, 178]. The next relative of GLUT 9 is the fructose transporter GLUT 5 [46].

GLUT 9 is expressed mainly in kidney, liver, placenta, and leukocytes, whereas GLUT9ΔN was detected only in kidney and placenta [178]. Both isoforms of GLUT 9 protein and mRNA are expressed in the epithelial of various tissues; however the two splice variants are expressed differentially within polarized cells, with GLUT 9 localized predominantly on the basolateral surfaces whereas GLUT9ΔN is expressed on apical surfaces [178, 179].

GLUT 9 appears to be a functional isoform with low affinity for deoxyglucose. The substrate specificity of GLUT 9 is unique since in addition to transporting hexose sugars, it also is a high capacity uric acid transporter. Caulfield and colleagues found that urate is transported by GLUT 9 (two splice variants of glucose transporter) at rates 45- to 60-fold faster than glucose, and demonstrated that urate transport is facilitated by glucose and, to a lesser extent, fructose [180].

The relationship between GLUT 9 and uric acid is highly clinically significant. Elevated uric acid levels have been associated with metabolic syndrome, obesity, diabetes, hypertension, and chronic renal failure. The uric acid may play a role in the pathogenesis of these diseases. GLUT 9 is expressed in articular cartilage and is a uric acid transporter thus it is possible that GLUT 9 plays a role in gout [179].

GLUT 10

GLUT 10 was described by McVie-Wylie and colleagues [181]. The human GLUT 10 gene is localized on chromosome 20q13.1, contains 5 of exons, and is approximately 27 bp in length [19, 46]. Human GLUT 10 is composed of 541 amino acids. It shares only 18 – 21% identity with human GLUT 1 – 11 [19] and exhibits highest sequence similarity with GLUT 8 [46]. GLUT 10 does not have the PESPR motif in loop 6. The lack of this motif is very surprising, because it is conserved in all other members of the GLUT family [46].

Although GLUT 10 does not contain a dileucine motif, its reported expression is in the insulin-sensitive tissues of skeletal muscle and heart [6, 181]. GLUT 10 mRNA is expressed at highest levels in the liver and pancreas. Low mRNA levels are also detected in placenta and kidney [181]. GLUT 10 expression is also found in human adipose tissue (subcutaneous and omental), human preadipocyte cell strain (SGBS) and 3T3-L1 adipocytes [182].

GLUT 10 is a transporter protein with a very high affinity for both deoxy-D-glucose (Km ~ 0,3 mM) and D-galactose [183], but not for fructose [45].

The association of GLUT 10 with a known type 2 diabetes mellitus susceptibility locus on chromosome 20 [181, 183] makes it a particular interesting target of study. Polymorphisms of GLUT 10, on the other hand, are not associated to type 2 diabetes mellitus in investigated human populations [184, 185, and 186]. The mutations in the GLUT 10 have been found to be associated with human arterial tortuosity syndrome [187].

GLUT 11

The human GLUT 11 (formerly designated GLUT 10) was isolated and described by Doege and colleagues [188]. The human GLUT 11 gene (*SLC2A11*) is 28 bp in length, contains of 10 – 13 exons, and is located on chromosome

22q11.2 [19, 188]. In human, three isoforms of GLUT 11 have been cloned, because the separate exons 1 (exon 1A, exon 1B, and exon 1C) of the *SLC2A11* gene generated mRNA of three GLUT 11 variants (GLUT 11-A, GLUT 11-B, and GLUT 11-C) which differ only at their N-terminal sequences [189]. The GLUT 11 isoforms are expressed in a tissue specific manner but do not appear to differ in their functional characteristics.

The GLUT 11 is comprised of 496 amino acids [19]. Human GLUT 11 exhibits similarity with the members of the GLUT family, and the closest relative of GLUT 11 is the fructose transporter GLUT 5 (sharing about 42% amino acid identity with GLUT 11) [188].

GLUT 11 appears to recognize fructose with comparable affinity to, possibly with even higher affinity than, glucose (Km ~ 0,2 mM) but not galactose [45, 188].

GLUT 11-A is expressed in heart, skeletal muscle, and kidney; GLUT 11-B in kidney, adipose tissue, and placenta; and GLUT 11-C in adipose tissue, heart, skeletal muscle, and pancreas [189].

Surprisingly, *SLC2A11* gene is not present in mice and rats [189].

GLUT 12

The cDNA of GLUT 12 (formerly designated GLUT 8) has been detected in breast cancer cell line, MCF-7, and was cloned from a human embryonic cDNA library [190]. The human GLUT 12 gene (*SLC2A12*) is located on chromosome 6q23.2. It is 65 bp in length and contains 5 exons [19, 43]. GLUT 12 cDNA encodes 617 amino acids [191]. Dileucine motifs are present in N termini. GLUT 12 exhibits 29% amino acid identity with GLUT 4 and 40% to the GLUT 10 [191].

GLUT 12 expression occurs in heart, skeletal muscle, adipose tissue, small intestine and chondrocytes [182, 191]. Differential expression of GLUT 12 was observed in human placenta. In first trimester tissue GLUT 12 was present predominantly in the syncytiotrophoblast, to a lesser extent in villous cytotrophoblast and in extra-villous trophoblast cells. At term, GLUT 12 was found predominantly in villous vascular smooth muscle and stromal cells and was not detected in syncytiotrophoblast [192].

GLUT 12 contains potential C-terminal and N-terminal targeting motif, in similar positions to the LL and FQQI targeting motifs of GLUT 4 [191]. When MCF-7 cells (breast cancer cell line) were grown in the absence of insulin, GLUT 12 was located to a perinuclear region. This localization is altered when the cells are grown continuously in the presence of insulin [191]. GLUT 12 was also localized to a perinuclear region and to the plasma membrane in cultured human prostate cancer lines [193]. In human muscle, insulin caused a shift of a portion of GLUT 12 from intracellular low density microsomes to the plasma membrane fraction.

Translocation of GLUT 12 in cultured myoblasts was dependent on activation of PI 3-kinase [194]. These findings, along with the potential targeting motifs present in the GLUT 12 protein, suggest that GLUT 12 could undergo regulated protein trafficking in a similar manner to plasma membrane in response to the insulin [79].

GLUT 12 protein expression occurs in human breast tumors. It was detected in eight of ten invasive tumors [195]. GLUT 12 protein is expressed also in human prostate carcinoma cells [196].

GLUT 12 exhibits transport activity for glucose (Km ~ 4 – 5 mM), galactose and fructose [45].

HMIT

Human HMIT gene (*SLC2A13*) is located on chromosome 22q12.3, contains 10 exons and is 351 bp in length [19]. The deduced amino acid sequence of human HMIT is 629 amino acid long [46]. HMIT is expressed predominantly in the brain where it is found as a glycosylated protein of molecular weight 83 kDa. It is present both with astrocytes and some neurons. The investigation revealed the presence of HMIT in intracellular compartments and on the plasma membrane [46]. It can be induced to move to cell surface following cell depolarization, activation of protein kinase C or increased intracellular calcium concentrations [197].

HMIT is a protein coupled myo-inositol transporter, making it the only GLUT that has been demonstrated to use a proton gradient to energize the movement of substrate [198]. HMIT is a H^+/myo-inositol co-transporter and exhibits transport activity only for myo-inositol. Transport is with high affinity (Km ~ 100 mM) and is increased by the low pH with a maximal rate being reached at pH = 5,0 [198]. No hexose transport activity was found [46].

GLUT 14

GLUT 14 was identified and cloned by Wu and Freeze [199]. The human GLUT 14 gene (*SLC2A14*) is located on chromosome 12p13.3, about 10 Mb upstream of GLUT 3. GLUT 14 gene contains 11 exons and exhibits a genomic organization similar to that of GLUT 3. GLUT 14 has two alternatively spliced forms. The shorter form of GLUT 14 (GLUT 14-S) consists of 10 exons and produces a 497 amino acid protein. It shares 94,5% identity with GLUT 3. The long form (GLUT 14-L) has an additional exon and codes for protein with 520 amino acids that differs from GLUT 14-S only at the N-terminus. Both isoforms of GLUT 14 are specifically expressed in testis. Interestingly, the ortholog of GLUT 14 is not found in mice [199].

PSEUDOGENES

1. *SLC2A3P1* (alias GLUT 6) is located on chromosome 5q33-35 and is a retroposon of *SLC2A3* [46]

2. *SLC2A3P2* is located on chromosome 1q31.3 and is a retroposon of *SLC2A3* [46]

3. *SLC2A3P3* is located on chromosome 12p13.3 and is a retroposon of *SLC2A3* [46]

4. *SLC2AXP1* is located on chromosome 2q11.2 and contains internal stop sequences [46]

REFERENCES

[1]   Riklis E, Quastel JH. Effects of cations on sugar absorption by isolated surviving guinea pig intestine. Can J Biochem Physiol 1958;36:347-362

[2]   Crane RK. Hypothesis for mechanism of intestinal active transport of sugars. Fed Proc 1962;21:891-895

[3]   Crane RK. Na$^+$-dependent transport in the intestine and other animal tissues. Fed Proc 1965; 24:1000-1006

[4]   Hediger MA, Coady MJ, Ikeda TS, Wright EM. Expression cloning and cDNA sequencing of the Na$^+$/glucose co-transporter. Nature 1987;330:379-381

[5]   Hediger MA, Turk E, Wright EM. Homology of the human intestinal Na$^+$/glucose and Escherichia coli Na$^+$/proline cotransporters. Proc Natl Acad Sci USA 1989; 86:5748-5752

[6]   Woods IS, Trayhurn P. Glucose transporters (GLUT and SGLT): expanded families of sugar transport protein. Br J Nutr 2003;89:3-9

[7]   Wright EM. Renal Na$^+$/glucose cotransporters. Am J Physiol 2001; 280:F10-F18

[8]   Wright EM, Turk E. The sodium/glucose cotransport family SLC5. Pflugers Arch – Eur J Physiol 2004;447:510-518

[9]   Wright EM, Loo DDF, Hirayama BA, Turk E. Surprising versatility of Na$^+$/glucose cotransporters: SLC5. Physiology 2004;19,6:370-376

[10]   Turk E, Wright EM. Membrane topology motifs in the SGLT cotransporters family. J Membrane Biol 1977;159:1-20

[11]   Drozdowski LA, Thomson ABR. Intestinal sugar transport. World J Gastroenterol 2006;12,11:1657-1670

[12]   Wright EM. Glucose galactose malabsorption. Am J Physiol 1998;275:G879-G882

[13]   Wright EM, Martin MG, Turk E. Intestinal absorption in health and disease – sugars. Best Prac Res Clin Gastroenterol 2003;17:943-956

[14]   Gagnon DG, Bissonnette P., Lapointe IY. Identification of a disulfide bridge linking the fourth and the seventh extracellular loops of the Na$^+$/glucose cotransporter. J Gen Physiol 2006;127,2:145-158

[15]   Turk E., Martin MG, Wright EM. Structure of the human Na$^+$/glucose cotransporter gene SGLT1. J Biol Chem 1994;269,21:15204-15209

[16]   Loo DDF, Hirayama BA, Gallardo EM, Lam JT, Turk E, Wright EM. Conformational changes couple Na$^+$ and glucose transport. Proc Natl Acad Sci USA 1998;95:7789-794

[17]   Meinild AK, Hirayama BA, Wright EM, Loo DDF. Fluorescence studies of ligand-induced conformational changes of the Na$^+$/glucose cotransporter. Biochemistry 2002;41:1250-1258

[18]   Takata K, Kasahara T, Kasahara M, Ezaki O, Hirano H. Localization of Na$^+$-dependent active type and erythrocyte/HepG2-glucose transporters in rat kidney: immunofluorescence and immunogold study. J Histochem Cytochem 1991; 39:287-298

[19]   Zhao F-Q, Keating AF. Functional properties and genomic of glucose transporters. Curr Genomics 2007;8,2:113-128

[20]   Diez-Sampedro A, Wright EM, Hirayama BA. Residue 457 controls sugar binding and transport in the Na$^+$/glucose cotransporter. J Biol Chem 2001; 276:49188-49194

[21]   Panayotova-Heiermann M, Loo DDF, Kong CT, Lever JE, Wright EM. Sugar binding to Na$^+$/glucose cotransporters is determined by the C-terminal half of the protein. J Biol Chem 1996;271:10029-10034

[22]   Panayotova-Heiermann M, Wright EM. Mapping the urea channel through the rabbit Na$^+$/glucose cotransporter SGLT1. J Physiol 2001;535:419-425

[23]   Panayotova-Heiermann M, Eskandari S, Turk E, Zampighi GA, Wright EM. Five transmembrane helices form the sugar pathway through the Na$^+$/glucose cotransporter. J Biol Chem 1997;272,30:20324-20327

[24]   Pajor AM, Wright EM. Sequence, tissue distribution and functional expression of a mammalian Na$^+$/nucleoside cotransporter. J Biol Chem 1992;267:3557-3560

[25]   Zhou L, Cryan EV, D'Andrea MR, Belkowski S, Conway BR, Demarest KT. Human cardiomyocytes express high level of Na$^+$/glucose cotransporter 1 (SGLT1). J Cell Biochem 2003;90,2:339-346

[26]   Elfeber K, Kohler A, Lutzenburg M, *et al.* Localization of the Na$^+$-D-glucose cotransporter SGLT1 in the blood-brain barrier. Histochem Cell Biol 2004;121:201-207

[27]   Hirayama BA, Lostao MP, Panayotova-Heiermann M, Loo DD, Turk E, Wright EM. Kinetic and specificity differences between rat, human, and rabbit Na$^+$/glucose cotransporters 1 (SGLT-1). Am J Physiol 1996;270:G919-G926

[28]   Zhao FQ, Zheng YC, Wall EH, McFadden TB. Cloning and expression of bovine sodium/glucose cotransporters. J Dairy Sci 2005;88:182-194

[29]   Wright EM, Loo DDF, Turk E, Hirayama BA. Sodium cotransporters. Curr Opinion in Cell Biol 1996;8:468-473

[30]   Loo DDF, Wright EM, Zeuthen T. Water pumps. J Physiol 2002;42:53-60

[31]   Leung DW, Loo DDF, Hirayama BA, Zeuthen T, Wright EM. Urea transport by cotransporters. J Physiol 2000,528,Pt2:251-257

[32]   Wells RG, Kanai Y, Pajor AM, Turk E, Wright EM, Hediger MA. The cloning of a human kidney cDNA with similarity to the sodium/glucose cotransporter. Am J Physiol Renal Fluid Electrolyte Physiol 1992;263:F459-F465

[33]   Wells RG, Mohandas TK, Hediger MA. Localization of the Na$^+$/glucose cotransporter gene SGLT2 to human chromosome 16 close to the centromere. Genomics 1993;17:787-789

[34]   Kanai Y, Lee WS, You G, Brown D, Hediger MA. The human kidney low affinity Na$^+$/glucose cotransporter SGLT2. Delineation of the major renal reabsorptive mechanism for D-glucose. J Clin Invest 1994;93:397-404

[35]   Mackenzie B, Loo DDF, Panayotova-Heiermann M, Wright EM. Biophysical characteristics of the pig kidney Na$^+$/glucose cotransporter SGLT2 reveal a common mechanism for SGLT1 and SGLT2. J Biol Chem 1996;271:32678-32683

[36]   You G, Lee WS, Barros EJ, *et al.* Molecular characteristics of Na-coupled glucose transporters in adult and embryonic rat kidney. J Biol Chem 1995;270:29365-29371

[37]   Van den Huevel LP, Assink K, Willemsen M, Monnens L. Autosomal recessive renal glucosuria attributable to a mutation in the sodium glucose cotransporter (SGLT2). Hum Genet 2002;111:544-547

[38]   Kleta R, Stuart C, Gill FA, Gahl WA. Renal glucosuria due to SGLT2 mutations. Mol Genet Metab 2004;82:56-58

[39]   Diez-Sampedro A, Eskanderi S, Wright EM, Hirayama BA. Na$^+$-to-sugar stoichiometry of SGLT3. Am J Physiol Renal Physiol 2001;280:F278-F282

[40]   Diez-Sampedro A, Hirayama BA, Oswald C, *et al.* A glucose sensor binding in a family of transporters. Proc Acad Sci USA 2002;100:11753-11758

[41]   Tazawa S, Yamato T, Fujikura H, *et al.* SLC5A9/SGLT4, a new Na$^+$-dependent glucose transporter, is an essential transporter for mannose, 1,5-anhydro-D-glucitol, and fructose. Life Sci 2005;76,9:1039-1050

[42]   Mueckler M, Caruso C, Baldwin SA, *et al.* Sequence and structure of a human glucose transporter. Science 1985;229:941-945

[43]   Joost H-G, Mueckler M, Bell GI, *et al.* Nomenclature of the GLUT/SLC2A of sugar/polyol transport facilitators. Am J Physiol 2002,282:E974-E976

[44]   Medina RA, Owen GI. Glucose transporters: expression, regulation and cancer. Biol Res 2002;35,1:9-26

[45]   Manolescu AR, Witkowska K, Kinnaird A, Cessford T, Cheeseman C. Facilitated hexose transporters: new perspectives on form and function. Physiology 2007;22:234-240

[46]   Joost H-G, Thorens B. The extended GLUT-family of sugar/polyol transport facilitators – nomenclature, sequence characteristics, and potential function of its novel members. Mol Membrane Biol 2001,18;247-256

[47]   Lachaal M, Rampal AL, Lee W, Jung CY. Transmembrane glucose channel: affinity labeling with a transportable D-glucose diazirine. J Biol Chem 1996;271:5225-5230

[48]   Zeng H, Parthasarathy R, Rampal AL, Jung CY. Proposal structure of putative glucose channel in GLUT1 facilitative glucose transporter. Biophys J 1996;70:14-21

[49]   Mueckler M. Facilitative glucose transporters. Eur J Biochem 1994;219:713-725

[50]   Jung CY. The facilitative glucose transporter and insulin action. Exp Mol Med 1996;28,4:153-160

[51]   Mueckler M, Weng W, Kruse M. Glutamine 161 of GLUT1 glucose transporter is critical for transport activity and exofacial ligand binding. J Biol Chem 1994;269:20533-20538

[52]   Doege H, Schürmann A, Ohnimus H, Monser V, Holman GD, Joost H-G. Serine 294 and threonine 259 in the exofacial loop domain between helices 7 and 8 of glucose transporters (GLUT) are involved in the conformational alterations during the transport process. Biochem J 1998;329: 289-293

[53]   Hruz PW, Mueckler MM. Structural analysis of the GLUT1 facilitative glucose transporter (Review). Mol Membrane Biol 2001,18:183-193

[54]   Longo N, Elsas LJ. Human glucose transporters. Adv Pediatr 1998;45:293-313

[55]   Olson AL, Pessin JE. Structure, function and regulation of the facilitative glucose transporter gene family. Annu Rev Nutr 1996;16:235-256

[56]   Maher F, Vannuci SJ, Simpson IA. Glucose transporter protein in brain. FASEB J 1994;8: 1003-1011

[57]   Maher F, Davies-Hill TM, Lysko PG, Henneberry RC, Simpson IA. Expression of two glucose transporters, GLUT1 and GLUT3, in cultured cerebellar neurons: Evidence for neuron specific expression of GLUT3. Mol Cell Neurosci 1991;2:351-360

[58]   McMahon RJ, Hwang JB, Frost SC. Glucose deprivation does not affect GLUT 1 targeting in 3T3-L1 adipocytes. Biochem Biophys Res Com 2000;273:859-864

[59]   Onetti R, Baulida J, Bassols A. Increased glucose transport in ras-transformed fibroblasts: a possible role for N-glycosylation of GLUT 1. FEBS Lett 1997;407:267-270

[60]   Pardridge WM, Boado RJ, Farrel CR. Brain-type glucose transporter (GLUT-1) is selectively localizes to the blood-brain-barrier. Studies with quantitative Western blotting and in situ hybrydization. J Biol Chem 1990;265:18035-18040.

[61]   Kumagai AK, Dwyer KJ, Pardridge WM. Differential glycosylation of the GLUT1 glucose transporter in brain capillaries and choroid plexus. Biochim Biophys Acta 1994;1193:24-30

[62]   Mueckler M, Makepeace C. Transmembrane segment 6 of the Glut 1 glucose transporter is an outer helix and contains amino acid side chains essential for transport activity. J Biol Chem 2008;283,17:11550-11555

[63]   Mueckler M, Makepeace C. Transmembrane segment 12 of the Glut 1 glucose transporter is an outer helix and is not directly involved in the transport mechanism. J Biol Chem 2006;281,48: 36993-36998

[64]   Takata K, Kasahara M, Ezaki O, Hirano H. Erythrocyte/HepG2-type glucose transporter is concentrated in cells of blood-tissue barriers. Biochem Biophys Res Commun 1990;173:67-73

[65]   Gould GW, Holman GD. The glucose transporter family: structure, function and tissue-specific expression. Biochem J 1993;295:329-341

[66]   Korgun ET, Demir R, Sedlmayr P, *et al.* Physiological leukocytosis during pregnancy is associated with changes in glucose transporter expression of maternal peripheral blood granulocytes and monocytes. Am J Reprod Immunol 2002;48:110-116

[67]   Gould GW, Bell GI. Facilitative glucose transporters: an expanding family. TIBS 1990;15: 18-22

[68]   Zorzano A, Wilkinson W, Kotliar N, *et al.* Insulin-regulated glucose uptake in rat adipocytes is mediated by two transporter isoforms present in at least two vesicle populations. J Biol Chem 1989; 264,21:1238-12363

[69]   Marette A, Richardson JM, Ramlal T, *et al.* Abundance, localization, and insulin-induced translocation of glucose transporters in red and white muscle. Am J Physiol 1992;263,2Pt1:C443- C452

[70]   Uldry M, Ibberson M, Hosokawa M, Thorens B. GLUT 2 is highly affinity glucoseamine transporter. FEBS Lett 2002;524:199-203

[71]   Wieczorke R, Dlugai S, Krampe S, Boles E. Characterisation of mammalian GLUT glucose transporters in a heterologous yeast expression system. Cell Physiol Biochem 2003;13,3:123-134

[72]   Sagun KC, Cárcamo JM, Golde DW. Vitamin C enters mitochondria via facilitative glucose transporter 1 (Glut 1) and confers mitochondrial protection against oxidative injury. FASEB J 2005; 19:1657-1667

[73]   Jin Q, Agrawal L, VanHorn-Ali Z, Alkhatib G. Infection of CD4[+] T lymphocytes by the human T cell leukemia virus type 1 is mediated by the glucose transporter GLUT1: Evidence using antibodies specific to the receptor's large extracellular domain. Virology 2006;349,1:184-196

[74]   Jones KS, Fugo K, Petrow-Sadowski C, *et al.* Human T-cell leukemia virus type1 (HTLV-1) and HTLV-2 use different receptor complexes to enter T cells. J Virol 2006;80,17:8291-8302

[75]   Manel N, Kinet S, Kim FJ, Taylor N, Sitbon M, Battini J-L. GLUT-1 est le récepteur des rétrovirus humains HTL. Méd Sci 2004;20,3:277-279

[76]   Warburg O. On the origin of cancer cell's. Science 1956;123:309-314

[77] Isslbacher KJ. Sugar and amino acid transport by cells in culture: differences between normal and malignant cells. N Engl J Med 1972;286:929-933

[78] Zhang JZ, Behrooz A, Ismail-Beigi F. Regulation of glucose transport by hypoxia. Am J Kidney Dis 1999;34:189-202

[79] Macheda ML, Rogers S, Best JD. Molecular and cellular regulation of glucose transporter (GLUT) proteins in cancer. J Cell Physiol 2005;202:654-662

[80] Noguchi Y, Marat D, Saito A, *et al.* Expression of facilitative glucose transporters in gastric tumors. Hepato-Gastroenterol 1999;46:2683-2689

[81] Boado RJ, Black KL, Pardridge WM. Gene expression of GLUT 3 and GLUT 1 glucose transporters in human brain tumors. Mol Brain Res 1994;27:51-57

[82] Yasushi N, Kuniaki T, Nobuso M, Yoshio A, Toshikazu M, Hiroshi H. Investigative urology: Immunohistochemical localization of glucose transporters in human renal cell carcinoma. J Urol 1995;153,3:798-801

[83] Grover-McKay M, Walsh SA, Seftor EA, Thomas PA, Hendrix MJC. Role for glucose transporter 1 protein in human breast cancer. Pathol Oncol Res 1998;4,2:115-120

[84] Parent P, Coli A, Massi G, Mangoni A, Fabrizi MM, Bigotti G. Immunohistochemical expression of the glucose transporters Glut-1 and Glut-3 in human malignant melanomas and benign melanocytic lesions. J Exp Clin Cancer Res 2008;27,1:34,doi:10.1186/1756-9966-27-34

[85] Cooper R, Sarioğlu S, Sökmen S, *et al.* Glucose transporter-1 (GLUT-1): a potential marker of prognosis in rectal carcinoma? Br J Cancer 2003;89:870-876

[86] De Vivo DC, Trifiletti RR, Jacobson RI, Ronen GM, Behmand RA, Harik SI. Defective glucose transport across the blood-brain barrier as a cause of persistent hypoglycorrhachia, seizures, and developmental delay. New Engl J Med 1991;325:703-709

[87] Pascual JM, Wang D, Lecumberri B, Yang H, Mao X, Yang R, De Vivo DC. GLUT1 deficiency and other glucose transporter diseases. Eur J Endocrinol 2004;150:627-633

[88] Fukumoto H, Seino S, Imura H, *et al.* Sequence, tissue distribution, and chromosome localization of mRNA encoding a human glucose transporter-like protein. Proc Natl Acad Sci USA 1988;85:5434-5438

[89] Thorens B, Sarkar HK, Kaback HR, Lodish HF. Cloning and functional expression in bacteria of a novel glucose transporter present in liver, intestine, kidney, and β-pancreatic islet cells. Cell 1988;55:281-290

[90] Thorens B, Cheng ZQ, Brown D, Lodish HF. Liver glucose transporter: a basolateral protein in hepatocytes and intestine and kidney cells. Am J Physiol 1990;259:C279-C285

[91] Thorens B, Lodish HF, Brown D. Differential localization of two glucose transporter isoforms in rat kidney. Am J Physiol 1990;259:C286-C294

[92] Lelup C, Arluison M, Lepetit N, *et al.* Glucose transporter 2 (GLUT 2) expression in specific brain nuclei. Brain Res 1994;638:221-226

[93] Johnson JH, Newgard CB, Milburn JL, Lodish HF, Thorens B. The high Km glucose transporter of islets of Langerhans is functionally similar to the low affinity transporter of liver and has an identical primary sequence. J Biol Chem 1990;265:6548-6551

[94] Colville CA, Seater MJ, Jess TJ, Gould GW, Thomas HM. Kinetic analysis of the liver-type (GLUT2) and brain type (GLUT3) glucose transporters in Xenopus oocytes: substrate specificities and effects of transport inhibitors. Biochem J 1993;290:701-706

[95] Orci L, Ravazzola M, Baetens D, *et al.* Evidence that down-regulation of beta-cell glucose transporters in non-insulin-dependent diabetes may be the cause of diabetic hyperglycemia. Proc Natl Acad Sci USA 1990;87:9953-9957

[96] Johnson JH, Ogawa A, Chen L, *et al.* Underexpression of beta cell high Km glucose transporters in noninsulin-dependent diabetes. Science 1990;250,4985:546-549

[97] Fanconi G, Bickel H. Die chronische aminoacidurie (Aminosaurediabetes oder nephrotisch-glukosurisscher Zwergwuchs) Cystinkrankheit. Helvetica Ped Acta 1949;4:359-396

[98] Santer R, Schneppenheim R, Dombrowski A, Gotz H, Steinmann B, Schaub J. Mutations in GLUT2, the gene for the liver-type glucose transporter, in patients with Fanconi-Bickel syndrome. Nature Genet 1997;17:324-326

[99] Santer R, Groth S, Kinner M, *et al.* The mutation spectrum of the facilitative glucose transporter gene SLC2A2 (GLUT2) in patients with Fanconi-Bickel syndrome. Human Genet 2002;110:21-29

[100] Nagamatsu S, Kornhauser JM, Burant CF, Seino S, Mayo KE, Bell GI. Glucose transporter expression in brain. cDNA sequence of mouse GLUT3, the brain facilitative glucose transporter isoform, and identification of sites of expression by in-situ hybridization. J Biol Chem 1992;267: 467-472

[101] Bondy CA, Lee W-H, Zhou J. Ontogeny and cellular distribution of brain glucose transporter gene expression. Mol Cell Neurosci 1992;3:305-314

[102] Gould GW, Brant AM, Kahn BB, Shepherd PR, Mc Coid SC, Gibbs EM. Expression of the brain-type glucose transporter is restricted to brain and neuronal cells in mice. Diabetologia 1992;35: 304-309

[103] Pantaleon M, Harvey MB, Pascoe WS, James DE, Kaye PL. GLUT3: ontogeny, targeting and role in the mouse blastocyst. Proc Natl Acad Sci USA 1997;94:3795-3800

[104] Burant CF, Davidson NO. GLUT3 glucose transporter isoform in rat testis: localization, effect of diabetes mellitus, and comparison to human testis. Am J Physiol 1994,267:R1488-R1495

[105] Heijnen HFG, Oorschot V, Sixma JI, Slot JW, James DE. Thrombin stimulates glucose transport in human platelets via the translocation of the glucose transporter GLUT-3 from α-granules to the cell surface. J Cell Biol 1997;138,2:323-330

[106] Immunolocalization of GLUT1 and GLUT3 glucose transporters in primary cultured neurons and glia. J Neurosc Res 1995;42:459-469

[107] Knott RM, Robertson M, Muckersie E, Forrester JV. Regulation of glucose transporters (GLUT1 and GLUT3) in human retinal endothelial cells. Biochem J 1996;318:313-317

[108] Haber RS, Weinstein SP, O'Boyle E, Morgello S. Tissue distribution of the human GLUT3 glucose transporter. Endocrinol 1993;132:2238-2243

[109] Burant CF, Sivitz WI, Fukumoto H, *et al.* Mammalian glucose transporters: structure and molecular regulation. Recent Prog Horm Res 1991;47:349-387

[110] Zhao FQ, Glimm DR, Kenelly JJ. Distribution of mammalian facilitative glucose transporter messenger RNA in bovine tissues. Int J Biochem 1993;25:1897-1903

[111] Yano H, Seino Y, Inagaki N, *et al.* Tissue distribution and species differences of the brain type glucose transporter (GLUT3). Biochem Biophys Res Commun 1991;174:470-477

[112] Colville CA, Seatter MJ, Jess TJ, Gould GW, Thomas HM. Kinetic analysis of the liver-type (GLUT2) and brain-type (GLUT3) glucose transporters in Xenopus oocytes: substrate specificities and effects of transport inhibitors. Biochem J 1993;290:701-706

[113] Kayano T, Fukumoto H, Eddy RL, *et al.* Evidence for a family of human glucose transporter-like proteins. Sequence and gene localization of a protein expressed in fetal skeletal muscle and other tissues. J Biol Chem 1988;263:15245-15248

[114] Baer SC, Casaubon L, Younes M. Expression of the human erythrocyte glucose transporter Glut1 in cutaneous neoplasia. J Am Acad Dermatol 1997;37,4:575-577

[115] Ogawa J, Inoue H, Koide S. Glucose-transporter-type-I-gene amplification correlates with sialys-Lewis-X synthesis and proliferation in lung cancer. Int J Cancer 1997;74,2:189-192

[116] Younes M, Brown RW, Mody DR, Fernandez L, Laucirica R. GLUT1 expression in human breast carcinoma: Correlation with known prognostic markers. Anticancer Res 1995;15,6B:2895- 2898

[117] Haber RS, Rathan A, Weiser KR, *et al.* GLUT1 glucose transporter expression in colorectal carcinoma: A marker for poor prognosis. Cancer 1998;83,1:34-40

[118] Cantuaria G, Fagotti A, Ferrandina G, *et al.* GLUT-1 expression in ovarian carcinoma: Association with survival and response to chemotherapy. Cancer 2001;92,5:1144-1150

[119] Kang SS, Chun YK, Hur MH, *et al.* Clinical significance of glucose transporter 1 (GLUT1) expression in human breast carcinoma. Jpn J Cancer Res 2002,93,10:1123-1128

[120] Pascoe W, Inukai K, Oka Y, Slot J, James DE. Differential targeting of facilitative glucose transporter in polarized epithelial cells. Am J Physiol 1996;271:C547-C554

[121] Huang S, Czech MP. The GLUT4 glucose transporter. Cell Metab 2007;5:237-252

[122] Kandror KV, Pilch PF. Compartmentalization of protein traffic in insulin-sensitive cells. Am J Physiol 1996;271:E1-E14

[123] Somwar R, Kim DY, Sweeney G, *et al.* GLUT4 translocation precedes the stimulation of glucose uptake by insulin in muscle cells: potential activation of GLUT4 via p38 mitogen-activated protein kinase. Biochem J 2001;359:639-649

[124] Sweeney G, Garg RR, Ceddia RB, *et al.* Intracellular delivery of phosphatidylinositol (3,4,5)-triphosphate causes incorporation of GLUT4 into the plasma membrane of muscle and fat cells without increasing glucose uptake. J Biol Chem 2004;279:32233-32242

[125] Thong FSL, Dugani CB, Klip A. Turning signals on and off: GLUT4 traffic in the insulin-signaling highway. Physiology 2005;20:271-284

[126] Foster LJ, Li D, Randhawa VK, Klip A. Insulin accelerated inter-endosomal GLUT4 traffic via phosphatidylinositol 3-kinase and protein kinase B. J Biol Chem 2001;276:44212-44221

[127] Govers R, Coster ACF, James DE. Insulin increases cell surface GLUT4 levels by dose dependently discharging GLUT4 into a cell surface recycling pathway. Mol Biol Cell 2004;24: 6456-6466

[128] Korylowski O, Zeigerer A, Cohen A, McGraw TE. GLUT4 is retained by an intracellular cycle of vesicle formation and fusion with endosomes. Mol Biol Cell 2003;15:870-882

[129] Asano T, Katagiri H, Takata K, *et al.* Characterization of GLUT3 protein expressed in Chinese hamster ovary cells. Biochem J 1992;288:189-193

[130] Nishimura H, Pallardo FU, Seidner GA, *et al.* Kinetics of GLUT1 and GLUT4 glucose transporters in Xenopus oocytes. J Biol Chem 1993;268:8514-8520

[131] Kasahara T, Kasahara M. Characterization of the rat Glut4 glucose transporter expressed in the yeast Saccharomyces cerevisiae: comparison with the Glut1 glucose transporter. Biochim Biophys Acta 1997;1324:111-119

[132] Shepherd PR, Kahn BB. Mechanisms of disease: glucose transporters and insulin action – implications for insulin resistance and diabetes mellitus. New Engl J Med 1999;341,4:248-257

[133] He J, Thamotharan M, Devaskar SU. Insulin-induced translocation of facilitative glucose transporters in fetal/neonatal rat skeletal muscle. Am J Physiol Regul Integr Comp Physiol 2003; 284:R1138-R1146

[134] Zorzano A, Muñoz P, Camps M, Mora C, Testar X, Palacin M. Insulin-induced redistribution of GLUT4 glucose carriers in the muscle fiber. In search of GLUT4 trafficking pathways. Diabetes 1996;45,Suppl.1:S70-S81

[135] Blot V, McGraw TE. Molecular mechanism controlling GLUT4 intracellular retention. Mol Biol Cell 2008;19,8:3477-3487

[136] Ing BL, Chen H, Robinson KA, Buse MG, Quon MJ. Characterization of a mutant GLUT4 lacking the N-glycosylation site: studies in transfected rat adipose cells. Biochem Biophys Res Commun 1996;218:76-82

[137] Heyward CA, Pettitt TR, Leney SE, Welsh GI, Tavare JM, Wakelam MJO. An intracellular motif of GLUT4 regulates fusion of GLUT4-containing vesicles. BMC Cell Biol 2008;9:25; doi:10.1186/1471-2121-9-25

[138] Hanpeter D, James DE. Characterization of the intracellular GLUT-4 compartment. Mol Membr Biol 995;12:263-269

[139] Malide D, St-Denis J-F, Keller SR, Cushman SW. Vp165 and GLUT4 share similar vesicle pools along their trafficking pathways in rat adipose cells. FEBS Lett 1997;409:461-468

[140] Ishiki M, Klip A. Minireview: Recent developments in the regulation of glucose transporter-4 traffic: new signals, locations, and partners. Endocrinol 2005;146,2:5071-5078

[141] Kirchhausen T. Adaptors for clathrin-mediated traffic. Annu Rev Cell Dev Biol 1999;15:705-732

[142] Chavrier P, Goud B. The role of ARF and Rab GTPases in membrane transport. Curr Opin Cell Biol 1999;11:466-475

[143] Burant CF, Takeda J, Brot-Laroche F, Bell GI, Davidson NO. Fructose transporter in human spermatozoa and small intestine is GLUT5. J Biol Chem 1992;267:14523-14526

[144] Kayano T, Burant CF, Fukumoto H, *et al.* Human facilitative glucose transporters. Isolation, functional characterization, and gene localization of cDNA encoding an isoform (GLUT5) expressed in small intestine, kidney, muscle, and adipose tissue and an unusual glucose transporter pseudogene-like sequence (GLUT6). J Biol Chem 1990;265:13276-13282

[145] Douard V, Ferraris RP. Regulation of the fructose transporter GLUT5 in health and disease. Am J Physiol Endocrinol Metab 2008;295:E227-E237

[146] Buchs AE, Sasson S, Joost HG, Cerasi E. Characterization of GLUT5 domains responsible for fructose transport. Endocrinol 1998;139,3:827-831

[147] Oka Y, Asano T, Shibosaki Y, *et al.* C-terminal truncated glucose transporter is locked into an inward-facing form without transport activity. Nature 1990; 345:550-553

[148] Davidson NO, Hausman AM, Ifkovits CA, *et al.* Human intestinal glucose transporter expression and localization of GLUT5. Am J Physiol 1992;262:C795-C800

[149] Stuart CA, Yin D, Howell MEA, Dykes RJ, Laffan JL, Ferrando AA. Hexose transporter mRNA for *GLUT4*, *GLUT5*, and *GLUT12* predominate in human muscle. Am J Physiol Endocrinol Metab 2006;291:E1067-E1073

[150] Bray GA. How bad is fructose? Am J Clin Nutr 2007;86:895-896

[151] Schürmann A. Insight into the „odd" hexose transporters GLUT3, GLUT5, and GLUT7. Am J Physiol Endocrinol Metab 2008;295:E225-E226

[152] Stuart CA, Howell ME, Yin D. Overexpression of GLUT5 in diabetic muscle is reversed by pioglitazone. Diabetes Care 200;30:925-931

[153] Dyer J, Wood IS, Palejwala A, Ellis A, Shirazi-Beechey SP. Expression of monosaccharide transporters in intestine of diabetic humans. Am J Physiol Gastrointest Liver Physiol 2002;282: G241-G248

[154] Cheeseman C. Fructose the odd man out. Why is the genomic control of intestinal GLUT5 expression different? J Physiol 2008;586:15,3563; doi:10.1113/jphysiol.2008.158667

[155] Barone S, Fussel SL, Singh AK, *et al.* Slc2a5 (Glut5) is essential for the absorption of fructose in the intestine and generation of fructose-induced hypertension. J Biol Chem 2009;284,8:5056-5066

[156] Grover-McKay M, Walsh SA, Seftor EA, Thomas PA, Hendrix MJ. Role of glucose transporter 1 protein in human breast cancer. Pathol Oncol Res 1998; 4,2:115-120

[157] Rivas CI, Vera JC, Guaiquil VH, *et al.* Increased uptake and accumulation of vitamin C in immunodeficiency virus-1-infected hematopoetic cell lines. J Biol Chem 1997;271:5814-5820

[158] Doege H, Bocianski A, Joost HG, Schürmann A. Activity and genomic organization of human glucose transporter 9 (*GLUT9*), a novel member of the family of sugar transport facilitators predominantly expressed in brain and leukocytes. Biochem J 2000;350:771-776

[159] Godoy A, Ulloa V, Rodriquez F, *et al.* Differential subcellular distribution of glucose transporters GLUT1-6 and GLUT9 in human cancer: ultrastructural localization of GLUT1 and GLUT5 in breast tumor tissues. J Cell Physiol 2006;207,3:614-627

[160] Kayano T, Burant CF, Fukumoto H, *et al.* Human facilitative glucose transporters. Isolation, functional characterization, and gene localization of cDNA encoding an isoform (GLUT5) expressed in small intestine, kidney, muscle, and adipose tissue and an usual glucose transporter pseudogene-like sequence (GLUT6). J Biol Chem 1990;265:13267-13282

[161] Lisinski Y, Schürmann A, Joost H-G, Cushman SW, Al-Hasani H. Targeting of GLUT6 and GLUT8 in rat adipose cells. Biochem J 2001;358:517-522

[162] Li Q, Manolescu A, Ritzel M, *et al.* Cloning and functional characterization of the human GLUT7 isoform *SLC2A7* from the small intestine. Am J Physiol Gastrointest Liver Physiol 2004; 287:G236-G242

[163] Chaseeman C. GLUT7: a new intestinal facilitated hexose transporter. Am J Physiol Endocrinol Metab 2008;295:E238-E241

[164] Ibberson M, Uldry M, Thorens B. GLUTx1, a novel mammalian glucose transporter expressed in the central nervous system and insulin sensitive tissues. J Biol Chem 2000;275:4607-4612

[165] Doege H, Schürmann A, Bahrenberg B, Brauers A, Joost H-G. GLUT8: A novel sugar transport facilitators with glucose transport activity. J Biol Chem 2000;275:16275-16280

[166] Schmidt S, Joost H-G, Schürmann A. GLUT8, the enigmatic intracellular hexose transporter. Am J Physiol Endocrinol Metab 2009;296:E614-E618

[167] Reagan LP, Gorovits N, Hoskin EK, *et al.* Localization and regulation of GLUTx1 glucose transporter in hippocampus of streptozotocin diabetic rats. Proc Natl Acad Sci USA 2001;98,5:2820-2825

[168] Carayannopoulos MO, Chi MM-Y, Cui Y, *et al.* GLUT8 is a glucose transporter responsible for insulin-stimulated glucose uptake in the blastocyst. Proc Natl Acad Sci USA 2000;97,13:7313-7318

[169] Schmidt U, Briese S, Leicht K, Schürmann A, Joost H-G, Al-Hasani H. Endocytosis of the glucose transporter GLUT8 is mediated by interaction of a dileucine motif with the β2-adaptin subunit of the AP-2 adaptor complex. J Cell Sci 2006;119:2321-2331

[170] Widmer M, Uldry M, Thorens B. GLUT8 subcellular localization and absence of translocation to the plasma membrane in PC12 cells and hippocampal neurons. Endocrinol 2005, doi:10.1210/en.2005-0668

[171] Schürmann A, Axer H, Sheepers A, Doege H, Joost H-G. The glucose transport facilitator GLUT8 is predominantly associated with the acrosomal region of mature spermatozoa. Cell Tissue Res 2002;307:237-242

[172] Henry DN, Busik JV, Botolin D, Grant MB, Gorovits N, Charron M. Glut8 expression in the blood retinal barrier. Invest Ophtalmal Vis Sci 2002;43:E-Abstract 904

[173] Gorovits N, Cui L, Busik JV, Ranalletta M, DE-Mouzon SH, Charron MJ. Regulation of hepatic GLUT8 expression in normal and diabetic models. Endocrinol 2003;144,5:1703-1711

[174] Goldman NA, Katz EB, Glenn AS, *et al.* GLUT1 and GLUT8 in endometrium and endometrial adenocarcinoma. Modern Pathol 2006;19:1429-1436

[175] Doege H, Bocianski A, Scheepers A, *et al.* Characterization of human glucose transporter (GLUT) 11 (encoded by SLC2A11), a novel sugar-transport facilitator specifically expressed in heart and skeletal muscle. Biochem J 2001;359:443-449

[176] Tartiglia LA, Weng X. Nucleic acid molecules encoding GLUTX and uses thereof. 1999, U.S. Patent no. 5,942,398

[177] Phay JE, Hussein HB, Moley JF. Cloning and expression analysis of a novel member of the facilitative glucose transporter family, *SLC2A9* (GLUT9). Genomics 2000;66:217-220

[178] Augustin R, Carayannopoulos MO, Dowd LO, Phay JE, Moley JF, Moley KH. Identification and characterization of human glucose transporter protein-9 (GLUT9): Alternative splicing alters trafficking. J Biol Chem 2004;279,16:16229-16236

[179] Doblado MA, Moley KH. Facilitative glucose transporter 9 (GLUT 9), a unique hexose and urate transporter. Am J Physiol Endocrinol Metab 2009, doi: 10.1152/ajpendo.00296.2009

[180] Caulfield MJ, Munroe PB, O'Neill D, *et al.* SLC2A9 is a high-capacity urate transporter in humans. PloS Med 2008,5(10):e197, doi: 10.1371/journal.pmed.0050197

[181] McVie-Wylie AJ, Lamson DR, Chen YT. Molecular cloning of a novel member of the GLUT family of transporters, SLC2A10 (GLUT10), localized on chromosome 20q13:1: A candidate gene for NIDDM susceptibility. Genomics 2001;72:113-117

[182] Wood IS, Hunter L, Trayhurn P. Expression of Class III facilitative glucose transporter genes (GLUT-10 and GLUT-12) in mouse and human adipose tissues. Biochem Biophys Res Commun 2003;308:43-49

[183] Dawson PA, Mychaleckyj JC, Fossey SC, Mihic SJ, Craddock AL, Bowden DW. Sequence and functional analysis of GLUT10: a glucose transporter in the Type 2 diabetes-linked region of chromosome 20q12-13.1. Mol Genet. Metab 2001;74:186-199

[184] Bento JL, Bowden DW, Mychaleckyj JC, *et al.* Genetic analysis of the GLUT10 glucose transporter (SLC2A10) polymorphism in Caucasian American type 2 diabetes. BMC Med Genet 2005;6:42, doi:10.1186/1471-2350-6-42

[185] Rose CS, Andersen G, Hamid YH, *et al.* Studies of relationships between the GLUT10 Ala206Thr polymorphism and impaired insulin secretion. Diabetes Med 2005;22:946-949

[186] Lin WH, Chuang LM, Chen CH. Association study of genetic polymorphisms of SLC2A10 gene and type 2 diabetes in Taiwanese population. Diabetologia 2006;49:1214-1221

[187] Coucke PJ, Willaert A, Wessels MW. Mutations in the facilitative glucose transporter GLUT10 alter angiogenesis and cause arterial tortuosity syndrome. Nat Genet 2006;38:452-457

[188] Doege H, Bocianski A, Scheepers A, *et al.* Characterization of human glucose transporter (GLUT) 11 (encoded by *SLC2A11*), a novel sugar-transport facilitator specifically expressed in heart and skeletal muscle. Biochem J 2001;359:443-449

[189] Scheepers A, Schmidt S, Manolescu A, *et al.* Characterization of the human *SLC2A11* (GLUT11) gene: alternative promoter, usage function, expression, and subcellular distribution of three isoforms, and lack of mouse orthologue. Mol Membr Biol 2005;22,4:339-351

[190] Rogers S, James DE, Best JD. Identification of novel facilitative transporter like protein-GLUT8. Diabetes 1998;47,Suppl.1:A45

[191] Rogers S, Macheda ML, Docherty SE, *et al.* Identification of a novel transporter-like protein-GLUT-12. Am J Physiol Endocrinol Metab 2002;283:E733-E738

[192] Gude NM, Stevenson JL, Rogers S, *et al.* GLUT12 expression in human placenta in first trimester and term. Placenta 2003;24:566-570

[193] Chandler JD, Williams ED, Slavin JL, Best JD, Rogers S. Expression and localization of GLUT1 and GLUT12 in prostate carcinoma. Cancer 2003;97,8:2035-2042

[194] Stuart CA, Howell MEA, Zhang Y, Yin D. Insulin-stimulated translocation of GLUT12 parallels that of GLUT4 in normal muscle. J Clin Endocrinol Metab 2009 (Epub ahead of print)

[195] Rogers S, Docherty SE, Slavin JL, Henderson MA, Best JD. Differential expression of GLUT12 in breast cancer and normal breast tissue. Cancer Letters 2003;193:225-233

[196] Chandler JD, Williams ED, Slavin JL, Best JD, Rogers S. Expression and localization of GLUT1 and GLUT12 in prostate carcinoma. Cancer 2003;97,8:2035-2042

[197] Uldry M, Steiner P, Zurich MG, *et al.* Regulated exocytosis of H^+/myo-inositol symporter at synapses and growth cones. EMBO J 2004;23:531-540

[198] Uldry M, Ibberson M, Horisberger J-D, Chatton JY, Riederer B, Thorens B. Identification of a mammalian H^+/*myo*-inositol symporter expressed predominantly in the brain. EMBO J 2001;20:4467-4477

[199] Wu X, Freeze HH. GLUT14, a duplication of GLUT3 is specifically expressed in testis as alternative splice forms. Genomics 2002;80:553-557.

CHAPTER 3

Glucose Homeostasis

Abstract: Glucose is the main and preferred source of energy for the body. Poly- and oligosaccharides contained in foods are broken down into glucose. The liver and kidney also make glucose in the process of gluconeogenesis. In order to ensure the euglycemia necessary for metabolic processes in the cells glucose levels are carefully regulated to around 90 mg/dL (5 mM). The process of maintaining blood glucose at a steady-state level is called glucose homeostasis. This maintenance is achieved through a balance of several factors, including the rate of consumption and intestinal absorption of dietary carbohydrate, the rate of utilization of glucose by peripheral tissues and the loss of glucose through the kidney tubule, and the rate of removal or release of glucose by the liver. To avoid postprandial hyperglycemia (uncontrolled increases in blood glucose levels following meals) and fasting hypoglycemia (decreased in blood glucose levels during periods of fasting), the body can adjust glucose levels by a variety of cellular mechanisms. Important signals are conveyed by hormones, cytokines, and fuel substrates and are sensed through of cellular mechanisms. The liver plays a major role in blood glucose homeostasis by maintaining a balance between the uptake and storage of glucose via glycogenesis and the release of glucose via glycogenolysis and gluconeogenesis.

INTRODUCTION

Most tissues and organs, such as the brain, need glucose constantly, as an important source of energy. The low blood concentrations of glucose can cause seizures, loss of consciousness, and death. On the other hand, long lasting elevation of blood glucose concentrations, can result in blindness, renal failure, cardiac and peripheral vascular disease, and neuropathy. Therefore, blood glucose concentrations need to be maintained within narrow limits. The process of maintaining blood glucose at a steady-state level is called glucose homeostasis [1]. This is accomplished by the finely hormone regulation of peripheral glucose uptake (glucose utilization), hepatic glucose production and glucose uptake during carbohydrates ingestion. This maintenance is achieved through a balance of several factors, including the rate of consumption and intestinal absorption of dietary carbohydrate, the rate of utilization of glucose by peripheral tissues and the loss of glucose through the kidney tubule, and the rate of removal or release of glucose by the liver and kidney. These organs produce a specific enzyme, glucose-6-phosphatase, that cleaves the glucose-phosphate bond. Regulation of balance between phosphorylation and dephosphorylation processes is crucial and determines the net direction of uptake or release of glucose in these organs.

To avoid postprandial hyperglycemia and fasting hypoglycemia, the body can adjust glucose levels by secreting two hormones, insulin and glucagon. These hormones work in opposition to each other.

During periods of hyperglycemia, the β-cells of pancreas secrete more insulin, the hormone that facilitates the transport of glucose into muscle cells, adipose tissue, and other cells and the suppression of gluconeogenesis, which decrease blood glucose levels. In addition, insulin inhibits glucagon secretion. During hypoglycemia, the α-cells of pancreas secrete more glucagon. Glucagon causes the liver to increase hepatic glucose production, which increases blood glucose levels.

After food ingestion, the digestion and absorption of nutrients are associated also with increased secretion of multiple gut hormones that act on distal targets. A majority of gut hormones are secreted within minutes after nutrient ingestion. Their concentrations rise transiently in the circulation with concentrations higher in the hepatoportal blood than the arterial blood [2]. These hormones are synthesized by specialized enteroendocrine cells located in the epithelium of the stomach, small bowel, large bowel and are secreted at low basal levels in the fasting state. The secretion of gut hormones is regulated, at least in part, by nutrients. Plasma levels of most gut hormones rise quickly within minutes of nutrient intake and fall rapidly thereafter, mainly because they are cleared by the kidney and are enzymatically inactivated [3].

The endocrine cells play important roles in glucose homeostasis through their actions on peripheral target organs. These hormones are among the first messengers signaling the new metabolic status to the body.

PANCREATIC HORMONES

Insulin

Insulin is synthesized in the β-cells of the pancreatic islets of Langerhans in response to an elevation in blood glucose and amino acid after a meal. The islets of Langerhans are roughly spheric structures of radius $50 - 250$ μm in which β-cells and other secretory cells are densely packed. The pancreas contains about 10^6 islets, and within each islet, there are $10^3 - 10^4$ β-cells and $100 - 200$ secretory cells of other types [11]. Insulin is secreted into the bloodstream; it is directly infused via the portal vein to the liver, where it exerts profound metabolic effects. The major function of insulin is to counter the concerned action of a number of hyperglycemia-generating hormones to maintain low blood glucose levels. This hormone also plays an important role in the regulation of glucose metabolism. Insulin regulates glucose metabolism at many sites reducing hepatic glucose output (via decreased gluconeogenesis and glycogenolysis) and increasing the rate of glucose uptake, primarily into striated muscle and adipose tissue. Insulin also stimulates in lipogenesis, therefore it also profoundly affects lipid metabolism,increasing lipid synthesis in liver and fat cells, and attenuating fatty acid release from triglycerides in fat and muscle. Insulin diminishes lipolysis, increases amino acid transport into cells, modulates transcription, altering the cell content of numerous mRNAs, thereby stimulating growth, DNA synthesis and cell replication.

The chromosomal location of the human insulin gene is mapped to 11p15. The primary translation of the insulin gene is preproinsulin (preprohormone), as a single chain precursor, composed of 110 amino acids [4]. By the removal of its signal peptide, processed by proteases, during insertion into the cisternae of the endoplasmic reticulum, proinsulin (prohormone) is generated. Within the endoplasmic reticulum, proinsulin is exposed to several specific endopeptidases to derive insulin (hormone). Specific protease activity cleaves the third center of the molecule, which dissociates as C peptide chain of 31 amino acids from the single-stranded polypeptide, leaving the amino terminal B peptide disulfide bonded to the carboxy terminal A peptide. The mature form of insulin is a 51-amino acid polypeptide, made of two chains (A and B) connected by 2 disulfide bonds, connecting the amino acid cysteine to cysteine. There is also a third disulfide bond that connects these same amino acids within chain A. Chain A consists of 21 amino acids and chain B contains 30 amino acids. Insulin is processed to the biologically active form inside the secretory granules. The granules are small membrane-bound secretory granules with a diameter of ~ 0,35 μm. Insulin can be stored within the granules for several days prior to its release [10]. Insulin has a half-life of about 5 minutes. Secretion of insulin is, therefore, difficult to measure. One can measure the level of C peptide, which has a half-life of about 30 minutes.

Insulin action is carefully regulated in response to circulating glucose concentrations. It is not secreted if the blood glucose concentration is ≤ 3 mM/l, but is secreted in increasing amounts as glucose concentrations increase beyond this threshold [5]. When blood glucose levels increase over about 5 mM/l the β-cells increase their output of insulin and C peptide. The glucagon producing α-cells remain quiet, and hold on to their hormone.

Postprandially, the secretion of insulin occurs in two phases. An initial rapid release of preformed insulin, followed by increased insulin synthesis and release in response to blood glucose. Long-term release of insulin occurs if glucose concentrations remain high [6, 7].

Insulin secretion from β-cells is principally regulated by plasma glucose levels. The secretion of insulin requires a high blood glucose levels. It is due to the activity of both glucose transporter 2 and hexokinase. GLUT 2 has a low affinity for glucose ($K_m \sim 17$ mM) and activity of pancreatic glucokinase is also very low ($K_m = 5,5$ mM) in comparison to various hexokinase enzymes in other tissues which have K_m values around 0,01 mM. Glucose exerts both concentration- and time-dependent effects in pancreatic β-cells. Upon stimulation by an abrupt and sustained increase in the ambient glucose concentration, insulin secretion occurs following a biphasic time course. The secretion rate initially accelerates markedly beforeslowing down (first phase), and eventually increases again at a slower rate or stabilizes depending on the preparation and the species (second phase) [8]. Glucose-stimulated biphasic insulin secretion involves at least two signalling pathways, the K_{ATP} channel-dependent and K_{ATP} channel-independent pathways, respectively [9]. The β-cells contain as many as 20 different ion channels, but two types of ion channels are particularly important for the initiation of insulin secretion: the K_{ATP} channels and Ca^{2+}-channels [10].

Glucose enters β-cell via facilitative glucose transporter 2 (GLUT 2). GLUT 2 is believed to play a role in glucose-stimulated insulin secretion. Glucokinase is a key enzyme of glucose metabolism that phosphorylates glucose to glucose-6-phosphate. This is the first step of glucose metabolism after the uptake of glucose by GLUT 2. Glucokinase is one of the hexokinases and is expressed in pancreatic β-cells, hepatocytes, gut and brain of humans.

Glucose equilibrates across the plasma membrane and is phosphorylated by glucokinase, which determines the rate of glycolysis and the generation of pyruvate. Pyruvate, once transported into the mitochondria, is a substrate both for pyruvate dehydrogenase and pyruvate carboxylase. These enzymes ensure, respectively, the formation of acetyl-CoA and oxaloacetate. The latter provides input to the Krebs cycle. Through activation of the tricarboxylic acid cycle, reducing equivalents (as for example NADH + H$^+$) are transferred to the electron transport chain resulting in generation of ATP. The ATP/ADP ratio is relatively low in β-cells exposed to fasting blood glucose levels. In the model of glucose-stimulated insulin secretion, oxidative phosphorylation in mitochondria increases the cytosolic ATP/ADP ratio. In other words, increased uptake of glucose by pancreatic β-cells leads to a concomitant increase in metabolism. The increase of metabolism leads to an elevation in the ATP/ADP ratio. Therefore, glucose-induced insulin secretion is determined by signals generated in the mitochondria [12].

The increase of cytosolic ATP/ADP ratio leads to the closure of an ATP-sensitive K$^+$ channels (K$_{ATP}$), inhibition of K$^+$ transport, and depolarization of the plasma membrane. The K$_{ATP}$ channel is a complex of eight polypeptides comprising four copies of the protein. The ATP-sensitive K$^+$ channels control K$^+$ efflux and, therefore, cellular K$^+$ levels according to the cell's energy state. [13]. As a consequence of depolarization of the plasma membrane, the cytosolic Ca^{2+} concentration is raised by the opening of voltage-sensitive Ca^{2+} channels [14], and uptake of Ca^{2+} ions over the cell's outer membrane. The Ca^{2+} channel responsiblefor this is regulated by the degree of polarization of the membrane. The cell's resting potential of about -60 mV does not activate the voltage-dependent Ca^{2+} channel nor insulin release. The depolarization to -40 mV or less causes the Ca^{2+} channel to open and increases the inward flow of Ca^{2+}. The increase in the cytosolic Ca^{2+} concentrations is the main trigger for exocytosis, the process by which the insulin-containing secretory granules fuse with the plasma membrane [15].

Not only glucose causes release of insulin from β-cells. It is also interesting to note that three amino acids, alanine, glycine, and arginine, also cause insulin release. They do this through the same basic mechanism as glucose.

Insulin has many actions, the most well-known being stimulation of glucose and amino acid uptake from the blood to various tissues and organs. Insulin helps control postprandial glucose in three ways: 1) it acts on the liver to promote glycogenesis, 2) this hormone simultaneously inhibits glucagon secretion from pancreatic α-cells, thus signaling the liver to stop producing glucose via glycogenolysis and gluconeogenesis, and 3) it signals the cells of insulin-sensitive peripheral tissues, primarily skeletal muscle and adipocytes, to increase their uptake of glucose [6] (Fig. 1).

Insulin also enhances the conversion of circulating pools of glucose, amino acids and free fatty acids into stored glycogen, protein and adipose tissue. It reduces the rate of release of glycerol/free fatty acids from adipose tissue, stimulates fatty acid synthesis and the conversion of free fatty acids to triglycerides in the liver. Insulin also has an effect on protein metabolism by the stimulation of uptake of amino acids into liver and muscle, stimulation of protein biosynthesis and reduction of release of amino acids from muscle. It increases the accumulation of K$^+$ and Mg^{2+} in muscle and adipose tissue. Insulin also acts on growth and development. It is particularly important in fetal development (Fig. **1**).

INSULIN ACTION IN GLUCOSE HOMEOSTASIS

Insulin Actions on the Liver

In 1849, the French physiologist Claude Bernard identified the liver as a reservoir for glucose. He also reported that pricking of the floor of the fourth ventricle of the brain in rabbits resulted in glucosuria, as an effect of hypoglycemia, and concluded that the central nervous system plays an essential role in the control of peripheral blood glucose levels [16]. The effect of insulin on hepatic fluxes may be divided into direct effects on the liver and indirect effect [17]. The direct effect mostly leads to rapid inhibition of glycogenolysis [18]. The indirect effects mediated through extrahepatic actions, are for example the inhibition of lipolysis and reduction of glucagon levels [19].

Most recently, insulin signaling in neuronal cells have been shown in life span, growth, reproduction, glucose production and energy homeostasis in many organisms; from primitive organisms as *Caenorhabditis elegans* (nematode) and *Drosophila melanogaster* (flies) to mammals [17, 20, and 21]. Therefore, it has been proposed that indirect effect of insulin on glucose production also include the activation of hypothalamic insulin signaling [22]. This work has led to the concept that besides regulating body weight homeostasis and reproductive endocrinology, hypothalamic insulin signaling also controls glucose utilization in the peripheral, possibly via its action on central K_{ATP} channels.

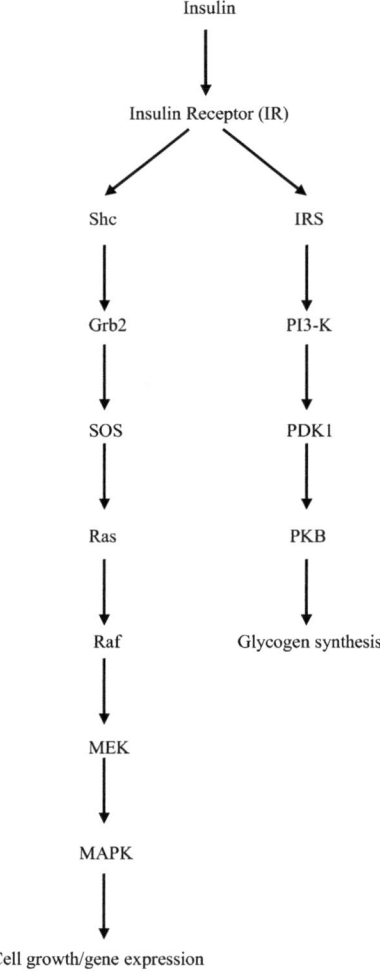

Figure 1: Intracellular insulin signaling. For details see text.

The activation of insulin receptors in the hypothalamus, in particular in the arcuate nucleus, plays an important role in the regulation of glucose homeostasis. The activation of insulin signaling in the absence of elevated systematic insulin levels, is sufficient to decrease blood glucose levels via a substantial inhibition of endogenous glucose production [22]. Peripherally circulating insulin crosses the blood-brain barrier in proportion to serum insulin levels via a saturable mechanism [25]. Insulin receptors are widely distributed in the brain, with the highest concentrations in the olfactory bulb, hypothalamus, cerebral cortex, cerebellum, and hippocampus [26]. The obtained findings suggest that hypothalamic action of insulin requires an intact insulin-signaling cascade involving the activation of the insulin receptor, insulin receptor substrate (IRS), PI 3-kinase and K_{ATP} channels in the arcuate nucleus. [22 – 24].

Pocai and colleagues [23] showed that insulin acts on K_{ATP} channels in hypothalamic neurons to control hepatic glucose production by decreasing glucose-6-phosphate and phosphoenolpyruvate kinase expression in the liver. This effect is mediated by the activation of efferent vagal fibers, which innervate the liver. Transection of the vagal nerve to the liver nullified this effect [24].

It has been shown that brain insulin action is responsible for the increase of hepatic IL-6 in the liver. It implicates the cytokine IL-6 as insulin's effector in the liver. It has been shown that insulin acting on unidentified neurons in the brain stimulates IL-6 secretion from uncharacterized cells in the liver [27]. IL-6 then activates, by phosphorylation, STAT3 in hepatocytes and inhibits glucose production. The obtained results indicate that IL-6 is essential for phosphorylation of hepatic STAT3 induced by brain-insulin action and inhibits the expression of gluconeogenic genes in cultured hepatocytes [27].

The other mode of action of insulin in the arcuate nucleus of the hypothalamus is the stimulation of secretion the anorexigenic neuropeptides (appetite-suppressing), resulting in a reduction in body weight [24].

The net glucose release is the result of two simultaneous ongoing pathways that are tightly regulated. Indeed, liver produces glucose by breaking down glycogen (glycogenolysis) and by *de novo* synthesis of glucose (gluconeogenesis) from non-carbohydrate precursors such as lactate, amino acids and glycerol [28, 29].

When glucose is directly available from external resources, gluconeogenesis and glycogenolysis are dispensable and consequently need to be shut off [30]. The regulation of hepatic glucose metabolism is an important process in the adjustment of the blood glucose levels.

The most important hormone that regulates glucose metabolism is insulin. It inhibits gluconeogenesis and glycogenolysis and induces a process of glycogenesis.

The rate of gluconeogenesis is controlled principally by the activities of enzymes such as phosphoenolpyruvate carboxykinase (PEPCK), fructose-1,6-bisphosphatase (FP$_2$ase) and glucose-6-phosphatase (G6Pase) [31]. Fructose-1,6-bisphosphatase and phosphoenolpyruvate carboxykinase are enzymes specific for gluconeogenesis and indirect glycogen synthesis [32]. PEPCK catalyzes the conversion of oxaloacetate to phosphoenolpyruvate, while G6Pase catalyzes the production of free glucose from glucose-6-phosphate (see Chapter 1, part: Gluconeogenesis). The genes of gluconeogenic enzymes are controlled at the transcriptional level, mainly insulin, glucagon, and glucocorticoids. Insulin decreases gluconeogenesis through specific transcriptional inhibition of PEPCK, FP$_2$ase, and G6Pase [33]. The transcriptional regulation of genes encoding for G6Pase and PEPCK involves complex interactions of a variety of transcription factors and other proteins. The G6Pase and PEPCK promoters are known to contain so-called insulin-responsive sequences [34, 35].

Stimulation of the insulin receptor results in the activation of two major pathways: 1) the phosphatidylinositol 3-kinase, and 2) the mitogen-activated protein (MAP) kinase cascade. The insulin signaling cascade is initiated by the binding of insulin to the extracellular α-subunits receptor. The insulin receptor is a tyrosine kinase that becomes activated after ligand binding. This binding leads to the autophosphorylation of the tyrosine residues at the intrecellular β-subunits. This leads to the phosphorylation of several intracellular substrates, including the family receptor substrate (IRS) proteins. There are 6 different IRS (5 in humans) with different tissue-specific distribution [36, 37]. The studies have demonstrated that IRS-2 has a predominant role in the signaling pathway that controls gluconeogenesis [38]. IRS proteins bind to the phosphorylated insulin receptor via their phosphotyrosine binding domain and are in turn phosphorylated on multiple tyrosine residues – thus creating docking sites for the src homology 2 domain containing proteins. The proteins that bind to tyrosine phosphorylated IRS proteins are the regulatory subunit of PI 3-kinase and the adaptor molecule growth factorreceptor-binding protein 2 (Grb2). The phosphorylation of IRS proteins result in the recruitment of the PI 3-kinase to the plasma membrane. It phosphorylates phosphatidylinositol-4,5-bisphosphate (PtdIns(4,5)P$_2$) to generate phosphatidylinositol-3,4,5-triphosphate (PtdIns(3,4,5)P_3), the lipid second messenger, which is necessary to recruit downstream kinases. The generation of PtdIns(3,4,5)P_3 is known to increase the activity of 3-phosphatidylinosito-dependent kinase-1 (PDK1) [39] that phosphorylates and activates several members of the AGC kinase superfamily. This superfamily contains the proteins kinase A (PKA), protein kinase G (PKG) and protein kinase C (PKC)-related kinases [30, 40]. Among substrates are the protein kinase B (Akt/PKB), p70 S6 kinase, and the two isoforms of protein kinase C: isoform PKCλ and isoform PKCζ [41]. Protein kinase B decreases PEPCK and G6Pase gene transcription [42]. Several proteins have also been identified that are able to mediate the observed suppression of PEPCK and G6Pase gene transcription by PKB, such as FOXO1 and cAMP response element binding protein (CREBP) [30]. Akt PKB phosphorylates the transcription factors forkhead box protein O1 (FOXO1) and peroxisome proliferator-activated receptor γ co-activator (PGC)-1α, which prevents the binding to their regulatory sequences in the PEPCK and G6Pase promoters and subsequently blocks the transcription of these genes [37].

Insulin modulates gluconeogenesis also by inhibition of the coactivator TORC2 [43]. Under fasting conditions, FOXO1 increases gluconeogenic gene expression in concert with the TORC2. Insulin disrupts TORC2 activity by induction of the Ser/Thr kinase SIK2 [43].

Activated PKB is also able to phosphorylate and thereby to inhibit glycogen synthase kinase-3 (GSK-3) [30] and to increase hepatic glycogen synthesis. Glycogen synthesis is induced by the activation of the PI 3-kinase-Akt PKB pathway. The Akt PKB phosphorylates and thereby inhibits glycogen synthase kinase-3 which enables the activation of glycogen synthase, the key enzyme responsible for the formation of glycogen. The decreased hepatic glucose production after inhibition of GSK-3 might be due to a suppression of PEPCK and G6Pase gene expression; however the molecular events underlying the regulation of PEPCK and G6Pase gene expression by GSK-3 are unclear [30].

The data obtained from experiments suggest that PKCλ does not appear to be involved in the suppression of PEPCK and G6Pase genes by insulin, and p70 S6 kinase does not significantly contribute to the effect of this hormone on the expression of these genes [30].

Insulin is also able to stimulate the Raf/MEK/ERK1/ERK2 pathway, but the obtained data suggest that insulin stimulation of ERK1/ERK2 might apparently be too weak to significantly contribute to the overall regulation of the G6Pase gene. Barthel and Schmoll [30] wrote that "… the Raf/MEK/ERK pathway is a redundant mechanism for the regulation of gluconeogenic enzyme activity and … the physiological significance of this pathway in the context of hepatic glucose production is largely unclear".

Insulin also stimulates AMP-activated protein kinase (AMPK) pathway. Activation of AMPK has been described to stimulate glucose uptake [44]. The activation of AMPK is able to suppress G6Pase and PEPCK gene expression [45]. There is no evidence for a direct regulation of AMPK by insulin. Recent evidence suggests that AMPK can phosphorylate IRS-1 in C_2C_{12} myotubes and that this phosphorylation correlates with an increase in insulin-stimulated IRS-1-associated PI 3-kinase activity [46]. Other data suggest that activation of AMPK can repress G6Pase gene expression and therefore inhibit gluconeogenesis in hepatoma cells by reducing the cellular level of FOXO1 [47].

In most nonhepatic tissues, insulin increases glucose uptake by increasing the number of plasma membrane facilitative glucose transporters, GLUTs. These transporters, especially GLUT 1 and GLUT 4, are in a continuous state of turnover. Increases in the plasma membrane content of transporters stem from an increase in the rate of recruitment of new transporters into the plasma membrane, deriving from a special pool of preformed transporters localized in the intracellular storage vesicles.

Skeletal muscles dominate in the fight for blood sugar after a meal, accounting for about 50% of the total glucose uptake. Approximately half of this is stored as glycogen. Muscle does not carry out gluconeogenesis, cannot dephosphorylate glucose-6-phosphate and, therefore, cannot generate glucose and stabilize blood sugar levels. Muscle lacks receptors for glucagon and does not react to the increases in glucagon levels seen postprandial. The energy stored as muscle glycogen can only be utilized in the muscle cells. Unlike the liver, skeletal muscle lacks fatty acid synthetase and cannot synthesize fatty acids and triglycerides.

Insulin regulates glucose homeostasis at many sites, as for example, reducing hepatic glucose output (via decreased gluconeogenesis and glycogenolysis) and increasing the rate of glucose uptake, primarily into striated muscle and adipocytes. The clearance of circulating depends on the insulin-stimulated translocation of the glucose transporter 4 (GLUT 4) from the cytoplasm to the cell surface. In unstimulated adipocytes or muscle cells (i. e. the basal state), 5 – 10% of GLUT 4 is located at the cell surface and > 90% is in intracellular compartment.

GLUT 4 is constitutively active for hexose transport, and glucose uptake is regulated by insulin, controlling the amount of GLUT 4 in the plasma membrane [48]. In unstimulated cells, GLUT 4 is rapidly removed from the plasma membrane to which it recycles only slowly, leading to a steady-state accumulation in intracellular storage vesicles. In the presence of insulin, the equilibrium of this recycling process is altered to favor the translocation of

GLUT 4 from cytoplasm to the plasma membrane. The net effect is a rise in the maximum velocity of glucose transport into the cell [49, 50]. Multiple studies are all consistent with a necessary role for PI 3-kinase activity in insulin-stimulated glucose uptake and GLUT 4 translocation.

Insulin Stimulation of GLUT 4 Translocation

Both insulin and contraction stimulate increased glucose uptake and GLUT 4 translocation in muscle cells, whereas only insulin stimulates glucose transport in adipocytes. Insulin exerts pleiotropic biologic effects. The major function of insulinis to counter the concerted action of a number of hyperglycemia-generating hormones and to maintain low blood glucose levels. Insulin stimulates lipogenesis, diminishes lipolysis, and increases amino acid and glucose transport into cells.

Insulin also modulates transcription, altering the cell content of numerous mRNAs. It stimulates growth, DNA synthesis, and cell replication.

There are at least two distinct signaling pathways that are necessary for insulin to induce translocation of GLUT 4. One pathway requires activation of PI 3-kinase (phosphatidylinositol 3-kinase) while another essential pathway involves activation of TC10 (a GTPase belonging to the rho family).

PI 3-Kinase Dependent Pathway

Insulin-stimulated intracellular movement of GLUT 4 is initiated by the binding of insulin to the extracellular portion of the transmembrane insulin receptor (Fig. **2**). The receptor is a transmembrane heterotetrameric glycoprotein with two extracellular α-subunits that serve as insulin-binding sites and two intracellular β-subunits that contain tyrosine residues. Binding of insulin to the α-subunit induces a conformational changes resulting in the autophosphorylation of a number of tyrosine residues present in the β-subunit [51]. After tyrosine phosphorylation of the insulin receptor β chains, adaptor proteins are recruited and in turn are tyrosine phosphorylated [52]. Several insulin receptor adaptor proteins have been identified including members of the insulin receptor substrate family (IRS-1, IRS-2, IRS-3, IRS-4), the Shc adaptor protein isoforms, SIRP family members, Gab-1, Cbl, andAPS. Both, IRS-1 and IRS-2, have been implicated in insulin-stimulated glucose transport. Tyrosine phosphorylation of the IRS proteins creates recognition sites for additional effector molecules containing Src homology 2 (SH2) domains. These include the small adaptor proteins Grb2 and Nck, the SHP2 protein tyrosine phosphatase and, most importantly, the regulatory subunit of the type 1A phosphatidylinositol 3-kinase (PI 3-kinase) [53, 54].

PI 3-kinase exists in the cytosol as a dimmer of a regulatory p85 subunit and a catalytic p110 subunit. Recruitment of the regulatory subunit brings the catalyticp110 subunit to the plasma membrane, where it catalyzes the phosphorylation of the 3' position in the inositol ring of phosphoinositide lipids. Once PI 3-kinase is activated, it produces lipid second messengers that stimulate downstream proteins. Type 1A PI 3-kinase catalyzes the formation of phosphatidylinositol-3,4,5-triphosphate (PI(3,4,5)-triphosphate) from phosphatidylinositol-4,5-bisphosphate, and phosphatidylinositol-3,4-phosphate (PI(3,4)-bisphosphate) from phosphatidylinositol-4-phosphate [55]. PI 3-kinase generates phosphatidylinositol-3,4-5-triphosphate in surface membranes, thereby providing a lipid-based platform for the recruitment of proteins containing PH domains. A key downstream effector of phosphatidylinositol-3,4,5-triphosphate is serine/threonine kinase B (PKB, also called Akt), which is recruited to the plasma membrane. Activation of PKB also requires the 3'-phosphoinositide-dependent kinase 1 and 2 (PDK1 and PDK2) [52]. There are three Akt isoforms, but only Akt2 isoform is involved in insulin action on glucose transport and GLUT 4 translocation in adipocytes [56, 58]. Atypical protein kinase C (aPKC) isoforms, PKCζ and PKC ζ/λ, have also been implicated in insulin action on glucose uptake in skeletal muscle and adipocytes, although these kinases lack PH-domains [57].

AS160 (Akt-substrate of 160 kDa or TBC1D4) is a GAP (GTPase-activating protein) for Rabs [59, 65]. Rabs are small G-proteins that, in their GTP form, function in vesicle movement by linking vesicles to microtubule and microfilament motors and in vesicle fusion to target membranes through interactions with the docking and fusion machinery. AS160 associates with GLUT 4 vesicles via its interaction with the insulin-responsive aminopeptidase (IRAP) cytosolic tail. AS160 is phosphorylated after insulin stimulation by the Akt or other kinases. The insulin-regulated phosphorylation of AS160 may somehow modify its GAP activity, and this step plays an important role in

GLUT 4 trafficking. Insulin-stimulated phosphorylation of AS160 induces 14-3-4 binding, which is critical for the insulin-regulated function of AS160 in GLUT 4 trafficking. In the unstimulated state AS160 maintains a Rab in its GDP-bound inactive state, thereby preventing GLUT 4 translocation. Phosphorylation of AS160 catalyzes 14-3-3 binding and this likely deactivates the GAP activity of AS160 facilitating activation of the Rab protein involved in GLUT 4 storage vesicles translocation [60]. Fusion of vesicles with target membranes is mediated by SNARE proteins. In the basal state, GLUT 4 vesicles arrive at the plasma membrane but do not dock, and that docking/fusion is an insulin-regulated event. Indeed, components of the exocyst complex, in particular Exo70, contribute to directing the vesicle to the precise site of fusion followed by SNARE complex formation between VAMP2 of the insulin-mobilized vesicles and the plasma membrane t-SNARE syntaxin4 and SNAP23. Additional accessory proteins regulate this process [61].

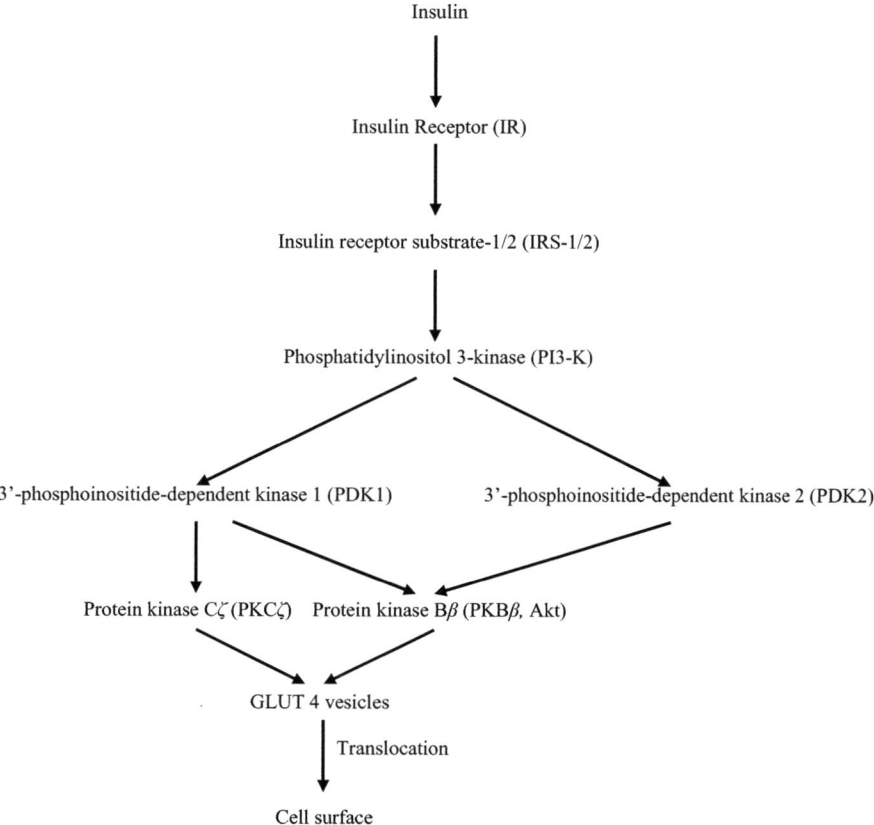

Figure 2: Intracellular signaling pathway (PI3-kinase-dependent) involved in translocation of GLUT 4 to the cell surface in skeletal muscle [54, modified].

TC10 Dependent Pathway (PI 3-Kinase Independent Pathway)

As described above, PI 3-kinase pathways are necessary for translocation of GLUT 4 vesicles from an intracellular compartment to the plasma membrane in response to insulin. The results obtained in numerous laboratories [62, 63], on the other hand, indicate the presence of an insulin signaling pathway that promotes GLUT 4 translocation independently of the phosphoinositol 3-kinase. A PI 3-kinase-independent mechanism for translocation of GLUT 4 may help to determine the specificity of insulin response [64] (Fig. **3**).

Khan and Pessin have proposed a model for a second pathway of insulin signaling required for GLUT 4 translocation and glucose uptake. The proposed model could proceed through a signaling pathway originating from lipid rafts and resulting in the ultimate activation of a small G-protein, TC10 [63]. A central point in this pathway is the CAP (Cbl-associated protein) and APS (the associated protein substrate) [64, 66]. In this model, the proto-oncogene c-Cbl is tyrosine phosphorylated in response to insulin in differentiated 3T3-L1 adipocytes. APS is an adaptor protein containing PH and SH2 domains and CAP (c-Cbl-associated protein) that stabilize and localize the

Cbl complex to the insulin receptor. Phosphotyrosine residues on Cbl provide docking sites for the CrkII/C3G complex [67]. CrkII is an adaptor protein that links Cbl to C3G, while C3G can function as a guanine nucleotide exchange factor for the small GTP binding protein, TC10 [68, 69]. CAP contains an amino terminal Sorbin homology domain, and 3 carboxyl terminal Src homology 3 (SH3) domains. The three SH3 of CAP form a complex with Cbl even in the absence of insulin stimulation [65]. The insulin receptor phosphorylates APS on Tyr[618]. This is required for the interaction with Cbl and CAP.

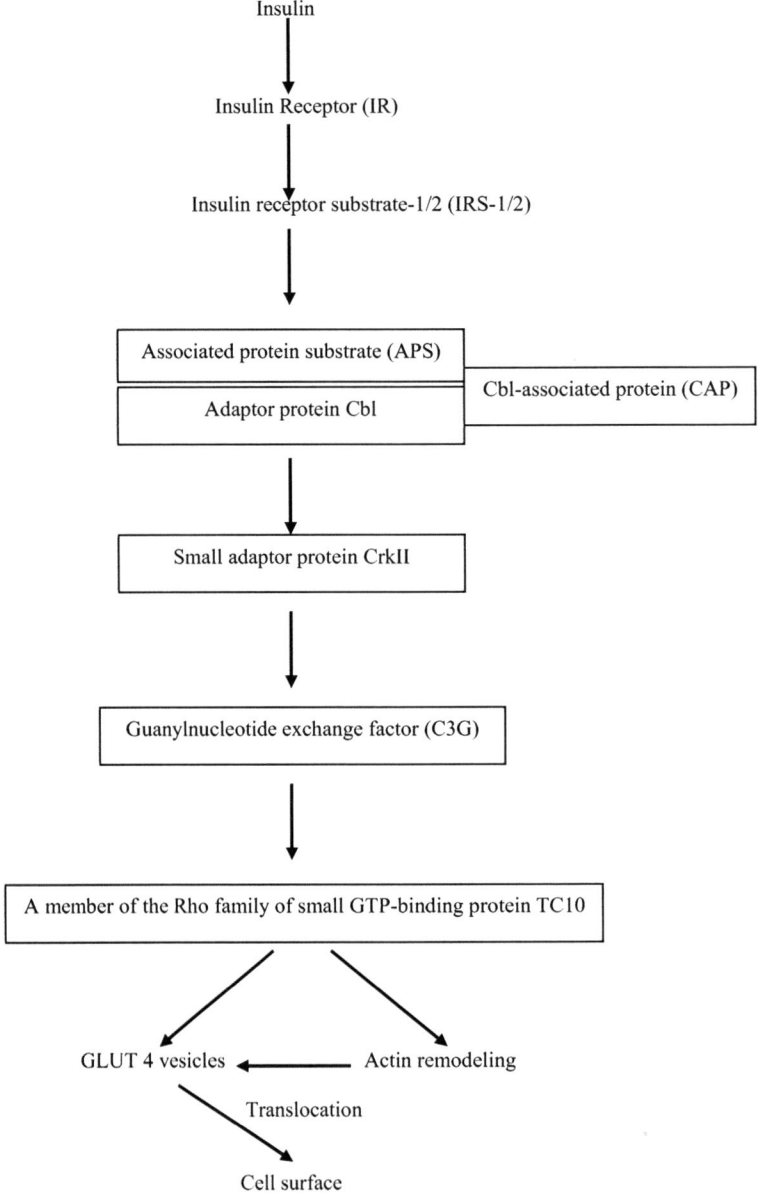

Figure 3: Intracellular signaling pathway (PI3-kinase-independent) involved in translocation of GLUT 4 to the cell surface in skeletal muscle [54, modified].

After Cbl is phosphorylated by the insulin receptor, some of the Cbl-CAP complex is released from the receptor and translocates to lipid rafts in the plasma membrane [62]. Lipid raft microdomains contain a unique set of membrane lipids, including sphingolipids and cholesterol, from their own liquid order phase in the plasma membrane [70]. Lipid rafts share a unique protein constituency relative to the non-lipid raft plasma membrane, including GPI-anchored proteins, caveolin, flotillin and palmitoylated proteins. Caveolae are a specific kind of lipid raft found in the greatest abundance in adipocytes, skeletal muscle and endothelial cells [63].

Numerous signaling and cytoskeletal proteins are found in these subdomains, suggesting that they may act as organizing centers for signal transduction, particularly for insulin. In the plasma membrane, the caveolar protein flotillin, a component of lipid rafts, forms a ternary complex with Cbl and the sorbin homology domain of CAP [68]. The phosphorylated Cbl-CAP complex then recruits the SH2-containing adaptor protein CrkII to lipid rafts, which in turn,recruits the guanyl-exchange protein C3G (exchange factor for the small G-protein) [69].

The recruitment of C3G lipid raft leads to activation of TC10, a Rho family GTPase. TC10 localizes to the caveolar donut structures. The insulin-mediated activation of TC10 only occurs when it is localized to lipid raft microdomains at the plasma membrane. The localization of TC10 may play an important role in inducing the actions of its downstream effectors. Both the insulin receptor and TC10 reside in lipid rafts and the mistargeting of TC10 to a nonlipid raft domain prevents its activation by insulin and blocks insulin action [71, 81].

TC10 is a member of the Rho family of small GTPases. The Rho family of GTPases is predominantly involved in regulating the actin cytoskeleton. A possible avenue of TC10 actin on insulin-stimulated GLUT 4 translocation is to regulate the actin cytoskeleton [63] and is required for insulin-stimulated glucose uptake in adipocytes [87]. Interestingly, while TC10 appears to be a key mediator of insulin-stimulated GLUT 4 translocation in adipocytes, it may not be required for this function in skeletal muscle [75, 82].

Downstream from TC10, variety effectors may be necessary to regulate insulin-stimulated glucose transport. CIP4/2 (Cdc42-interacting protein 4/2) and TCGAP (TC10/cdc42 GTPase activating protein) are two effector molecules that translocate from an intracellular compartment to the plasma membrane in response to insulin and interact directly with TC10 [72, 73]. The some downstream effectors of TC10 are likely to interact with actin directly. Two candidates are the actin-regulatory neural Wiskott-Aldrich syndrome protein (N-WASP) and actin-related protein-3 (Arp3) [74]. Both of these proteins localize to cortical actin upon insulin stimulation and cause F-actin polymerization [62].

The exocytosis, docking, and fusion of GLUT 4 containing vesicles with the plasma membrane are essential for insulin stimulated glucose uptake [62]. Recently, the exocyst complex that directs GLUT 4 vesicles to fusion sites has been identified [76]. The exocyst is a multisubunit complex that has been implicated in the transport of vesicles from the Golgi complex to the plasma membrane. Exo70, one of the components of the exocyst complex, translocates to lipid rafts and interacts with TC10 upon insulin stimulation [77]. It exists in a multiprotein complex with the proteins Sec6 and Sec8. However, the results obtained by Lizunov andcolleagues suggest that insulin regulates fusion of GLUT 4 vesicles independent of Exo70-mediated tethering [78].

The central component of the mammalian exocyst complex is Exo70, demonstrating specific interactions with almost all of the other subunits, including Sec5, Sec6, Sec8, Sec10, and Exo84. Exocyst complex regulates the compartmentalization of GLUT 4-containing vesicles at lipid raft domains in adipocytes. Exo70 is recruitedby the 6 protein TC10 after activation by insulin and brings with it Sec6 and Sec8 [79]. According to results obtained by Inoue and colleagues [79], their targeting to lipid rafts required for glucose uptake and GLUT 4 docking at the plasma membrane. The assembly of this complex also requires the PDZ domain (structural domain in the signaling proteins) protein SAP97, a member of the MAGUKs family (membrane associated guanylate kinase), which binds to Sec8 upon its translocation to the lipid raft. The TC10/exocyst complex/SAP97 axis, plays an important role in the tethering of GLUT 4 vesicles to the plasma membrane [79, 83].

Bao and colleagues have described an interaction between the Exo70 subunit of the exocyst and Snapin. Snapin is a ubiquitous protein known to associate with two t-SNAREs: SNAP23 and SNAP25. SNAP23 is a major t-SNARE regulating GLUT 4 vesicle trafficking. The interaction between Exo70 and Snapin is mediated via an N-terminal domain in Exo70 and C-terminal region in Snapin. Exo70 competes with SNAP23 for Snapin binding. The insulin-regulated trafficking of GLUT 4 to the plasma membrane serves to facilitate glucose uptake in adipocytes, and both SNAP23 and exocyst have been implicated in this process [81].

Insulin stimulates the translocation of GLUT 1 from cytoplasm to plasma membrane. For example, in cells, such as 3T3-L1 adipocytes, GLUT 1 is distributed between an intracellular compartments and the plasma membrane. Insulin increases the amount of membrane-bound GLUT 1 transporters from 20% to 50% of the total cellular GLUT 1 transporters [84, 85]. Insulin also regulates neuronal glucose uptake by promoting translocation of GLUT 3 to the plasma membrane. However, what regulates translocation of GLUT 3 to the plasma membrane is not completely understood; what signal transduction events underlie insulin-stimulated translocation of GLUT 3 [86].

Insulin has been shown to stimulate translocation of GLUT 1, GLUT 3, and GLUT 4 in L6 myotubes [87].

Glucagon

Glucagon was described by Kimball and Murlin in 1923 [88]. It is the principal hormone responsible for maintaining plasma glucose at appropriate levels during periods of increased functional demand [89]. This hormone counteracts hypoglycemia and opposes insulin actions by stimulating hepatic glucose synthesis. Glucagon induces a catabolic effect, mainly by activating liver glycogenolysis and gluconeogenesis, which results in the release of glucose to the bloodstream, thereby increasing blood glucose concentrations. Glucagon-secreting α-cells are on of the main endocrine cell populations that coexist in the islet of Langerhans along with insulin-secreting β-cells, somatostatin-secreting δ-cells, and pancreatic polypeptide-secreting PP-cells (also called F-cells or γ-cells). The α-cells comprise a small fraction (15 – 2-%) of the pancreatic islet cells. Despite the importance of the α-cells and glucagon secretion in the regulation of glycemia and nutrient homeostasis, little is known about the physiology of these cells in comparison with the information about β-cells [90].

The regulation of glucagon gene expression has not been studied as extensively as the insulin gene. Glucagon is a hormone consisting of 29 amino acids. The preproglucagon gene is expressed in the central nervous system, intestinal L cells and pancreatic α-cells. The preproglucagon-derived peptides glucagon, glucagon-like peptide-1 (GLP1) and glucagon-like peptide-2 (GLP2) are encoded by the preproglucagon gene. The chromosomal location of the human gene was mapped to 2q36-37. A post-translational cleavage by prohormone convertases (PC) is responsible for the maturation of the preprohormone that generates these peptides [90]. In α-cells, the predominance of PC2 (PCSK2) leads to a major production of glucagon together with the other derivatives [90, 92].

Control of glucagon secretion is not as well understood as that of insulin. Secretion of glucagon is clearly linked to the α-cell's metabolism. As in case of the β-cell's release of insulin, it has become clear that regulation of the membrane potential is decisive for control of glucagon secretion. In contrast to the β-cell, the "glucose sensor" of the α-cell is comprised of GLUT 1 and glucokinase (the "glucose sensor" of the β-cell is comprised GLUT 2 and glucokinase). This implies that glucose entry to the α-cell will occur at lower levels than in the β-cell. The K_m for human pancreatic glucokinase is 5,5 mM and GLUT 1 has a K_m of about 1 mM. The mentioned values suggest that uptake of glucose and initiation of glycolysis will start at lower blood glucose levels.

Multiple studies have determined the ion channel composition of α-cells. Pancreatic α-cells are equipped with a special set of channels. These channels generate action potentials of Na^+ and Ca^{2+} in the absence or at low levels of glucose [93, 94].

Such as in β-cells, ATP-dependent K^+ (K_{ATP}) channels play a fundamental role in α-cells. These channels couple variations in extracellular glucose concentrations to changes in membrane potential and electric activity [90].

Two ion channels determine the membrane potential of the α-cell, a K_{ATP} and tetrodotoxin-sensitive Na^+ channel. The Na^+ channels are fundamental for the generation of action potentials in α-cells. These channels are activated at voltages above -30 to -20 mV [95]. Action potentials occur when the membrane potential is lower than -50mV [96].

Glucose increases intracellular free ATP in α-cells, although reports vary as to the ability to inhibit α-cell K_{ATP} channels. These channels can be closed by ATP [97].In the absence of glucose or at low glucose levels, the activity of K_{ATP} channels in α-cells renders a membrane potential of about -60 mV. At this voltage, T-type Ca^{2+} channels open, and depolarize the membrane potential. Activation of the T-typeCa^{2+}-channels brings the membrane potential to levels where Na^+ channels begin toopen (-30 mV), leading to regenerative opening of these channels [98]. When the membrane potential exceeds -20 mV, N-type Ca^{2+} channels open, resulting in Ca^{2+}-influx and exocytotic release of glucagon [90, 98].

The increase of glucose in extracellular levels rises the cytosolic ATP/ADP ratio. The elevated cytosolic ATP/ADP ratio blocks K_{ATP} channels, depolarizing membrane potential of α-cells to a range where the channels involved in action become inactivated. These events cause electrical activity. Ca^{2+} signals and become inactivated. These events cause electrical activity. Ca^{2+} signals and glucagon secretion are inhibited [90].

Glucagon activates glucose formation and release from the liver to stabilize blood glucose between meals and under physical work [28, 90, and 100]. It does this through activation of the cyclic AMP/protein kinase A system. This pathway is also activated by pituitary adenylate cyclase-activating polypeptide (PACAP) [102], glucagon-like peptide-1 (GLP-1) [103], glucose-dependent insulinotropic polypeptide (GIP) and corticotropin-releasing factor (CRF) [104].

Glucagon stimulates gluconeogenesis and glycogenolysis, which increases hepatic glucose output, and at the same time, it decreases glycogenesis and glycolysis. Glucagon regulates gluconeogenesis mainly by the up-regulation of key enzymes such as glucose-6-phosphatase and phosphoenolpyruvate carboxykinase through the activation of the cAMP response element-binding protein and peroxisome proliferator-activated receptor γ-coactivator-1 [101].

The glucagon receptor belongs to the secretin-glucagon receptor II class family of G protein-coupled receptors [105]. It is present in multiple tissues, as for example liver, pancreas, heart, kidney, brain and smooth muscle [90]. Hormone binding to this receptor is coupled to GTP-binding heterotrimeric G proteins of the $G_{αs}$ type that leads to activation of adenylate cyclase, cAMP production and protein kinase A (PKA).

Key and fundamental roles in the guconeogenesis have three enzymes: phosphoenolpyruvate carboxykinase (PCK2), glucose-6-phosphatase (G6P), and fructose-1,6-biphosphatase (FBP1). The conversion of oxaloacetate is mediated by PCK2, G6P regulates glucose production from glucose-6-phosphate, while FBP1 catalyzes the conversion of fructose-1,6-biphosphate into fructose-6-phosphate. Glucagon decreases the intracellular levels of an allosteric inhibitor of fructose-1,6-biphosphatase, fructose-2,6-biphosphate. The decrease in an inhibitor reduces the activity of phosphofructokinase-1, down-regulating glycolysis. The glycolytic pathway is inhibited by glucagon at the pyruvate kinase level [90, 106].

Glycogen metabolism, and indirect blood glucose levels, are mainly determined by activity glycogen synthase and glycogen phosphorylase. Glucagon phosphorylates (activation) glycogen phosphorylase and inhibits glycogen synthase function by phosphorylation and its conversion into an active form of the enzyme [107].

Glucagon also stimulates gluconeogenesis by stimulation of uptake of amino acids in the liver. This hormone increases the release of glycerol from adipose tissue that can further be used in the liver during gluconeogenesis. However, the existence of a lipolytic action of glucagon observed in several animal models is still controversial in humans. An elevated glucagon to insulin ration accelerates gluconeogenesis as well as fatty acid β-oxidation and ketone bodies formation [90, 108].

Somatostatin

Somatostatin, also known as somatotropin release-inhibiting factor (SRIF) or growth hormone inhibiting hormone (GHIH) is a neuropeptide family that is produced by neuroendocrine, inflammatory, and immune cells in response to different stimuli. It was first discovered in hypothalamic extracts and identified as a hormone that inhibited secretion of growth hormone (GH) [110]. To date, somatostatin has been shown to inhibit the secretion of number hormones such as glycagon, growth hormone, and insulin, and in rodents it also inhibits TSH, prolactin, ACTH, and exocrine pancreas secretion [110 – 113]. Somatostatin was found to be secreted by broad range tissues, including pancreas, δ-cells, intestinal tract and regions of the central nervous system outside hypothalamus.

There are two forms of somatostatin: somatostatin-14 (SRIF-14, SS-14) and somatostatin-28 (SRIF-28, SS-28), reflecting their amino acid chain length.

The chromosomal location of the human gene was mapped to 3q28 [114], however, the nucleotide sequence and chromosomal location of both peptides clearly indicate that they are the products of two separate genes [132]. Both forms of hormone are generated by proteolytic cleavage of prosomatostatin, which itself is derived from preprosomatostatin. Two cysteine residues in somatostatin-14 allow the peptide to form an internal disulfide bond.

The relative amounts of somatostatin-14 versus somatostatin-28 secreted depend upon the tissue. The shorter form is the predominant form produced in the nervous system and apparently the sole form, secreted from pancreas, whereas the intestine mostly secretes the longer form. Somatostatin is released in large amounts from storage pools of secretory cells, or in small amounts from activated immune and inflammatory cells [115]. The blood concentration of somatostatin which mainly comes from gastroenteric system, is too low to affect the target cells inside islets.Thus, somatostatin released from δ-cells is considered to be potentially important as a local inhibitor of insulin and glucagon secretion from adjacent β- and α-cells [116].

If little is known about the regulation of glucagon release from α-cells, even less is known about δ-cells. This is mainly the consequence of the scarcity of δ-cells in the islet and the difficulties associated with their isolation and identification [98]. On the other hand, several features suggest that the mechanisms of glucose sensing in δ-cells are similar to those in β-cells [95]. Somatostatin release is increased in response to glucose stimulation [117, 118]. The omission of extracellular Ca^{2+} inhibits somatostatin secretion. These observations suggest that release of somatostatin is Ca^{2+} dependent. The regulation of somatostatin release from the δ-cells was reviewed by Kanno et al [98].

Acute administration of somatostatin to animals either systemically [119] or directly into the brain [120] reduces food intake. As in the case of several other satiety signals, the ability of systemic somatostatin to reduce food intake requires an intact vagus nerve [119, 121].

Somatostatin also regulates pancreatic insulin and glucagon secretion. It potently inhibits insulin and glucagon release from pancreatic islets. Somatostatin has been reported to have no direct effect on basal glucose production (gluconeogenesis or glycogenolysis) in isolated hepatocytes [122]. Similarly, *in vivo* studies have demonstrated that somatostatin does not alter the basal glucose production rate when the levels of insulin and glucagon are maintained [123, 124].

In addition to tissue-specific differences in secretion of somatostatin-14 and somatostatin-28, the two forms of this peptide can have different biological potencies. For example, only somatostatin-28 regulates glucose metabolism during the postprandial state [125]. Somatostatin-28 is a potent inhibitor of insulin release, both *in vivo* and *in vitro* [126, 127]. The pancreatic somatostatin-14 does not have a hormonal role in the control of insulin secretion [125]. In the pancreas somatostatin-14 is a more potent inhibitor of glucagon secretion from the pancreatic α-cells, whereas somatostatin-28 preferentially inhibits insulin secretion from the β-cells [128, 130]. The longer form of peptide is ten-fold more potent in the inhibition of growth hormone secretion, but less potent that shorter form of peptide in inhibiting glucagon release. Because both forms of somatostatin inhibit insulin and glucagon release with different potencies from pancreatic α-cells and β-cells, it has been postulated that each cell type expresses different somatostatin receptor subtypes [129].

The effects of somatostatin are mediated by a family of seven transmembrane domain G-protein-coupled receptors that comprise five distinct subtypes (termedSSTR1 – SSTR5) that are encoded by separate genes segregated on differentchromosomes [115, 131, 133, and 134]. At least two (SSTR2 and SSTR5) have been proposed to regulate pancreatic endocrine function [135]. At the cellular level, SSTR2 colocalizes strongly with glucagon while SSTR5 and SSTR1 quantitavely predominate in β-cells [136].

It is also interesting to note that four of these genes are intronless, the exception being sstr2, which is alternatively spliced in rodents to generate two isoforms, named sstr2A and sstr2B, which diverge in their C-terminal sequence [137, 138]. Four of the five receptors do not differentiate somatostatin-14 from somatostatin-28. They all bind both forms of peptide with similar high affinity only sstr5 displays a 10-fold higher affinity for somatostatin [131].

Each of the receptors activates distinct signaling pathway within cells as the inhibition of adenylate cyclase, activation of phosphotyrosine phosphatase and modulation of mitogen-activated protein kinase (MAPK) through G-protein-dependent mechanism. All five SSTRs are functionally coupled to inhibition of adenylate cyclase via a perfusion-toxin sensitive protein and this effect may participate in the antisecretory action of somatostatin.

If one had to summarize the effect of somatostatin on glucose homeostasis, it would be "somatostatin inhibits the secretion of insulin and glucagon from pancreatic islet cells". The portal vein insulin and glucagon levels were significantly decreased by somatostatin infusion. These hormonal changes were associated with a significant decrease in glucose levels in the portal circulation. It seems that hypoglycemia induced by somatostatin is associated with a significant decrease in the portal vein glucagon levels [124].

Amylin

The chromosomal location of the human amylin gene was mapped to 12p12.3-p12.1. Amylin (or islet amyloid polypeptide) is a 37 amino acid polypeptide produced by β-cells and stored in their secretory granules. It is co-secreted with insulin from pancreatic β-cells in response to glucose as same as insulin [139] (in a roughly about 10:100 amylin:insulin ratio) [121]. Plasma amylin levels are low during fasting and increase during meals and following glucose administration, and the levels are directly proportional to body fat [121].

Amylin participates in glucose homeostasis by two mechanisms, retarding gastric emptying in dose-response manner [140, 141] and suppressing postprandial glucagon secretion [141, 142].

Amylin crosses the blood-brain barrier, and widespread amylin binding sites have been described within central nervous system [143]. Plasma amylin is thought to function as a satiety signal by accessing receptors in the area postrema in the hindbrain. Therefore, the area postrema of the hindbrain appears to play a predominant role in mediating the anorectic effect of amylin [143]. Peripheral injection of amylin causes increased c-fos expression within the area postrema/nucleus tractus solitarus region, the lateral parabrachial nucleus [144, 145].

Little is known of the postreceptor intracellular signaling mechanisms elicited by amylin. Its anorectic action has been linked to the formation of cGMP in area postrema [144]. There is no unique amylin receptor gene. Rather, the functional amylin receptor in the area postrema utilizes a calcitonine receptor [146]. The amylin signal interacts with other signals controlling energy homeostasis at the level of the lateral hypothalamus. There is also evidence that amylin functions as an adiposity signal in additional to a satiety signal.

Pancreatic Polypeptide (PPY)

The pancreatic polypeptide (PP) belongs to the PP-fold family together with a second gut hormone, peptide YY (PYY) and neuropeptide Y (NPY). These peptides share a similar structure known as the PP-fold. All three peptides are 36 amino acids long with an amidated carboxy-terminus. NPY is one of the most evolutionary conserved peptides known. Only two of 36 amino acids of NPY are variable between different orders of mammals. PYY has eight variable amino acids between different orders of mammals, whereas the third member of the PP-fold family of peptides is one of the least-conserved peptides known [147].

The genes for PP and PYY are located only 10 kb apart from one another on chromosome segment 17q21.1 in humans [148].

Pancreatic polypeptide (PP) is a 36-amino acid peptide produced predominantly by F-cells (PP-cells) located in the periphery of pancreatic islets of Langerhans at the head of the pancreas. Circulating PP concentrations increase following nutrient ingestion in a biphasic manner in proportion to the caloric load [149]. The secretion of PP during meals requires an intact vagus nerve.

Like the other endocrine pancreatic hormones, PP exerts a variety of regulatory functions including inhibition of pancreatic secretion, gall bladder activity, intestinal motility, and modulation of gastric motility [150]. Pancreatic polypeptide has been found to inhibit ileum contractions [151], and to stimulate colon contractions [152]. It also affects metabolic functions including glycogenolysis, and decreases fatty acid levels [153]. However, binding sites for PP have been found in several rat brain regions [154, 155], suggesting that PP may also have direct effects on brain function. The nutrient ingestion is the main stimulus for PP release. On the other hand, other factors alter circulating PP levels, as for example: adrenergic stimulation following hypoglycemia, exercise and the cholecystokinin stimulate PP release. Pancreatic polypeptide reduces activity of both afferent and efferent vagal neurons. It suggests a fundamental role for the vagus in mediating the anorectic actions of PP.

Five PP-fold family receptors have been cloned from mammals, including humans (Y1, Y2, Y4, Y5, and y6) [147]. These receptors belong to a large and very heterogeneous family of G-protein-coupled receptors (GPCRs) belonging to the rhodopsin like superfamily (class 1) of receptors. PP binds to all of the Y receptors family subtypes but exhibits the greatest affinity for the Y4 subtype and this receptor subtype is thought to mediate the anorectic effects of PP [156].

The activation of PP-fold receptors involves pertussis toxin-sensitive phosphorylation of extracellular signal-regulated protein kinase 1 and 2 in Chinese hamster ovary cells (CHO cells), confirming that these receptors couple to Gi/Go [157]. The Y1 receptor has been shown to activate mitogen-activated protein kinase (MAPK) in gut epithelial cells [158]. Protein kinase C seems to be necessary for Y5 receptor signaling. A protein kinase C-independent pathway may also be involved in Y1, Y2 and Y4 receptors [157]. All of these receptors, excluding y6, can also couple to phospholipase C to provoke release of Ca^{2+} from intracellular compartment [158, 159]. For details see [147].

Gut Hormones

The gut is the most exciting endocrine organ in the body. Currently, the neuroendocrine role of the gut in energy homeostasis is a dynamic and rapidly expanding field of scientific investigation. The concept of the gut as an endocrine organ is hardly new. There are more than 50 gut hormones and peptides synthesized and released from the gastrointestinal tract, of which only a small proportion have been vigorously investigated for their role in glucose homeostasis.

Incretin Hormone

Perley and Kipnis, by the late 1960s, demonstrated that ingest food caused a more potent release of insulin than glucose infused intravenously [161]. In normal subjects, the augmentation is three- to four fold [162]. Similar increases are noted for arterial C-peptide concentrations, ruling out that differences in hepatic insulin uptake are responsible for the differences [163]. This effect, termed the "incretin effect", suggests that signals from the gut are important in the hormonal regulation of glucose disappearance.

Specific criteria have to be fulfilled for an agent to be called an incretin: 1) it must be released in response to oral nutrient ingestion, especially glucose, and 2) reach physiological concentrations *in vivo* to cause insulin release [164]. They have a number of important biological effects, as for example, release of insulin, inhibition of glucagon and somatostatin, maintenance of β-cell mass, delay of gastric emptying, and inhibition of feeding. Several incretin hormones have been characterized, but currently, GLP-1 and GIP are the only known incretins. Both GLP-1 and GIP are secreted in a nutrient-dependent manner and stimulate glucose-dependent insulin secretion.

Incretin hormones are peptide hormones secreted from the gut.

Glucagon-Like Peptide-1 (GLP-1)

Glucagon-like peptide-1 was discovered after sequential analysis of the pre-proglucagon gene [165].

Glucagon-like peptide-1 (GLP-1) is derived from the product of the glucagon gene. This gene encodes a preproprotein that is differentially cleaved dependent upon the tissue in which it is synthesized. GLP-1 is produced and secreted by L cells in the distal ileum and colon [166]. It is also expressed in neurons in the nucleus tractus solitarius [167].

GLP-1 is produced as an inactive 37-amino acid peptide whose C-terminal end contains glycine. The active form is produced by post-translational cleavage of six amino acids from the N-terminal end of GLP-1. This truncated form of GLP-1 can be amidated at the glycine end of the C-terminal end [164]. GLP-1 circulates as 2 equipotent forms; GLP-1$_{7-37}$ and GLP-1$_{7-36}$ amide [168, 169], but GLP-1$_{7-36}$ amide is the major circulating form [170]. Glucagon-like peptide-1 has approximately a 50% structural homology to glucagon [171]. The circulating half-life of GLP-1 is very short (less than 2 minutes). It is mainly a result of action of the dipeptidyl peptidase IV (DPP-IV), which removes the first 2 amino acids of the N-terminal end [172]. Glucagon-like peptide-1 is released 5 – 30 min after food ingestion in proportion to energy content. It is released in response to intake of carbohydrates and fats (a slower, more sustained release), while proteins and mixed amino acids also have an effect [173].

The original physiological role described for GLP-1 was that of an incretin hormone that stimulates insulin secretion in a glucose-dependent manner [174, 175]. Glucagon-like peptide-1 stimulates insulin and inhibits glucagon secretion acting on islet β- and α-cell receptors during hyperglycemia [176]. The inhibition of glucagon secretion may be direct via GLP-1 receptors expressed on α-cells or indirect via stimulation of insulin and somatostatin secretion. Secretion of a GLP-1 plays key role in the regulation of oral-glucose enhanced insulin secretion. GLP-1 inhibitsgastric emptying and food intake [177]. GLP-1 also replenishes insulin stores viastimulation of proinsulin gene expression [178]. These effects are mediated via increases in proinsulin gene transcription and mRNA stability through cAMP-dependent PKA-independent mechanisms.

The human GLP-1 receptor (GLP-1R) is a 463 amino acid hepta-helical G protein-coupled receptor [179]. The receptor was first cloned by Bernard Thorens. It was subsequently found that the GLP-1 receptor belongs to the same family as the glucagon receptors [180]. The GLP-1R is widely distributed in pancreatic islets, brain, heart and the gastrointestinal tract. Within pancreatic islets, the GLP-1 receptor is predominantly localized to β-cells, although GLP-1R expression on islet α-cells and δ-cells has also been reported [179].

Binding of glucagon-like peptide-1 to the receptor causes activation, via a stimulatory G protein, of adenylate cyclase, resulting in the formation of cAMP. Elevated levels of intracellular cAMP result in the activation of protein kinase A and the cAMP-regulated guanine nucleotide exchange factor II (cAMP-GEFII, also known as Epac 2). Consequence of this is a plethora of events including altered ion channel activity and elevation of intracellular calcium concentrations in the target cells [163, 180].

The effects of GLP-1 on pancreas can be divided into two categories: effects on the pancreatic secretions, insulin in particular, and effect on pancreatic cells. The insulinotropic activity of GLP-1, which is strictly glucose dependent, is exerted via interaction with a GLP-1R located on the cell membrane of the pancreatic β-cells. A certain level of glucose must be present for GLP-1 to have any effect on insulin secretion.

GLP-1 binds to GLP-1R and causes activation, via a stimulatory G protein, of adenylate cyclase, producing an increase of cAMP which in turn activates protein kinase A (PKA) [181]. Through this pathway GLP-1 promotes the phosphorylation of GLUT 2 and the K_{ATP} and Ca^{2+} channels [181 – 183]. Acting in concert with glucose, GLP-1 facilitates membrane depolarization resulting in the closure of ATP-sensitive K^+ (K_{ATP}) channels. These channels are sensitive to the intracellular ATP levels and, thereby, to glucose metabolism of the β-cells. This enhances Ca^{2+} influx and exocytotic release of insulin [163, 184] (See also Chapter "Glucose homeostasis" part "Insulin"). GLP-1 also up regulates the genes involved in insulin secretion, as for example glucokinase and GLUT 2 genes [185] and stimulates all steps of insulin biosynthesis as well as insulin gene transcription [186].

The specific functions in pancreatic cells include proliferation, differentiation and inhibition of apoptosis of cells. It is to note that GLP-1 mediated stimulation of islet cell proliferation occurs via a PI 3-kinase-dependent pathway [180].

GLP-1 also lowers glucose levels via inhibition of glucagon secretion from islet α-cells. Although, probably, there are no receptors for GLP-1 on the α-cell, intra-islet insulin released from β-cells in response to GLP-1 locally inhibits glucagon secretion [164].

Glucose-Dependent Insulinotropic Polypeptide (GIP)

Glucose-dependent insulinotropic polypeptide (formerly called gastric inhibitory peptide) was discovered in 1973, but its insulinotropic properties were discovered soon after [187]. It belongs to the family of secretins, presenting homology with some of its members, as for example secretin, glucagon, GLP-1. The human GIP gene has been assigned to chromosome 17q21.3-q22. Glucose-dependent insulinotropic peptide is derived from a 153-amino acid proprotein and circulates as a biologically active 42-amino acid peptide [189]. The sequence of GIP is highly conserved across species, with over 90% of the amino acid sequence being identical between human, rat, mouse, porcine, and bovine GIP [179]. GIP is synthesized and secreted from specific endocrine cells, the so-called K cells whose locations are primarily in the duodenum and proximal jejunum, which exhibit the highest density in the duodenum. It is expressed also in stomach.

Once released, GIP is rapidly degraded by dipeptidyl peptidase IV (DPP-IV) to an inactive truncated derivative. The half-life of biological active GIP is approximately 7 minutes [190]. GIP is cleared through the kidney.

The original activity associated with GIP was the inhibition of gastric acid secretion and was thus, originally called gastric inhibitory peptide. Its main effect is insulinotropic; therefore, it was renamed glucose-dependent insulinotropic polypeptide. The dominant action of GIP is the stimulation of glucose-dependent insulin secretion. GIP also promotes insulin biosynthesis and stimulates GLUT 2 and glucokinase gene expression [193]. GIP affects hepatic glucose production, glucose uptake by muscle and glucose transport in adipose tissue [194, 195]. It has significant effect on fat metabolism exerted at the level of adipocytes. These actions include stimulation of lipoprotein lipase activity leading to increased uptake and incorporation of fatty acids by adipocytes.

GIP secretion is greatly increased in response to meal ingestion. Secretion is stimulated by absorbable carbohydrates and by lipids. It is also interesting to note that in humans, the stimulatory effect of fat is higher than that of carbohydrates [191].

The GIP receptor (GIPR) is a seven-transmembrane glycoprotein associated to a G protein which activates adenylate cyclase with the subsequent increase of cAMP. The chromosomal location of the human GIPR gene was mapped to 19q13.2-13.3 [192]. The GIP receptor is a type II G-protein coupled receptor belonging to a superfamily of receptors the ligands of which are constituted by the members of the secretin-glucagon family of peptides [163, 194]. GIPR is expressed in the pancreatic islets. GIP presents also functional extrapancreatic receptors in liver, muscle, adipose tissue, intestine, adrenal cortex, heart, pituitary, several regions of the brain and in symphatetic nervous system. Its functions in many of those locations are generally unknown.

Interaction of GIP with its receptor on the pancreatic β-cells causes an elevation of cAMP levels. The increase in cAMP acts through a PKA-dependent and a PKA independent pathway. It also acts in opening voltage-dependent Ca^{2+} channels, thus increasing the intracellular calcium concentration and inhibits ATP-sensitive K^+ channels, which together induces the exocytosis of insulin-containing granules [195]. A number of other signaling pathways may also by activated (presumably secondarily to the rise in cAMP), including the phosphatidylinositol 3-kinase/protein kinase B as well as the MAP kinase pathway [197 – 199].

Other Gut Hormones

Ghrelin

The name "ghrelin" is derived from **g**rowth-**h**ormone **rel**ease or by Wu and Kral [213] from "ghre" in the Proto-Indo-European language meaning "grow", and the suffix "relin" as in "release".

Ghrelin is a gastric hormone recognized in 1999 as a mediator of growth hormone release. It was initially discovered as a ligand for the growth hormone secretagogue receptor [200]. Ghrelin is currently the only known orexigenic gut hormone. It is the first identified hormone that acts as a food-intake stimulatory signal originating from the stomach [201].

The human ghrelin gene is located on chromosome 3p25-26. A revised exon-intron structure demonstrates that the human ghrelin gene consists of six [202] rather than five exons [203]. This gene encodes a preproghrelin, containing 117 amino acids. Beside ghrelin, des-Gln[14]-ghrelin is also produced, although in smaller quantities [204].

Ghrelin is a 28-amino acid lipophylic peptide derived from preproghrelin. During post-translational modification, the serine-3 residue is covalently linked to octanoic acid. This acylation is unique to ghrelin and is necessary for ghrelin to bind to ghrelin receptor and to cross the blood-brain barrier [205, 206]. The desoctanoyl form of ghrelin without this side chain does not displace ghrelin from its hypothalamic and pituitary receptors, and does not stimulate growth hormone [207].

Ghrelin is principally synthesized in endocrine cells of the stomach termed X/A-like, now designated ghrelin-secreting cells. About 60% - 75% of circulating ghrelin is the gastric origin [208], and most of the remainder originates in the intestine. In the intestine, ghrelin concentration gradually decreases from the duodenum to the colon [209]. It has been suggested that low-level ghrelin expression also occurs in several tissues, including hypothalamus (arcuate nucleus and paraventricular neuron groups), pituitary, lung, adrenal cortex, kidney and bone [210 – 212]. The pancreas is also a ghrelin-producing organ. In the pancreatic islets, the cell type of ghrelin cells remains controversial. Is ghrelin secreted from α-cells, β-cells, ε-cells or novel cell type? [214 – 216].

It is not clear what factors are involved in the regulation of ghrelin secretion. Plasma ghrelin levels are increased by fasting, before meals and at night and are rapidly suppressed by high-calorie or high-carbohydrate meals [214 – 217]. Blood glucose levels may be critical: oral or intravenous administration of glucose decreases plasma ghrelin concentration [209, 218]. Similar results were obtained in the case insulin, glucagon, growth hormone and somatostatin [214, 219 – 221]. On the other hand, the results obtained by other authors suggest that plasma ghrelin levels are not affected by glucose or insulin levels in healthy subjects [230].

Ghrelin has been found in the hypothalamic arcuate nucleus, an important region controlling appetite [222]. In humans ghrelin infusion that leads to an increase in plasma ghrelin to preprandial levels stimulates hunger and spontaneous food intake [223]. The experiments indicated that ghrelin stimulates the release of insulin [224]. In rats, intravenously administrated ghrelin also resulted in an increase of serum insulin levels [225]. In the other experiments ghrelin has been shown to inhibit insulin secretion in perfused pancreases of the rat and mouse [226, 227] and subsequent *in vivo* studies in several species suggest also an inhibitory, rather than a stimulatory effect of ghrelin on insulin secretion. Ghrelin inhibits the effects of insulin on glycogen synthesis and gluconeogenesis *in vitro* [228]. In human, ghrelin administration induces hyperglycemia and reduces insulin secretion [229].

The half-life of circulating ghrelin is 30 min [231]. The inactivation and degradation processes involve proteases and tissue esterases [232].

The human ghrelin receptor (GHS-R) is encoded by a single gene found at chromosomal location 3q26.2 [233]. The GHS-R gene consists of two exons: the first exon encodes transmembranes 1-sty to 5-th and the second exon encodes transmembranes 6-th and 7-th.

Ghrelin receptor is a typical G protein-coupled receptor with seven transmembrane domains (7-TM) [234]. This receptor is well conserved among several species, five of seven predicted transmembrane domains, it is thus a COOH-terminal truncated including mammals, chickens, and fish [235]. Two distinct ghrelin receptor cDNA have been isolated [236]. The first, GHS-R type 1a, encodes a 7-TM G protein-coupled receptor with binding and functional properties with its role as ghrelin's receptor. This type of receptor consisting of 366 amino acids with 7 transmembrane regions. GHS-R type 1b is produced by an alternative splicing mechanism [236]. This type of receptor is derived from only the first exon and encodes only the form of the type 1a receptor and is pharmacologically inactive [205, 209]. GHS-R type 1b consists of 289 amino acids with only 5 transmembrane domains [213].

The GHS-R type 1a is prominently expressed in the hypothalamic arcuate nucleus and ventromedial nuclei and in the hippocampus [237]. The GHS receptors (type 1a) have been found in other tissues including thyroid, pancreas, spleen, heart, and adrenal glands [238, 239]. GHS-R type 1b is found most commonly in the skin, myocardium, and pituitary gland, and its tissue distribution is comparable to ghrelin [238, 239]. This widespread distribution is likely to explain the many endocrine and non-endocrine effects of ghrelin.

Stimulation of GHS-R type 1a by ghrelin activates the phospholipase C signaling pathway, leading to increased inositol phosphate turnover and protein kinase C activation, resulting in the release of calcium from intracellular stores and an increase of intracellular Ca^{2+} [240]. The activation of ghrelin receptor also inhibits K channels, allowing the entry of calcium through voltage-gated L- and T-type channels [241].

Ghrelin upregulates several activities that are also potentiated by insulin, as for example tyrosine phosphorylation of insulin receptor substrate-1, association of the adaptor molecule growth factor receptor-bound protein 2 with IRS-1 and stimulates mitogen-activated protein kinase (MAPK) activity. Ghrelin also inhibits Akt kinase and partially reverses the downregulating effect of insulin on phosphoenolpyruvate carboxykinase mRNA expression, a key enzyme of gluconeogenesis. Blocking the function of endogenous ghrelin markedly lowered fasting glucose concentrations, attenuated glycemic excursion, and enhanced insulin responses during a glucose tolerance test. These results suggest an inhibitory role for ghrelin in the control of insulin secretion. On the other hand, exogenous ghrelin increases glycemic excursion and reduced insulin secretion in rodent *in vivo*, and ghrelin seems to directly inhibit insulin secretion in isolated islets *in vitro* [280].

Cholecystokinin (CKK)

Cholecystokinin (CCK) was discovered in 1928 by Ivy and Oldberg, as a hormone which contracted gall bladder [242]. The human cholecystokinin gene is located on chromosome 3p22-p21.3 [243].

Cholecystokinin is structurally related to gastrin. It exists in several molecular forms with differing numbers of amino acids, as for example CCK-8, CCK-33, CCK-39, and CCK-54 [244], of which an octapeptide (8 amino acids) is the most active. All these molecular forms derive from a single CCK gene through posttranslational processing and have the same C-terminal five amino acid sequence. The different forms are all carboxyamidated and *O*-sulfated and are all ligands for CCK-1 receptor [249].

Cholecystokinin is the prototypical satiety hormone [208]. CCK is widely distributed with the gastrointestinal tract, but the majority is synthesized in the duodenum by endocrine I cells acting via CCK-1 receptors on vagal afferent nerve [248]. It is also widely distributed in the brain, functioning as a neurotransmitter in different regions of brain [245, 246]. It is to note that brain and gut contain different molecular forms of cholecystokinin. This is because pro-cholecystokinin is processed by different isoforms of the prohormone convertase [250]. Prohormone convertase 1 is present in the intestines, whereas prohormone convertase 2 processes pro-cholecystokinin in the brain [251].

Cholecystokinin is rapidly released into the surrounding tissues and circulation in response to nutrients in the gut. Dietary fat and protein in the small intestine are the main stimulants of cholecystokinin release, with carbohydrates only providing a weak stimulus [246]. Cholecystokinin has a very short half life of only 1 – 2 minutes, and it is not effective at reducing meal size if the peptide is administrated more than 15 minutes before a meal [252]. This may depend on the molecular form of cholecystokinin, and is most accurate for CCK-8 [167]. Cholecystokinin is inactivated by enzymes including tripeptidyl peptidase II [253].

Cholecystokinin acts via two receptors CCK-1 and CCK-2 (formerly known as CCK-A and CCK-B, for "Alimentary" and "Brain"). The distribution of CCK-1 and CCK-2 receptors is tissue dependent.

The human CCK-1 receptor gene is located on chromosome 4p15-p15.2 [254] and the CCK-2 receptor gene – on chromosome 11p15.4-p15.5 [255]. The genes encoding the CCK-1 receptor and the CCK-2 receptor in humans are organized in a similar manner consisting of five exons and four introns [256].

The CCK-1 receptor was purified to homogeneity from rat pancreas. Hydropathy analysis predicts seven transmembrane-spanning domains as expected for a member of the G protein-coupled receptor superfamily [257]. The sequence contains at least three consensus sites for *N*-linked glycosylation. The CCK-1 receptor is highly conserved among different mammalian species, with an overall amino acid homology of 80% and a pairwise amino acid sequence identity of 87% to 92% in humans, guinea pig, rat and rabbit [256]. It is to note that CCK-1 receptor is capable of coupling to both phospholipase C and adenylate cyclase at physiological concentrations in native cells.

The CCK-2 receptor, similar to the CCK-1 receptor, hydropathy analysis predicts seven transmembrane-spanning domains as expected of a member of the G protein- coupled receptor superfamily [257], and the sequence contains at least three consensus sites for *N*-linked glycosylation. The CCK-2 receptor is highly conserved in humans, canine, guinea pig, calf, rabbit, and rat, with an overall amino acid identity of 72% and pairwise amino acid sequence identities of 84 to 93%, respectively [256].

The CCK-1 receptors in the periphery are primarily localized in the pancreas, gallbladder, pylorus, intestine, and vagus nerve [256]. In human pancreas, CCK-1receptor mRNA is ~ 30 times lower than CCK-2 receptor [261]. In the pancreas, cholecystokinin acts at CCK-1 receptors on acinar cells to stimulate the secretion of the enzyme amylase [258], and in the gallbladder, cholecystokinin acts at CCK-1 receptors to stimulate gallbladder contraction [259]. The CCK-2 receptors in the periphery are primarily localized in the stomach and on the vagus nerve [256]. Cholecystokinin stimulates gastric acid secretion [260].

Cholecystokinin signals its satiety effects to the hypothalamus through a neural pathway to the brainstem. CCK-1 receptor is involved in satiety whereas CCK-2 receptor is not. This effect is mediated through CCK-1 receptors on vagal afferents [262]. Cholecystokinin also plays a role in the control of glucose homeostasis. CCK-2 receptor mediates the effect of cholecystokinin on the control of glucose homeostasis by the pancreas [3]. On the other hand, results obtained by other authors demonstrate the importance of CCK-1 receptor in the control of insulin and glucagon release along with glycemia [264]. The absence of CCK-1 receptors impairs functions of the endocrine pancreas, although pancreatic insulin content is not affected in CCK-1 receptor deficient rats. Its release in response to CCK-8 remained at basal level. CCK-8 failed to induce glucagon secretion while it increased its release in normal rats. In response to a meal, plasma insulin was reduced and associated with transient hyperglycemia in CCK-1 receptor deficient rats [266]. CCK administration to patients with type 2 diabetes mellitus reduces postprandial hyperglycemia, thus suggesting increased insulin secretion [263]. Cholecystokinin has been shown to stimulate glucagon release from human islets *in vitro* and stimulates insulin secretion in rodents in a glucose-dependent manner.Infusion of CCK-8 increases plasma insulin concentration and reduces glucose excursion in healthy subjects and type 2 diabetic patients [265].

Oxyntomodulin

Oxyntomodulin (OXM) was originally isolated from porcine jejuno-ileal cells [267].

It was named after its inhibitory action on the oxyntic glands of the stomach [268].

Oxyntomodulin is a 37-amino acid peptide and contains the 29 amino acid structure of glucagon, followed by an octapeptyde C-terminal extension [269]. It is one of the products of the glucagon gene. Proglucagon is cleaved by prohormone convertases 1 and 2 into different breakdown products dependent on the tissue. Within the gut and brain, post-translational processing of proglucagon results in the production of glicentin, glucagon-like peptide 1 and glucagon-like peptide 2. Glicentin, also known as enteroglucagon, is broken down to produce oxyntomodulin.

Oxyntomodulin is expressed in the central nervous system, the intestinal L cells and the pancreas [270]. Significant amounts of oxyntomodulin have been found in human distal intestine [271].

Oxyntomodulin is rapidly released, 5 – 10 min after food intake in proportion to calorie intake. The release of oxyntomodulin is stimulated particularly by fatty acids in the gut lumen, produced by hydrolysis of fat [272]. Levels rise within 30 min and stay elevated for several hours [273]. Independently of food intake, the hormone also exhibits a diurnal variation with levels highest in the evening and lowest in the early morning [274].

Oxyntomodulin binds to the GLP-1 receptor, but with lower affinity (OXM has a 50-fold lower affinity for binding at this receptor) [275]. Therefore it is possible that its effects are mediated by other specific receptors [276].

The mechanism of anorexigenic action of oxyntomodulin is not known but it may involve the suppression of plasma ghrelin levels; it reduces circulating ghrelin by around 44% in human subjects [277]. Oxyntomodulin may also act directly on hypothalamic appetite centers [279]. Oxyntomodulin promotes meat-induced insulin secretion [278]. Acute oxyntomodulin infusion in humans reduces food intake, without affecting plasma glucose. The infusion of OXM has no effect on fasting or post-prandial levels of insulin and glucagon. Intravenous administration of oxyntomodulin reduced calorie uptake by 19% in healthy humans, and subsequent cumulative 12-h energy intake was reduced [277]. Oxyntomodulin released after ingestion of meal inhibits gastric secretion and emptying, decreases pancreatic secretion and stimulates intestinal glucose uptake [277]. It was shown that oxyntomodulin stimulates insulin release in perfused rat pancreas [281].

The half-life of oxyntomodulin in human plasma is 8,4 ± 2 min. Oxyntomodulin is inactivated by the enzyme dipeptidyl peptidase IV (DPP-IV) [282].

Peptide YY (PYY)

Peptide YY (PYY, peptide tyrosine-tyrosine) was initially isolated by Tatemoto and Mutt in 1980 from porcine jejunal mucosa [283]. The chromosomal location of the human peptide YY gene was mapped to 17q21.1 [284].

The gut hormone peptide YY belongs to the pancreatic polypeptide (PP) family along with PP and neuropeptide Y (NPY). These peptides have the PP fold structural motif and mediate their effects through the NPY receptors. Peptide YY was originally named in light of two tyrosine residues at the N- and C-terminus of protein [285]. PYY shares considerable homology with the peptide sequences of PP and NPY, and its amino acid structure is highly conserved between species.

The gut hormone PYY is a 36-amino acid peptide. Two main endogenous forms of PYY have been identified: PYY1-36 and PYY3-36, the latter being the predominant circulating form [286]. PYY3-36 is produced by the action of the enzyme dipeptidyl peptidase IV (DPP-IV), which hydrolyzes PYY at the Pro-Ile bond. DPP-IV preferentially cleaves substrates with an N-terminal praline or alanine residue at position two. Removing the NH_2-terminal tyrosine-proline markedly changes the three-dimensional conformation of PYY, altering its receptor specificity and biological effects [287, 288]. Whereas PYY1-36 binds to all of the Y receptors, with lesser affinity to Y4 receptor, PYY3-36 has a high affinity for the Y2 receptor and some affinity for Y1 and Y5 receptors [289].

PYY is mainly produced by endocrine L cells of the colon and rectum, although it is present at higher concentrations in more distal sections [290]. Peptide YY is released into the circulation after a meal, in a nutrient-dependent manner, and is reduced by fasting. PPY levels increase within 15 min of ingesting meal, with levels rising to a plateau after 1 – 2 h and remaining elevated for up to 6 h [291]. These levels are influenced not only by caloric intake but also by a meal composition, and higher levels are seen following fatty meals compared with meals containing high protein or carbohydrates [292, 293]. Interestingly, PYY levels are reported to be decreased in obese subjects [294].

Members of the PP-fold family mediate their effects via Y-receptors belonging to the G protein-coupled receptor family. There are five different subtypes in mammals, Y1 – Y5 [295]. They are all seven transmembrane domain receptors coupled to G_1 resulting in inhibition of adenylate cyclase. However, Y1 also increases intracellular calcium, and Y2 regulates both calcium and potassium channels [278]. The receptors differ in distribution and function, and are classified according to their affinity for PYY, PP, and NPY.

The studies on the actions of peripherally administered PYY demonstrated numerous effects on the gastrointestinal tract. It significantly delayed gastric emptying, gastric and pancreatic secretion [278]. Intraperitoneal administration ofPYY3-36 reduced both dark-phase food intake and feeding following a 24 h fast in rats, and in normal-weight human subjects peripheral infusion of PYY3-36 reduced appetite (food intake was reduced by > 30%), and 24 h caloric intake, without any alteration in gastric emptying [296]. The actions of peripheral PYY3-36 on satiety appear to be mediated by the Y2 receptor expressed in the hypothalamic arcuate nucleus [278].

Peptide YY administration to the central nervous system has opposite actions to patients seen with peripheral PYY. PYY injections into the third, lateral, or four cerebral ventricles [297], paraventricular nucleus [298] or hippocampus, potently stimulated food intake in rodents [299]. Similarly, intracerebroventricular injection of PYY3-36 increased food intake [300]. Administration of PYY in the dorsal vagal complex stimulated gastric acid secretion, again being the opposite effect to that seen following peripheral administration [278].

Peptide YY also has an effect on glucose homeostasis. PYY1-36 has an important role in glucose-stimulated rather than basal insulin secretion. Intravenously administered PYY1-36 inhibits glucose-stimulated insulin secretion in mice [301]. *In vitro* studies also demonstrate that PYY dose-dependently inhibits glucose-stimulated but not basal insulin secretion [302]. Studies using perfused islets isolated from rats suggest that this is a direct action of PYY1-36 on islets [303]. Results obtained by Boey and colleagues suggest that PYY1-36 has an important regulatory role in insulin secretion *in vivo*, and that PYY1-36 importantly modulates glucose-stimulated insulin secretion from the islets of Langerhans [304].

The mechanism by which PYY1-36 inhibits insulin secretion is still unclear. Several studies have led to an understanding that PYY1-36 acts on Y1 receptors to influence insulin secretion, and that Y2 and Y5 receptors are not involved in the inhibitory effect of PYY on 2-deoxyglucose-induced insulin secretion [305]. It is likely that PYY1-36 acts directly on Y1 receptors in the pancreas to inhibit insulin secretion, because only the Y1 receptor subtype has been detected on pancreatic islets [306]. These Y1 receptors have been detected on β-cells that produce insulin [307] and δ-cells that produce somatostatin that inhibits insulin and glucagon secretion [308]. PYY1-36 may also act on and influence other cells in pancreatic islets to inhibit insulin release by β-cells [304].

Peptide YY1-36 may also exert its effects on the central nervous system to inhibit insulin secretion [304]. It is likely that PYY1-36 binds to the Y1 and Y2 receptors located in the brainstem to modulate vagal output and regulating insulin secretion [309]. It was shown that PYY1-36 blocks β-adrenergic-stimulated insulin secretion in dogs [310].

PYY3-36 has less of a role on basal and glucose-stimulated insulin secretion, however, recent studies suggest a role for PYY3-36 in regulating insulin sensitivity [311, 312]. The results obtained by Pittner and colleagues [311] suggest that endogenous PYY3-36 may influence insulin sensitivity and glucose uptake. A possible mechanism by which PYY3-36 could influence insulin sensitivity is via the hypothalamic Y2 receptor [304]. However, the downstream pathways by whichPYY3-36 leads to changes in glucose uptake by muscle and adipose tissue are not well characterized [312].

Neuropeptide Y (NPY)

Neuropeptide Y (NPY) was discovered by Tatemoto and Mutt in 1982. It was isolated from porcine brain [313]. As mentioned in previous part (Peptide YY), NPY is a member of a peptide family consisting of NPY and two gut hormones, peptide YY and pancreatic polypeptide. Its name derives from the single-letter code (Y) for the amino acid tyrosine since it contains several tyrosine residues including an amidated C-terminal tyrosine residue. It is one of the most conserved peptides during evolution [314]. When comparing the amino acid sequences from a variety of mammals, only 2 of the 36 amino acids of NPY are variable [315].

The gene for human NPY maps to chromosome 7p15.1 [316]. It consists of four exons. The encoded pre-pro NPY is comprised of 97 amino acids. This is in turn proteolytically processed into the C-terminal peptide of NPY (CPON) and NPY. The C-terminus of NPY is amidated and this is essential for its biological activity. Dipeptidyl peptidase IV and aminopeptidase P can further process NPY – NPY3-36 and NPY2-36, respectively. The functional significance of CPON is unknown. The C-terminal fragments of NPY have some selectivity for the Y2 receptor subtype [315].

Neuropeptide Y is one of the most potent orexigenic peptides found in the brain. NPY is abundant in cerebral cortex, hippocampus, thalamus, hypothalamus and brainstem [317]. In the periphery, neuropeptide Y is found in the peripheral nerves and circulation. It is present in most sympathetic nerve fibers, particularly in the dense plexuses around the blood vessels [318]. The adrenal medulla is the primary source of circulating NPY [319] though it is also expressed in liver, heart, spleen, and in endothelial cells of blood vessels [320]. In the sympathetic nervous system NPY is co-stored and co-released with norepinephrine [321], and in brainstem neurons, NPY is colocalized with epinephrine or norepinephrine [322].

Neuropeptide Y is also expressed in pancreatic islets and is implicated in the regulation of islet function [323, 324].

The widespread distribution of NPY is associated with diverse biological actions [325]. Neuropeptide Y participates, for example, in the body temperature regulation[326], sexual and emotional behavior [327, 328], cardiovascular functions [329], hormone secretion [330] etc. It stimulates food intake with a preferential effect on carbohydrate uptake [331, 332]. Within the hypothalamus, neuropeptide Y plays an essential role in the control of food intake and body weight [325]. NPY also modifies the motivation to eat [334]. Its effect is comparable to that of a 36 – 48 hour food deprivation [335]. NPY increased the intake of the different sucrose solutions as well as the preferred saccharin solution [336]. Orosensory mechanisms might therefore play a role on the stimulatory effects of NPY on carbohydrate intake [332]. NPY injected into the brain induced feeding response [333]. Food intake is increased several fold and the effect lasts 6 – 8 hours. The orexigenic effect of neuropeptide Y has been noted in numerous species. No effect has been described after peripheral infusion.

Neuropeptide Y is also expressed in pancreatic islets and is implicated in the regulation of islet function. Here, neuropeptide Y is colocalized in glucagon, somatostatin, and insulin-producing cells [324, 337]. Neuropeptide Y decreases glucose-stimulated insulin secretion from the rat and mouse pancreas and islet [338, 339], and also from human islets [340]. Although studies indicated that application of NPY to pancreatic islets inhibits insulin secretion, its physiological role in the regulation of insulin secretion is not fully understood. Imai and colleagues [341] hypothesized that NPY in islets tonically suppresses insulin secretion and the reduction of islet NPY increases insulin secretion. On the other hand, little is known whether islet NPY has a physiological role in the regulation of glucose homeostasis [341].

All known NPY receptors belong to the large superfamily of G protein-coupled, heptahelical receptors [160, 342, and 343].

Adrenaline (Epinephrine)

The regulation of glucose homeostasis is also influenced by counter-regulatory hormones to insulin, a group of catabolic hormones, such as glucagon, adrenaline, growth hormone or cortisol [344, 345]. Secretion of these hormones increases between meals or during stress or aggression. As a whole, they decrease glucose uptake in insulin-sensitive tissues and stimulate hepatic glucose production.

Glucose metabolism is regulated by the balance between insulin and catabolic hormones [346].

First isolated and identified in 1895 by Polish physiologist Napoleon Cybulski, epinephrine was again discovered in 1897 by John Jacob Abel, and in 1900 by Jokichi Takamine and his assistant Keizo Uenaka, where mentioned scientists were not aware that it was the same hormone, and instead named it adrenaline [347, 348].

In 1901 Takamine successfully isolated and purified the hormone from the adrenal glands of sheep and oxen. Epinephrine was first synthesized by Friedrich Stolz and Henry Drysdale Dakin, independently, in 1904 [349].

Epinephrine is a hormone and neurotransmitter of the sympathetic nervous system [350]. Adrenaline participates in the "fight or flight" response of the sympathetic nervous system. It is a catecholamine, a sympathomimetic monoamine produced by the adrenal glands from the amino acids phenylalanine and tyrosine. Adrenaline is synthesized from noradrenaline in a synthetic pathway shared by all catecholamines.

It is synthesized via methylation of the distal amine of noradrenaline by phenylethanolamine N-methyltransferase (PNMT) in the cytosol of adrenergic neurons and cells of adrenal medulla (so-called chromaffin cells). It is released from the adrenal glands.

Epinephrine synthesis is solely under the control of the central nervous system. Sympathetic nervous system stimulates the synthesis of epinephrine precursors by enhancing the activity of enzymes involved in catecholamine synthesis. The sympathetic nervous system, acting via splanchnic nerves to the adrenal medulla, stimulates the release of epinephrine.

Adrenocorticotropic hormone (ACTH) also has an effect on norepinephrine synthesis. It stimulates the adrenal cortex to release cortisol, which increases the expression of PNMT in chromaffin cells, enhancing adrenaline synthesis. This is most often done in response to stress.

Renelase is a secreted amine oxidase that specifically degrades circulating catecholamines [350]. It is secreted into the blood by the kidney, and metabolizes circulating catecholamines [351]. The renalase protein has been very well conserved thought evolution, with orthologs not only in chimpanzee (95% amino acid identity) but also in Cyanobacteria (23% identity) [350]. It degrades catecholamines *in vitro* with a distinct substrate specificity.

Epinephrine's actions are mediated through adrenergic receptors. Adrenaline is receptor ligand to either α_1, α_2 or β-adrenergic receptors (β_1 and β_2 receptors). Adrenaline binds to α_1 receptors of liver cells, which activate inositol-phospholipids signaling pathway, signaling the phosphorylation of glycogen synthase and phosphorylase kinase (inactivating and activating them, respectively), leading to the later activation of another enzyme, glycogen phosphorylase, which catalyzes glycogenolysis (breakdown of glycogen) so as to release glucose to the bloodstream.

α_1–adrenergic receptors are the members of the G protein-coupled superfamily that plays an important role in the regulation of physiological responses mediated by epinephrine. There are 3 subtypes of human α_1 receptors (α_{1A}, α_{1B} and α_{1D}) [352, 353]. Adrenaline also binds to α_2 receptors. There are 3 highly homologous subtypes of α_2 receptors: α_{2A}, α_{2B} and α_{2C}. Specific actions of α_2 receptor include, for example, inhibition of insulin release in pancreas and induction of glucagon release from pancreas. Epinephrine also activates β-adrenergic receptors of the liver and muscle cells, thereby activating the adenylate cyclase signaling pathway, which will in turn increase glycogenolysis. Specific actions of the β_1 receptor include lipolysis in adipose tissue, and specific actions of the $\beta2$ receptor include, as for example, insulin release from pancreatic beta cells.

Carbohydrate metabolism is increased in human skeletal muscle with elevated adrenaline as a result of a twofold increase in glycogen utilization and increased flux through pyruvate dehydrogenase [354]. Pyruvate dehydrogenase regulates the entry of carbohydrate into oxidative pathway by catalyzing the decarboxylation of pyruvate to acetyl-CoA. Epinephrine increases pyruvate dehydrogenase activation and carbohydrate oxidation during moderate exercise. It also increases skeletal muscle glycogenolysis [354 – 356], because catecholamines can stimulate glucagon release [357]. Catecholamine infusions stimulate glucose production in human [358 - 360]. Epinephrine has been considered to inhibit insulin-mediated muscle glucose transport [361]. It inhibits insulin-mediated muscle glucose uptake [362]. Epinephrine attenuated glucose uptake by reducing the rate of glucose phosphorylation. Adrenaline also blocks insulin-stimulated insulin receptor substrate-1 (IRS-1)-associated phosphatidylinositol 3-kinase (PI 3-kinase) activity. It is possible that the reduction in insulin-stimulated glucose uptake by epinephrine is due to an attenuation in glucose transport rather than or in addition to the inhibition of glucose phosphorylation [361, 364]. Epinephrine has been shown to translocate GLUT 4 while increasing glucose transport in the absence of insulin, but to inhibit glucose transport in its presence [363]. On the other hand, epinephrine reduces insulin-stimulated GLUT 4 translocation to the plasma membrane. The results obtained by Mulder and colleagues [376] show that β-adrenergic stimulation inhibits insulin-induced glucose uptake in 3T3-L1 adipocytes, probably via the β_2- and β_3-adrenoceptor by interfering with GLUT 4 translocation (from intracellular compartment to the plasma membrane). Epinephrine can inhibit insulin-stimulated muscle glucose transport, but only when insulin is within a low to moderate physiological range [361]. The effect of catecholamines on glucose uptake during exercise appears to differ from their effects at rest, becoming stimulatory rather than inhibitory [365]. During moderate intensity exercise, adrenaline infusion increases glucose uptake and production [366]. Adrenaline does not appear to play a major role in matching hepatic glucose production to the increase in glucose clearance during exercise. On the other hand, adrenaline infusion results in a mismatch by simultaneously enhancing glucose production and inhibiting glucose clearance [367]. Catecholamines stimulate glucose uptake through phosphatidylinositol 3-kinase in the isolated rat heart [368]. This is in contrast to results obtained by addition of epinephrine *in vivo* [369]. The observed decrease in glucose uptake on catecholamine addition *in vivo* may be due to catecholamine effects on other metabolically active tissues [368].

The effects of cAMP on exocytosis are similar in α- and β-cells. It is important to emphasize that adrenergic stimulation has opposite effects on glucagon and insulin secretion. Adrenaline activates different signal pathways within the glucagon- and insulin-secreting cells. It potentates exocytosis in rat pancreatic α-cells by a mechanism involving activation of protein kinase A [370]. Adrenaline, via binding to β-receptors and stimulation of adenylate cyclase, accelerates exocytosis in the α-cells. It inhibits insulin secretion from isolated pancreatic β-cells [371]. The latter effect is mediated by α_2-receptors (α_{2A} and α_{2C}) [372] and culminates in the activation of the protein phosphatase calcineurin [373].

Adrenaline has been reported to induce glucose uptake in several cells other than vascular smooth muscle cells [374]. This is in contrast to results obtained by Kandaand Watanabe [375] that adrenaline increases glucose transport in rat vascular smooth muscle cells.

To summarize, adrenaline (epinephrine) plays an important role in glucose homeostasis.

Role of the Liver in the Carbohydrate Homeostasis

The liver plays a unique role in controlling carbohydrate metabolism and therefore plays a major role in blood glucose homeostasis by maintaining a balance between the uptake and storage of glucose via glycogenesis and the release of glucose via glycogenolysis and gluconeogenesis. Key enzymes in opposing metabolic pathways, glycolysis and glycogenesis, must be regulated in order for net flux in the appropriate direction to be achieved. Two enzymes specific for gluconeogenesis, phosphoenolpyruvate carboxykinase and fructose-1,6-bisphosphatase, are opposed by the glycolytic enzymes, pyruvate kinase and 6-phosphofructo-1-kinase. The glycogenolytic-specific enzyme glycogen phosphorylase is opposed by the glycogenic enzyme glycogen synthase [28]. The enzyme glucose-6-phosphatase is opposed by the glycolytic enzyme glucokinase [28, 385]. Hepatocytes express dozens of enzymes that are alternatively turned on or off depending on whether blood glucose levels are either rising or falling out of the normal rate.

In the post-absorptive state hepatic glucose production ensures a sufficient supply of glucose to the central nervous system and at the same time it regulates fasting plasma glucose concentrations. In the post-prandial period, the liver takes up a portion of ingested carbohydrates to restore glycogen stores [31]. The net glucose release is the result of two simultaneously ongoing pathways that are tightly regulated. Glycogenolysis occurs within 2 – 6 hours after a meal in humans, and gluconeogenesis has a greater importance with prolonged fasting [31].

The rate of gluconeogenesis is controlled principally by the activities of gluconeogenic enzymes. The genes of these enzymes are controlled at the transcriptional level by hormones, mainly insulin, glucagon and glucocorticoids. The interleukin-6 family of cytokines is also implicated in the regulation of these genes [31].

Hepatic glycogen metabolism is controlled by the coordination of two enzymes, glycogen synthase and glycogen phosphorylase, both of which are regulated by phosphorylation and allosteric modulation [377]. Although glucose and its metabolites can modulate their enzymatic activity and localization, two, above mentioned enzymes are principally regulated by phosphorylation.

The newborn mammals are in a transitional state of glucose homeostasis [378]. The fetus is dependent on the continuous provision of nutrients (in particular, glucose), by the maternal circulation via the placenta. The neonate is subject to a more variable and intermittent exogenous oral intake of nutrients in the form of a low-carbohydrate, high-fat milk diet. The transitional period of birth is a particularly sensitive time since the neonate must depend on the mobilization and oxidation of stored liver glycogen which is synthesized in the final days of gestation [378]. The initiation of hepatic glycogenolysis and gluconeogenesis in the first postnatal hours is critical for the maintenance of glucose homeostasis at this time [379]. Fetal life is characterized by chronic hyperinsulinemia which is an important condition for anabolic pathways of metabolism such as hepatic glycogen deposition. At birth hyperinsulinemia continues briefly and is one of the factors involved in the natural delay in hepatic glycogenolysis [380]. Counter-regulatory hormone (to insulin, such as glucagon, adrenaline, growth hormone) actions are vital for the reversal of the postnatal hypoglycemia and for establishing glucose homeostasis at this time. It has been assumed that glucagon, presumptively released in response to the postnatal hypoglycemia, is responsible for initiating glycogenolysis and switching on hepatic gluconeogenesis [379].

It has been suggested that catecholamine secretion at birth may be a critical event in establishing normal glucose homeostasis in the newborn [381, 382]. In contrast to the unresponsiveness of glycogenolysis to glucagon in hepatocytes, adrenalin is able to stimulate glycogen breakdown and increase hepatocytes glucose production[378]. The adrenaline-mediated effect on glycogenolysis in hepatocytes from newborn rats is due to a stimulus-response coupling via the β_2-adrenergic receptor, and this is in contrast to hepatocytes from adult rats which show a predominantly α-adrenoceptor-mediated glycogenolytic response [383].

At birth the mobilization of energy stores in the form of hepatic glycogen requires a decrease in plasma insulin levels, and follows the development of hypoglycemia due to continuing glucose utilization in the absence of glucose supply. Thehypoglycemia acts as a stimulus for catecholamine secretion which is then able to stimulate hepatic glycogenolysis unopposed by the previously high insulin levels at birth [378].

In the lactating rat there is an enhanced turnover of glucose imposed by the biosynthetic demands of the mammary gland and the liver in relation to the synthesis of milk constituents [384]. In the liver, the increased utilization of glucose is channeled towards fatty acid synthesis.

In summary, the control of glucose homeostasis by metabolic actions at the liver is under the influence of insulin. However, there is an essential and additional dependence on modulations of counter-regulatory hormonal responses to effectively control glucose homeostasis. The counter-regulatory hormones involved are different in two situations: catecholamines in hepatic glycogenolysis at birth and glucagon in hepatic lipogenesis during maternal lactation [378].

Shimazu and colleagues showed that autonomic nerves from the hypothalamus control glycogen metabolism in the liver [386, 387]. After receiving information from afferent nerves, the hypothalamus sends signals to peripheral organs, including the liver, to keep homeostasis. There are two ways for the hypothalamus to signal to the peripheral organs: by stimulating the autonomic nerves and by releasing hormones from the pituitary gland [388].

There are two types of neurons in the hypothalamus and the liver: efferent and afferent nerves. Efferent nerves consist of sympathetic and parasympathetic nerves. Efferent neural pathways from three major areas in the hypothalamus are involved in the autonomic regulation of the liver.

Stimulation of sympathetic nerve pathway causes glucose output from the liver through rapid activation of glycogen phosphorylase, the glycogenolytic enzyme, which results in hyperglycemia and a marked reduction of glycogen content in the liver [389, 390]. Stimulation of this pathway also causes an increase in the activity of phosphoenolpyruvate carboxykinase (a key gluconeogenic enzyme), and marked suppression of pyruvate kinase (a key glycolytic enzyme), of the liver [391].

Stimulation of parasympathetic nerve pathway leads to hepatic glycogen synthesis through activation of the enzyme, glycogen synthase (a key glycogenic enzyme) in the liver [390 – 392]. Stimulation of this pathway results in a decrease or complete inactivation of phosphoenolpyruvate carboxylase activity and pyruvate kinase activity [391]. Signals from parasympathetic nerves downregulate gluconeogenesis in the liver [388].

There are two afferent nerve pathways: vagal afferent nerve pathway and spinalafferent pathway. Vagal afferent nerves are function as sensor for circulating cytokines and metabolites such as glucose, amino acids, lipids etc [393 – 395]. Spinal afferent nerves are thought to transmit nociceptive information from the liver to the brain and contribute to the occurrence of pathological pain states such as inflammation and nerve injury [388].

The distribution of nerves in liver tissue is highly species-dependent. Among mammals, man has the highest density of intralobular nerves. These nerves contain classical neurotransmitters (adrenaline and acetylcholine) as well as neuropeptide (substance P, calcitonin gene-related peptide (CGPR), neuropeptide Y, vasoactive intestinal polypeptide (VIP), somatostatin, glucagon-like peptide etc) [388]. It has been reported that noradrenaline (norepinephrine) can affect glucose metabolism of hepatocytes via α_1-adrenergc receptors [396]. As to the function of acetylcholine, it has been reported that acetylcholine affects metabolic functions, including glucose production via type 3 muscarinic receptors [397].

Autonomic nerves can influence indirectly liver function via intervention of pancreas and adrenal gland. Sympathetic outflow from hypothalamus stimulates release of catecholamines (adrenaline and noradrenaline) from the medulla of the adrenal glands, release of the glucagon from α-cells in the pancreas and parasympathetic signals from hypothalamus stimulate the release of insulin from β-cells in the pancreas. These three hormones are intensively involved in the liver regulation of glucose homeostasis [388].

Role of the Hypothalamic-Pituitary Axis in the Carbohydrate Homeostasis

In 1849, Claud Bernard suggested that the central nervous system regulates blood glucose levels. In the early 1950s, it was first postulated that food intake is closely linked to the amount of stored energy (fat mass) in the body. In most humans, body weight remains stable for long periods of time, despite large fluctuations in food intake and physical activity because energy intake ad expenditure are matched through a neuroendocrine complex mechanism of energy homeostasis. Energy homeostasis is maintained by adapting meal size to current energy requirements. This control is achieved by communication between the digestive system and central nervous system. Generally, there are two systems that operate in the regulation of the quantity of food intake; short-term regulation, that is concerned primarily with preventing overeating at each meal, and long-term regulation, which is primarily related with the maintenance of normal quantities of energy stores in the form of fat in the body [248].

Several regions of the brain are involved in regulation of food intake and energy homeostasis. The hypothalamus is a brain region thought to play a critical role in the regulation of energy homeostasis. The hypothalamus is the most important locus involved in the neural control peripheral metabolism through the modulation of autonomic nervous system activity. The autonomic nervous system modulates hormone secretion (i.e. insulin and glucagon) and metabolic activity of several tissues and organs (i.e. liver, adipose tissue, and muscle). The hypothalamus is in turn informed of the energy status of the organism by several metabolic and hormonal signals establishing a feed back loop between the brain and periphery.

There are two ways for hypothalamus to signal to the peripheral organs: by stimulating the autonomic nerves and by releasing hormones from the pituitary gland. The hypothalamus consists of three major areas: lateral, medial, and paraventricular. Each are has some nuclei. Different experiments identified the lateral hypothalamus (LH) as an important region regulating the cessation of feeding [420] while the paraventricular nucleus of hypothalamus (PVN) was involved in the initiation of feeding [421]. In addition to direct neural connections, the hypothalamus can affect metabolic functions by neuroendocrine connections [388]. In the hypothalamus-pancreas axis, autonomic nerves release glucagon and insulin, which directly enter the liver and affect liver metabolism. In the hypothalamus-adrenal axis, autonomic nerves release catecholamines (adrenaline and noradrenaline) from the adrenal medulla, which also affects liver metabolism. In the hypothalamus-pituitary axis, release of glucocorticoids and thyroid hormones is stimulated by pituitary hormones. The hypothalamus-pituitary axis, which consists of neuroendocrine pathways from the hypothalamus, can also regulate liver functions. The hypothalamus sends signals to the pituitary gland, which release different hormones. Among them, three are thought to be intensely involved in the regulation of liver glucose metabolism [388].

The hypothalamic-pituitary-adrenal (HPA) axis referees to a complex set of homeostatic interactions between the hypothalamus, the pituitary gland, and the adrenal gland. The core of the HPA axis is the paraventricular nucleus of the hypothalamus. The PVN contains neurocrine neurons, which synthesize and secrete vasopressin (AVP) and corticotropin-releasing hormone (CRH). These two peptides can stimulate the secretion of the adrenocorticotropic hormone (ACTH) from anterior pituitary. In turn, ACTH enters peripheral circulation where is reaches the adrenal cortex to induce glucocorticoid hormones production (cortisol in humans, corticosterone in rodents). Glucocorticoids exert a negative feedback on the paraventricular nucleus of the hypothalamus and pituitary to suppress CRH and ACTH production, respectively.

ACTH is produced from a larger precursor namely the proopiomelanocortin protein, and stimulates the synthesis and release of cortisol by the adrenal cortex. In the circulation, cortisol is bound to corticosteroid-binding globulin with high affinity, facilitating transport of cortisol in blood, followed by conversion at the peripheral level by isoenzymes of 11 β-hydroxysteroid dehydrogenase types 1 and 2 [422 – 424].

Cortisol acts via two types of intracellular receptors, the mineralocorticoid receptor (MR) and glucocorticoid receptor (GR). MR and GR have different affinities to glucocorticoids with MR showing a greater affinity (10 fold higher) than GR. As a consequence, MR is fully occupied under basal circulating levels whereas GR becomes occupied only when glucocorticoids levels rise above normal. The GR initiates or represses gene transcription, and induces negative feedback of the hypothalamic-pituitary-adrenal axis through GR on the hypothalamus and pituitary level. The MR regulates basal activity of the hypothalamic-pituitary-adrenal axis.

Administration of glucocorticoids *in vivo* causes activation of glycogen synthase and inactivation of phosphorylase, resulting in glycogen synthesis [398]. Glucocorticoids lead to lipolysis in adipose tissue and proteolysis in skeletal muscle by inhibiting glucose uptake by these tissues, resulting in release of glycerol from adipose tissue and amino acids from muscles [399, 400, and 425]. In turn, glycerol and amino acids are used as substrates for the production of glucose in the liver [388]. Glucocorticoids stimulate hepatic gluconeogenesis and antagonize actions of insulin in liver and muscle, thus tending to increase glucose levels [28, 426, and 427]. The effect of glucocorticoids *in vivo* appears to include both impaired insulin-dependent glucose uptake in the periphery and enhanced gluconeogenesis in the liver [428, 429]. The expression of GLUT 4 (or Glut 4 in animals) is increased by glucocorticoids in skeletal muscle and adipose tissue [430 – 433]. Glucocorticoid actions in target tissues are determined not only by circulating hormone levels, but also by intracellular concentrations, which can be modulated by interconversion between active 11-hydroxylated steroids (cortisol in humans and corticosterone in rodents) and their inactive 11-keto forms [434, 435].

Increased lipolysis may be important in glucocorticoid-induced insulin resistance, since this is reversed by inhibiting lipolysis or lipid oxidation [436, 437]. Glucocorticoids inhibit insulin secretion from pancreatic β-cells [438, 439]. On the other hand, central actions of glucocorticoids may enhance vagal stimulation of insulin secretion [440]. According to Andrews and Walker [441], the balance of these effects may be important in determining whether insulin resistance is accompanied by compensatory hyperinsulinemia or hyperglycemia.

One mechanism by which hypothalamic peptides could influence energy efficiency (metabolic rate) independently of effects on food intake is by actions on the hypothalamo-pituitary-thyrotropic axis, which is an important regulator of metabolic rate in animals and humans [442]. Thyroid hormone is of critical importance to support protein synthesis and metabolic activity in peripheral tissues, but also for the regulation of thermogenesis.

Approximately 30% of resting energy expenditure is dependent upon thyroid hormone [443]. Maintenance of thyroid function is dependent on a complex interplay between the hypothalamus, anterior pituitary and thyroid gland (HPT) as well as other factors that influence the function of the HPT axis [444]. The thyroid gland is controlled by the activity of the hypothalamic-pituitary-thyroid axis. The hypothalamic peptide primarily responsible for regulating the HPT axis by stimulating the biosynthesis and release of thyrotropin (TSH) from the anterior pituitary gland pituitary gland is thyrotropin-releasing hormone (TRH) [445, 446].

TRH is a tripeptide widely expressed in the central nervous system [447]. Thyroid-releasing hormone released from hypophysiotropic neurons has two primary functions, including regulation of anterior pituitary thyroid stimulating hormone (TSH) and prolactin secretion [447, 448]. Indeed, thyrotropes and lactotropes comprise approximately 90% of the total cell population in the anterior pituitary that bind TRH [449]. TRH increases the synthesis and secretion of TSH from anterior pituitary that bind TRH [449] and is ultimately responsible for activation of the thyroid gland [447, 450].

Thyroid-stimulating hormone stimulates the release of thyroxine (T4) and triiodothyronine (T3) from the thyroid gland into the circulation [451]. The activity of the thyroid gland is regulated by a neuroendocrine negative feedback loop, in which thyroid hormone interacts with specific receptors on pituicytes to inhibit TSH secretion and at the hypothalamus to inhibit TRH secretion [446, 452 – 454]. Thyroid hormone causes a dose-related decrease in the TSH response to TRH [455]. The interactions along the hypothalamus-pituitary-thyroid axis maintain a stable amount of thyroid hormones in the circulation.

The thyroid gland synthesizes and releases thyroid hormones which have diverse physiologic effects including cardiac, pulmonary, hematopoietic, gastrointestinal, skeletal, neuromuscular, and endocrine effects. Thyroid hormone synthesis is mediated by an enzyme called thyroperoxidase (TPO) which mediates both the oxidation of iodine and their incorporation into tyrosyl residues on thyroglobulin. The thyroid gland produces two hormones, the prohormone thyroxine (T4) and the biologically active triiodothyronine (T3). The predominant T4 is converted to the biologically active T3 by specific deiodinases. Because 80% of serum T3 is derived from the deiodination of T4 in organs such as the liver and the kidney, and as the thyroid hormone receptor preferentially recognizes T3, T4 is considered a prohormone [456]. More than 99% of T4 and T3 circulate bound to transport protein. Less than 1& amount of thyroid hormone is unbound or free. Once T4 and T3 are released into the circulation, they are bound by 3 important plasma protein: thyroxine binding globulin (TBG), transthyretin (thyroxine binding prealbumin), and albumin. It is generally accepted that only the free (unbound) fraction is able to bind to specific thyroid hormone receptors in peripheral tissues and possesses biologic activity. Normally, approximately 0,03% of T4 and 0,5% of T3 is free [457]. Most of the biologic activity of thyroid hormones is due to the cellular effects of T3, which has a greater affinity for the thyroid hormone receptor and is approximately 4 – 10 times more potent than T4 [455, 458]. Free thyroid hormone is transported through the cell membrane by specific carriers and binds to the thyroid receptors in the nucleus. After the coupling of T3 to nuclear receptors, the transcriptionally active complex binds to thyroid-hormone responsive elements and thus increases gene expression (DNA transcription), accordingly synthesis of mRNA and proteins [459].

Thyroid receptor belongs to the nuclear receptor superfamily that also induces the receptors for lipophilic signaling molecule that includes steroid hormone, vitamin derivatives such as retinoic acid and vitamin D_3, fatty acids and cholesterol metabolites and xenobiotics [460]. Two thyroid hormone receptor gene, designated alpha and beta, have been identified, and although both receptors are highly homologous, they are encoded by genes on separate chromosomes and have different affinity for T3 [461, 462]. Two mRNA splice variants have been identified for each gene: TR-α1, TR-α2, TR-β1 and TR-β2. Because TR-α2 does not bind T3, there are three functional TRs [461, 463]. Whereas pituitary, liver, and kidney express high concentrations of thyroid hormone nuclear receptors, spleen and gonads exhibit low levels.

Thyroid hormones directly affect basal metabolic rate, appetite and body weight. In hyperthyroidism, body weight is often decreased, and basal metabolic rate and thermogenesis are increased and vice versa for hypothyroidism. The mechanisms responsible for the production of the physiological effect of thyroid hormones on weight and energy homeostasis are complex and have not yet been fully elucidated [464].

TH action has been long recognized as a significant determinant of glucose homeostasis [401 – 405]. A number of authors have speculated on a plausible interaction between insulin and TSH regulatory mechanisms [465, 467]. Available evidence suggests that glucose homeostasis appears to be the result of the T3 and insulin synergistic regulation of gene transcription involved metabolic pathways of glucose and lipids [468, 469]. T3 regulates a wide range of gene expression of glucose transporters, which include all of the regulatory enzymes essential for oxidation of glucose and lipids, glucose storage, glycolysis, cholesterol synthesis, cholesterol transfer, and glucose-lipid metabolism [470]. It is known that TH can stimulate the expression and activate a number of proteins that are candidates for regulating insulin sensitivity [471, 472]. A functional TH response element in the promoter region of GLUT 4 gene, which contributes to impaired insulin-stimulated glucose disposal, has been described [467]. Other authors have shown that Glut 4 expression in rats is under TH control [473]. The studies have demonstrated that T3 directly stimulates basal and insulin-mediated glucose uptake in rat skeletal muscle [474 – 476]. The mechanism for this induction was shown to be due primarily to an increase in Glut 4 protein expression [474]. Weinstein and colleagues demonstrated that Glut 4 protein and mRNA were coordinately regulated by T3 in rat skeletal muscle [476]. According to results obtained by Torrance and colleagues [473] *Slc2a4* gene expression in the rat is stimulated via transcriptional induction in red muscle, and a separate translational/posttranslational mechanism in white skeletal muscle. These studies also demonstrated the ability of T3 to stimulate *Slc2a4* gene expression in insulin-resistant skeletal muscle, and that T3 had a marked beneficial effect on hyperinsulinemia, but not glycemia in obese Zucker rats [473]. There is a strong indication that T3 regulates insulin secretion via transcription of glucokinase and ATP-sensing K^+ and Ca^{2+} channels of the pancreas [469]. Thyroid hormone modulates glucose production via a sympathetic pathway from the hypothalamus to the liver [477].

The association between thyroid disease and changes in glucose homeostasis is well described [478]. Several investigators have shown that hyperthyroidism results in an unopposed activation of gluconeogenesis. Gluconeogenesis from glycerol was decreased by 63% in hypothyroid rats and increased by 35% in several hyperthyroid rats [479]. Thyrotoxicosis is associated with an increase in endogenous glucose production, hepatic insulin resistance, and concomitant hyperglycemia [480, 481]. In obese males, insulin resistance is significantly related with impairment of thyroid function [482]. For more details see Chapter 4.

Human growth hormone (GH) is a 191 amino acid peptide, which is secreted from the pituitary gland [483, 484]. In the circulation various molecular forms of GH exist. About 50% of circulating growth hormone is bound to binding proteins. These include a high affinity growth hormone binding protein (GHBP) which actually represents the extracellular portion of the GH receptor [485, 486]. Circulating GH levels, both in the basal state and after provocative stimuli, are higher in females than in males [487]. Circulating GH levels are higher in adolescent than in prepubertal children and young adults [488]. The secretion of GH is maximal during puberty [489].

Secretion of GH from the pituitary somatotroph is controlled by at least one stimulatory and one inhibitory factor released from the hypothalamus into the hypothalamic-hypophyseal portal venous system. The production and release of the peptide GH by somatotrophs of the anterior pituitary is stimulated by growth hormone-releasing hormone ((GHRH), also known as growth hormone releasing factor (GRF), binding to specific receptors that utilize increased cAMP as a second messenger; the GHRH receptor activates the adenylate cyclase-cAMP system [492]. Under GHRH stimulation pituitary GH production is enhanced. It has been demonstrated *in vitro* that GHRH stimulates not only GH secretion but also transcription of the GH gene [493]. Another important hormone in this system is somatostatin (growth hormone release-inhibiting hormone or growth hormone-inhibiting hormone (GHIH)). Hypothalamic somatostatin, produced by the paraventricular nucleus, arrives at the pituitary through the portal system, where it activates somatostatin receptors. Somatostatin then inhibits GH secretion. The stimulatory effect of GHRH on GH can be inhibited by somatostatin decreasing cAMP levels upon receptor binding [490]. Growth hormone release is determined by a dynamic equilibrium between the inhibitory and stimulatory hypothalamic peptides, somatostatin and growth hormone-releasing hormone. The hypothalamic release of GHRH and somatostatin is, in turn, controlled through a complex network of neurotransmitters, and the hypothalamo-pituitary response may be influenced by age, sex, GH feedback, insulin, thyroid and steroid hormones and nutritional status [491].

Once pituitary GH has been synthesized and released, a key target for this hormone is the liver, which produces insulin-like growth factor-I (IGF-I), a chemical that carries out many of the actions of GH (e.g. protein formation and cell growth) at the tissue level. IGF-I is critical for promoting the protein anabolic effects of GH [494]. IGF-I also feeds back at the hypothalamus and the pituitary to reduce GH synthesis and secretion [495]. Most of GH promoting effects are mediated by IGF-I. GH also has effects independent of IGF-I. Although GH and IGF-I exert opposite effects on glucose metabolism, the precise role of these hormones in controlling normal glucose homeostasis is unknown [49].

The growth hormone receptor (GHR) belongs to class I of the hematopoietin superfamily of cytokine receptors, which includes more than 30 members, among others prolactin, erythropoietin, leptin, granulocyte stimulating factor, IL-2, IL-3, and IL-6 [497]. GHRs have been identified in many tissues and organs including muscle, adipose tissue, liver, kidney, brain, and the pancreas [498].

The intracellular GH signaling cascade is complex and not fully understood [499]. Activation of receptor-associated Janus kinase 2 (JAK2) is considered the critical step in initiating GH signaling [499]. Phosphorylated residues on GHR and JAK2 form docking sites for different signaling molecules including STAT1, STAT3, STAT5a, STAT5b, the MAPK pathway and the PI3-kinase pathway [500]. Down-regulation or attenuation of JAK2-associated GH signaling is mediated by a family of cytokine-inducible suppressors of cytokine signaling (SOCS), of which there are eight members: SOCS1 – SOCS7, and the cytokine-inducible SH2-domain-containing domain [501].

Growth hormone is an essential regulator of carbohydrate and lipid metabolism, participating in glucose uptake and usage, accelerating fat expenditure, preventing triglyceride accumulation, and facilitating lipid mobilization in adipose tissues. Growth hormone, released from pituitary gland, increases indirectly the production of glucose in the liver. It increases the sensitivity of the adipocytes to the lipolytic action of the catecholamines [406] and decreases its sensitivity to the lipogenic action of insulin [407]. Glycerol released into the blood acts as a substrate for gluconeogenesis in the liver. Growth hormone plays a significant role in protein synthesis and antagonizes insulin action. Acknowledging that GH decreases glucose oxidation and muscle glucose uptake in the presence of unchanged endogenous glucose production and plasma glucose concentration implies that GH must promote nonoxidative glucose utilization in some nonmuscle compartment of the body [499]. In both healthy subjects and those with type 1 diabetes, a pulse of GH increases fasting hepatic glucose output, by increasing hepatic gluconeogenesis and glycogenolysis, and decreases peripheral glucose utilization through the inhibition of glycogen synthesis and glucose oxidation [503 – 506]. GH stimulates lipolysis with the release of glycerol and non-esterified fatty acids. This provides a further mechanism for the diabetogenic properties of growth hormone through the effect of non-esterified fatty acids to increase hepatic glucose output and decrease peripheral glucose oxidation according to the glucose-fatty acid cycle [507, 508]. GH possesses direct and indirect, via IGF-I and insulin, protein anabolic effect. According to Møller and colleagues [502], "During conditions of energy excess GH, together with IGF-I and insulin, promotes nitrogen retention and when food is sparse, GH diverts fuel consumption from the use of carbohydrates and protein to the use of lipids, thereby allowing conservation of vital protein stores".

In animal diabetes, there is a decrease in the gene expression of the hypothalamic somatostatin and GHRH as well as the pituitary GH and GHR [509]. The circulating levels of growth hormone are suppressed [510, 511]. In humans, poorly controlled type 1 diabetes is associated with high plasma levels of GH [512]. Growth hormone concentrations are up to two to three times higher in individuals with diabetes compared with healthy subjects [513]. The coexistence of hyperglycemia, which should suppress the release of GH, and elevated GH levels suggests an abnormality of GH regulation in diabetes mellitus [514]. For details see Chapter 4.

The hypothalamus plays a central role in the hormonal regulation of the female and male reproductive system. The main regulatory factor of reproductive functions is gonadotropin releasing hormone (GnRH), a decapeptide secreted by the ventral medial nucleus of the hypothalamus. Production and further release of GnRH to the portal pituitary system are induced and controlled through stimuli received from other regions of the brain via mediators of different origins [550].

Gonadotropin releasing hormone is a primary stimulator of luteinizing hormone (LH) and follicle-stimulating hormone (FSH) release. LH and FSH control the production of the sex hormones. Synthesis and release of LH and FSH are suppressed by estrogen and testosterone. Progesterone has inhibitory direct effects on GnRH neurons. The effects of LH and FSH depend on sex. In women LH stimulates ovarian follicular development and ovulation. It stimulates the now-empty follicle to develop into the corpus luteum, which secretes progesterone during the latter half of the menstrual cycle. In men, LH acts on the interstitial cells (also known as Leydig cells) of the testes stimulating them to synthesize and secrete the male sex hormone, testosterone.

In women, FSH acts on the follicle to stimulate it to release estrogens. In men, FSH acts on Sertoli cells and on spermatogonia stimulating (with the aid of testosterone) the production of sperm.

Estrogens secreted by ovary, are hormones to be considered in blood glucose homeostasis. Evidence that high 17 β-estradiol concentrations are detrimental for blood glucose homeostasis has existed for a long time. Clinical administration of estrogens has long had a poor reputation with regard to carbohydrate metabolism [551]. This dates back to the 1960s, when glucose tolerance was seen to detoriate in women on high-estrogen oral contraceptives [552], some of whom developed a reduced early insulin response to glucose and diabetic plasma glucose levels [553]. There is a persistent perception that estrogens have an adverse effect on carbohydrate metabolism.

The effect of estrogens on the pancreas was originally examined in the search for agents that might be effective in treating diabetes. Early work showed that administration of estrogens increased the insulin content of the pancreas in rats [554]. Houssay and colleagues used a partially pancreatectomised rat model to show that administration of various estrogens was associated with hypertrophy and regeneration of the islets [555]. Receptor binding for estrogen is present in islets [556] and direct effects on insulin secretion have been reported [557]. Estrogen receptor in β-cell has a crucial role in increasing proinsulin biosynthesis in response to physiological concentrations of estrogens. This may be an important mechanism for the islet of Langerhans to adapt to a high demand of insulin during pregnancy. During pregnancy, estrogen receptor integrates information from estrogen, glucose and other nutrients in the blood to regulate insulin gene expression and, therefore, contributes to the maintenance of insulin and glucose homeostasis [562]. There is evidence of a positive correlation between the control of glycemia and the menstrual cycle in diabetic women. Irregulaties, most frequently amenorrhoea and oligoamenorrhoea [558] are expected only in the first 2 years following menarche in healthy, non-diabetic adolescent [559], but are present in about 20 – 30% of diabetic patients [560, 561].

Shi and Simpkins demonstrated that estrogen increased expression of glucose transporter subunits and increased glucose transport in blood brain barrier endothelium [563]. In the non-human primates, estrogen treatment induced two- to fourfold increases in Glut 3 and Glut 4 mRNA and protein [564]. Analysis of cellular localization indicated that estrogen-induced a marked rise in neuronal Glut 1 mRNA levels with no appreciable effect on vascular Glut 1 gene expression [565]. In cellular energetics, estrogen induced two-fold increases in key enzymes required for glycolysis; increased expression of the pyruvate dehydrogenase, increased activity of glycolytic enzymes – hexokinase, phosphofructokinase and phosphoglycerate kinase in rodent brain [566]. Estrogen increased expression and activity of protein required for oxidative phosphorylation electron transfer, a result that was consistent with a coordinated response that optimizes glucose metabolism in brain [567].

The effect of estrogens on glucagon secretion and action has received little attention in humans [551]. In animals, glucagon-induced hyperglycemia was diminished by estrogen [568].

Association between hyperandrogenism and insulin resistance is well recognized in women with polycystic ovary syndrome [569]. On the other hand, more recent studies demonstrated that antiandrogen treatment does not alter insulin resistance in polycystic ovary syndrome [570 – 572].

Androgens can influence body composition, which is associated with insulin sensitivity. It is conceivable that testosterone might indirectly influence insulin sensitivity via its effects on body composition. According to Volpi and colleagues [573], testosterone may affect insulin sensitivity both directly and indirectly, through changes in body composition. Yialamas and colleagues suggested that testosterone modulates insulin sensitivity directly and this pathway is not mediated by changes in body composition. Patients treated with androgen deprivation therapy had elevated glucose and increased insulin resistance, as measured by HOMA index levels; these findings were independent of age, and BMI [575]. Testosterone treatment in hypogonadal men reduces fasting insulin and insulin resistance by HOMA. Increased insulin sensitivity is negatively and significantly correlated with baseline testosterone levels [576, 577]. Apart from testosterone's effect on insulin sensitivity, it may have a direct effect of the pancreas and the β-cell [578]. Early apoptotic damage induced by streptozotocin in castrated animals was reversed by testosterone replacement, suggesting a protective effect on the pancreas. For further details see [579]. Testosterone activates the glucose metabolism-related signaling pathway in skeletal muscle. The addition of testosterone to cultured skeletal muscle induced the elevation of GLUT 4 protein expression and also accelerates its translocation from cytosol to the plasma membrane. The addition of testosterone to cultured skeletal muscle enhanced both Akt and PKC-ζ/λ phosphorylations, which have critical roles in GLUT 4-regulated signaling pathways. Moreover, the main glycolytic enzyme (hexokinase and phosphofructokinase) activities were enhanced with the addition of testosterone to skeletal muscle [580]. Testosterone improves fasting insulin sensitivity in men with chronic heart failure [581].

Androgens have been shown to regulate lipolysis and lipogenesis in the adipose cells of women. The study has demonstrated that testosterone induces selective insulin resistance in cultured subcutaneous adipocytes of women. Chronic testosterone treatment significantly impaired insulin action on glucose metabolism, as assessed by glucose uptake. The testosterone-induced defect in glucose transport was associated with impaired insulin-stimulated phosphorylation of PKC-ζ [582], a PKC isoform downstream of PI3-kinase, which mediates the effects of insulin on glucose transport in human adipocytes [583].

At present the mechanism by which androgens influence the insulin-glucose axis is uncertain [581]. There is considerable evidence that body composition governs insulin sensitivity and that excess visceral fat may induce insulin resistance by flooding hepatic metabolism with fatty acids leading to hepatic and systemic insulin resistance. On the other hand, testosterone has well documented effects on body metabolism including an increase in lean mass and a reduction in fat mass [584].

Renal Gluconeogenesis

Studies conducted over the last 70 years in animals and *in vitro* have provided considerable evidence that the mammalian kidney can make glucose and release under various conditions. Gluconeogenesis involves the formation of glucose-6-phosphate from precursors such as lactate, glycerol, and amino acids with its subsequent hydrolysis by glucose-6-phosphatase to free glucose. Liver and skeletal muscles contain most of the body's glycogen stores. However, because only the liver contains glucose-6-phosphatase, the breakdown of muscle glycogen leads to the release of lactate. This lactate and the lactate generated via glycolysis of glucose can be absorbed by gluconeogenic organs and re-formed into glucose [408]. Only two organs in human body, the liver and the kidney, possess sufficient gluconeogenic enzyme activity and glucose-6-phosphatase activity to enable them to release glucose into the circulation as a result of gluconeogenesis.

The kidney can be considered two separate organs because glucose utilization occurs predominantly in the renal medulla, whereas glucose release is confined to the renal cortex [409, 410]. The cells in the renal medulla have appreciable glucose-phosphorylating and glycolytic enzyme activity and they are obligate users of glucose [411]. They can take up, phosphorylate, glycolyse, and accumulate; they cannot release free glucose into the circulation [409, 410]. Cells in the renal cortex possess gluconeogenic enzymes, and thus they can make and release glucose into the circulation [408].

The main precursor for renal gluconeogenesis is lactate, followed by glutamine, alanine and glycerol [408]. Lactate accounted for approximately 50% of renal gluconeogenesis. It can be calculated that renal glucose release from lactate is equivalent to 50% of overall lactate conversion to glucose [408]. These data underline the major role of the kidneys in the Cori cycle. One-half of glucose production within the Cori cycle actually takes place in the kidney [412]. The largest study indicated that lactate was the most important renal gluconeogenic substrate, followed by glutamine and glycerol [413]. Renal conversion to glucose of these precursors accounted for ~ 50, 70, and 35% respectively, of their overall systemic gluconeogenesis [408]. It appears that glutamine is a preferential gluconeogenic substrate for the kidney, whereas alanine is preferentially used by the liver [414].

Insulin, growth hormone, cortisol, and catecholamines influence renal glucose release. Cersosime and colleagues showed that insulin suppressed renal glucose release while stimulating renal glucose uptake [415]. The other results showed that during a 180-min insulin infusion, a rapid suppression of endogenous glucose production was observed. Such an early decrease of endogenous glucose release was due to the simultaneous inhibition of liver glycogenolysis and renal gluconeogenesis. It was observed that the net renal uptake of lactate decreased earlier than the splenchnic uptake of lactate and alanine, and that both renal and splenchnic glycerol uptake decreased after 90 min of insulin infusion [416]. It can be deduced from these studies that renal gluconeogenesis is more sensitive to insulin than liver gluconeogenesis.

Mc Guinness and colleagues demonstrated that an infusion with glucagon increased renal glucose release in dogs [417]. On the other hand, glucagon was shown to increase systemic and hepatic glucose release but to have no effect on renal glucose release [418]. This effect of glucagon on glucose production was mainly attributed to an increase of liver gluconeogenesis from glutamine. During the infusion of glucagon, renal glucose production from glutamine was unaffected.

Epinephrine infusion was conversely shown to induce a greater than twofold increase in renal glucose production, and to stimulate overall glutamine and alanine incorporation into glucose [419] and increased renal glucose release in dogs [417].The stimulation of systemic glucose production from glutamine was mainly related to renal gluconeogenesis (90% of total glutamine gluconeogenesis). The stimulation of renal gluconeogenesis during the epinephrine infusion may involve free fatty acids [412].

It was demonstrated that an infusion with cortisol increased renal glucose release in dogs [417]. Data in humans are limited to the effects of insulin, glucagon and epinephrine [408].

Based on available evidence, it would appear likely that the release of glucose by the kidney may play a significant role in the regulation of glucose homeostasis. The reappraisal of renal gluconeogenesis together with studies on gluconeogenic substrates provided evidence for a key role of the kidney in interorgan glucose metabolism, and particularly in the Cori cycle and in gluconeogenesis from glutamine. These findings may help the understanding of abnormal glucose homeostasis during chronic renal failure [412].

The Role of Microvasculature in the Regulation and in the Mediation of Insulin

An exact definition of the microcirculation is elusive. Morphologically, the microcirculation is widely taken to encompass vessels < 100 μm in diameter. It therefore includes arterioles, capillaries, and venules [515]. Nowadays, a definition based on arterial vessel physiology rather than diameter or structure has been proposed, depending on the response of isolated vessel to increased internal pressure. By this definition, all vessels that respond to increasing pressure by a myogenic reduction in lumen diameter would be considered of the microcirculation [516]. A primary function of the microcirculation is to optimize the delivery of nutrients and removal of waste products from all cells of the body in response to variations in demand [517]. A second important function is to avoid large fluctuations in hydrostatic pressure at the level of the capillaries that otherwise would impair capillary exchange [516].

DeFronzo and colleagues [518] studied the relationship between exercise and insulin on muscle glucose uptake and suggested that the synergism was the result of increased blood flow and increased capillary surface area for enhanced insulin delivery to exercising muscle. However, Baron and colleagues must be given credit for being the first to show an independent action of insulin to increase limb blood flow that hat the potential to increase capillary recruitment. Baron and colleagues [519 – 521] pioneered concept that insulin acts as a vasodilator and can thereby control access of glucose as well as insulin to skeletal muscle and fat. Indeed, they showed a remarkable correlation between the effect of insulin on whole body glucose uptake and the effect of insulin on leg blood flow over a broad range of insulin sensitivities in normal and insulin-resistant states [522 – 524]. Insulin enhances both skeletal muscle glucose disposal and total leg blood flow in a time- and dose-dependent fashion [521, 525]. However, the observations that in most, but not all, studies insulin-induced increases in total muscle blood flow temporally lag significantly behind the stimulation of muscle glucose uptake [525] and that this flow effect requires relatively high insulin concentrations have led to controversy regarding physiological significance of insulin-induced flow increases [525 – 527]. Zhang and colleagues reported [528] that insulin exerts two vascular actions in muscle; it both increases blood flow and recruits capillaries. Authors conclude that the precapillary arterioles that regulate microvascular recruitment are more sensitive than resistance arterioles that regulate total flow. Other reported that insulin recruits microvascular vessels in skeletal muscle separate from any effect on total flow [529] and have suggested that insulin's microvascular action contributes to its overall effect on nutrient and hormone delivery to muscle [530].

Early studies using the perfused rat hindlimb showed that increasing glucose delivery with or without insulin raises glucose uptake [531, 532]. It was demonstrated that increasing glucose concentration within the physiological range increased glucose uptake in a linear fashion. On the other hand, with a constant glucose level the relationship between flow and glucose uptake was hyperbolic [531]. Grubb and Snarr [531] proposed that this saturation of glucose uptake might be due to flow being shunted into a parallel network with low nutrient exchange.

Concentration-dependent increases in total limb blood flow in response to intravenous insulin infusion spanning the physiological to pharmacological range is well documented in humans and animals [535, 536]. Studies in cultured human umbilical vein endothelial cells (HUVEC) also demonstrate that insulin increasesL-arginine transport [533] and stimulate the production of nitric oxide (NO) [534]. Insulin infusion at physiological concentrations under euglycemic glucose-clamp conditions causes a dose-dependent doubling in skeletal blood flow that is NO dependent [537, 538]. Vasodilation leading to increased blood flow is a major physiological consequence of insulin stimulated production of NO in vascular endothelium. However, within muscle, nitric oxide synthase (NOS) is present in both myocytes (µNOS, a variant of the neuronal NOS (nNOS) isoform) [539, 540] and endothelium (eNOS) [541], and the locus of the NO production that mediates insulin-dependent increases of total blood flow and glucose uptake is unknown [542]. Summarizing, the effects of insulin on both capillary recruitment [543], and larger resistance vessels that regulated total blood flow to muscle [538] are the result of insulin-induced nitric oxide-dependent relaxation process.

The metabolic action of insulin to stimulate glucose uptake in skeletal muscle and adipose tissue is mediated through stimulation of PI3-kinase-dependent signaling pathways. The vasodilator actions of insulin require highly parallel PI3-kinase-dependent insulin-signaling pathways. In addition to its vasodilator actions, insulin also has vasoconstrictor effects. These vasoconstrictor effects are mainly mediated by the vasoconstrictor peptide endothelin-1 (ET-1) [544]. ET-1 is produced in the vascular endothelium through stimulation of the intracellular MAP-kinase signaling pathway and the extracellular signal-regulated kinase-1/2 (ERK1/2). The PI3-kinase pathways are not involved. According to Jonk and colleagues [516], insulin has opposing endothelial-derived vasodilating and vasoconstrictor effect, with the net effect being dependent on the balance between these two. Normally, the net result is either neutral or vasodilatory.

It is now recognized that the endothelium plays an important role in the regulation of vessel permeability and proliferation as well as blood fluidity and the adhesion of blood cells to the vascular wall. Therefore, a range of complications can potentially result from a dysfunctional endothelium. This is a consequence, because it is also believed that endothelial dysfunction plays a key role in the development of the microvascular complications of type 2 diabetes, which include retinopathy, nephropathy, and neuropathy. Endothelial dysfunction is also central to the macrovascular complications of atherosclerosis and thrombosis, which lead to coronary artery, cerebrovascular, and peripheral vascular disease [545, 548]. Abnormalities in vascular reactivity in micro- and macrocirculation are well established in type 2 diabetes. However, little is known about changes in vascular reactivity in those at risk for developing type 2 diabetes [546]. Insulin's action to increased microvascular perfusion (capillary recruitment) of muscle is impaired in insulin resistance and reflects early-onset vascular dysfunction and results in diminished delivery of glucose. In addition, insulin resistance is characterized by blood flow being carried predominantly by nonnutritive vessels in connective tissue where intrafibriller adipocytes can grow [547]. It is widely accepted that endothelial dysfunction precedes and may cause diabetic microangiopathy in type 1 diabetes mellitus receiving standard insulin therapy. Endothelial dysfunction and early structural atherosclerotic changes are common manifestations in type 1 diabetes mellitus, and endothelial dysfunction is thought to be an early event in the atherosclerotic process and important in the pathogenesis of microvascular complications [549].

REFERENCES

[1]   DeFronzo RA. The triumvirate: beta cell, muscle, liver; a conclusion responsible for NIDDM. Diabetes 1988;37:667-684
[2]   Berculin R, Cani PD, Knauf C. Glucagon-like peptide-1 and energy homeostasis. J Nutr 2007;137:2534S-2538S
[3]   Drucker DJ. The role of gut hormones in glucose homeostasis. J Clin Invest 2007;117:1:24-30
[4]   SAD, Datta SP, Smith GH, Campbell PN, Bentley R, McKenzie HA. Oxford dictionary of biochemistry and molecular biology. Oxford University Press, Oxford; 1997:740 p
[5]   Gerich JE. Control of glycemia. Bailliers Best Pract Res Clin Endocrinol Metab 1993;7:551-586
[6]   Aronoff SL, Berkowitz K, Shreiner B, Want L. Glucose metabolism and regulation: beyond insulin and glucagon. Diabetes Spectrum 2004;17,3:183-190
[7]   Cryer PE. Glucose homeostasis and hypoglycemia. In William's Textbook of Endocrinology. Wilson JD, Foster DW, Eds. Philadelphia, Pa., W.B. Saunder Company, 1992; 1223-1253
[8]   Henquin J-C, Ishiyama N, Nenquin M, Ravier MA, Jonas J-C. Signals and pools underlying biphasic insulin secretion. Diabetes 2002;51,Suppl.1:S60-S67
[9]   Straub SG, Sharp GWG. Glucose-stimulated signaling pathways in biphasic insulin secretion. Diabetes Metab Res Rev 2002;18:451-463
[10]   Rorsman P. Insulin secretion: function and therapy of pancreatic beta-cells in diabetes. Br J Diabetes Vasc Dis 2005;5:187-191
[11]   Bertram R, Pernarowski M. Glucose diffusion in pancreatic islets of Langerhans. Biophys J 1998;74:1722-1731
[12]   Maechler P, Wollheim CB. Mitochondrial signals in glucose-stimulated insulin secretion in the beta cell. J Physiol 2000;529,1:49-56
[13]   Nichols CG. K_{ATP} channels as molecular sensor of cellular metabolism. Nature 2006;440:470-476
[14]   Rorsman P. The pancreatic beta-cell as a fuel sensor: an electro-physiologist's viewpoint. Diabetologia 1997;40:487-495
[15]   Kennedy ED, Rizzuto R, Theler JM, *et al.* Glucose-stimulated insulin secretion correlates with changes in mitochondrial and cytosolic Ca^{2+} in aequorin-expressing INS-1 cells. J Clin Invest 1996;98:2524-2538
[16]   Bernard C. Leçons de physiologie expérimentale appliquée à la médecine faites au Collège de France. Baillère et Fils. Paris, France. 1855:296-313
[17]   Puglianiello A, Cianfarani S. Central control of glucose homeostasis. Rev Diabetic Stud 2006;3:54-60
[18]   Sindelar DK, Chu CA, Venson P, Donahue EP, Neal DW, Cherrington AD. Basal hepatic glucose production is regulated by the portal vein insulin concentration. Diabetes 1998;47,4:523-529
[19]   Boden G, Chen X, Ruiz J, White JV, Rossetti L. Mechanisms of fatty acids induced inhibition of glucose uptake. J Clin Invest 1994;93:438-446
[20]   Rulifson EJ, Kim SK, Nusse R. Ablation of insulin-producing neurons in flies: growth and diabetic phenotypes. Science 2002;296:1118-1120
[21]   Wolkow CA, Kimura KD, Lee MS, Ruvkun G. Regulation of C. elegans life-span by insulinlike signaling in the nervous system. Science 2000;290:147-150
[22]   Obici S, Zhang BB, Karkanias G, Rossetti L. Hypothalamic insulin signaling is required for inhibition of glucose production. Nat Med 2002;8:1376-1382
[23]   Pocai A, Lam TK, Gutierrez-Juarez R, *et al.* Hypothalamic $K_{(ATP)}$ channels control hepatic glucose production. Nature 2005;434:102-1031
[24]   Plum L, Belgardt BF, Brüning JC. Central insulin action in energy and glucose homeostasis. J Clin Invest 2006;116,7:1761-1766
[25]   Margolis RU, Altszuler N. Insulin in the cerebrospinal fluid. Nature 1967; 215:1375-1376
[26]   Havrankova J, Roth J, Brownstein M. Insulin receptors are widely distributed in the central nervous system of the rat. Nature 1987;272:827-829
[27]   Inoue H, Ogawa W, Asakawa A, *et al.* Role of hepatic STAT3 in brain-insulin action on hepatic glucose production. Cell Metab 2006;3,4:267-275
[28]   Nordlie RC, Foster JD, Lange AJ. Regulation of glucose production by the liver. Annu Rev Nutr 1999;19:379-406

[29] Saltiel AR, Kahn CR. Insulin signalling and the regulation of glucose and lipid metabolism. Nature 2001;414:799-806

[30] Barthel A, Schmoll D. Novel concepts in insulin regulation of hepatic gluconeogenesis. Am J Physiol Endocrinol Metab 2003;285:E685-E692

[31] Postic C, Dentin R, Girard J. Role of the liver in the control of carbohydrate and lipid homeostasis. Diabetes Metab 2004;30:398-408

[32] Wu C, Okar DA, Kang J, Lange AJ. Reduction of hepatic glucose production as a therapeutic target in treatment of diabetes. Curr Drug Targ Immune Endocrine Metab Disord 2005;5:51-59

[33] O'Brien RM, Granner DK. Regulation of gene expression by insulin. Physiol Rev 1996;76:1109-1161

[34] O'Brien RM, Lucas PC, Rorest CD, Magnuson MA, Granner DK. Identification of a sequence in the PEPCK gene that mediates a negative effect of insulin on transcription. Science 1990;249:533-537

[35] O'Brien RM, Streeper RS, Ayala JE, Stadelmaier BT, Hornbuckle LA. Insulin-regulated gene expression. Biochem Soc Trans 2001;29:552-558

[36] Taniguchi CM, Emanuelli B, Kahn CR. Critical nodes in signalling pathways: insights into insulin action. Nat Rev Mol Cell Biol 2006;7:85-96

[37] Fritsche L, Weigrt C, Häring H-U, Lehman R. How insulin receptor substrate proteins regulate the metabolic capacity of the liver-implications for health and disease. Curr Med Chem 2008;15:1316-1329

[38] Kubota N, Tobe K, Terauchi Y, *et al.* Disruption of insulin substrate 2 causes type 2 diabetes because of liver insulin resistance and lack of compensatory beta-cell hyperplasia. Diabetes 2000;49:1880-1889

[39] Lizcano JM, Alessi DR. The insulin signalling pathway. Curr Biol 2002;12:R236-R238

[40] Storz P, Toker A. 3'-phosphoinositide-dependent kinase-1 (PDK-1) in PI 3-kinase signaling. Front Biosci 2002;7:d886-d902

[41] Belham C, Wu S, Avruch J. PDK1 – a kinase at the hub of things. Curr Biol 1999;9:R93-R96

[42] Agati JM, Yeagley D, Quinn PG. Assessment of the roles of mitogen-activated protein kinase, phosphatidylinositol 3-kinase, protein kinase B, and protein kinase C in insulin inhibition of cAMP-induced phosphoenolpyruvate carboxykinase gene transcription. J Biol Chem 1998;273:18751-18759

[43] Dentin R, Liu Y, Koo S-H, *et al.* Insulin modulates gluconeogenesis by inhibition of the coactivator TORC2. Nature 2007;449:366-370

[44] Winder WW, Hardie DG. AMP-activated protein kinase, a metabolic master switch: possible roles in type 2 diabetes. Am J Physiol Endocrinol Metab 1999;277:E1-E10

[45] Lochhead PA, Salt IP, Walker KS, Hardie DG, Sutherland C. 5-Aminoimidazole-4-carboxyamide riboside mimics the effects of insulin on the expression of the 2 key gluconeogenic genes PEPCK and glucose-6-phosphatase. Diabetes 2000;49:896-903

[46] Jakobsen SN, Hardie DG, Morrice N, Tornqvist HE. 5'-AMP-activated protein kinase phosphorylates IRS-1 on Ser-789 in mouse C2C12 myotubes in response to 5-aminoimidazole-4-carboxyamide riboside. J Biol Chem 2001;276:46912-46916

[47] Barthel A, Schmoll D, Krüger KD, Roth RA, Joost HG. Regulation of the forkhead transcription factor FKHR (FOXO1a) by glucose starvation and AICAR, an activator of AMP-activated protein kinase. Endocrinol 2002;143:3183-3186

[48] Huang S, Czech MP. The GLUT4 glucose transporter. Cell Metab 2007;5:237-252

[49] Gould GW, Holman GD. The glucose transporter family: structure, function and tissue-specific expression. Biochem J 1993;295:329-341

[50] Kandror KV, Pilch PF. Compartmentalization of protein traffic in insulin-sensitive cells. Am J Physiol 1996;271:E1-E14

[51] Van Obberghen E, Baron V, Delahaye L, *et al.* Surfing the insulin signaling web. Eur J Clin Invest 2001;31:966-977

[52] Watson RT, Kanzaki M, Pessin JE. Regulated membrane trafficking of the insulin-responsive glucose transporter 4 in adipocytes. Endocr Rev 2004;25:177-204

[53] Saltiel AR, Kahn CR. Insulin signalling and the regulation of glucose and lipid metabolism. Nature 2001;414:799-806

[54] Zorzano A, Palacín M, Gumà A. Mechanisms regulating GLUT4 glucose transporter expression and glucose transport in skeletal muscle. Acta Physiol Scand 2005;183:43-58

[55] Fruman DA, Meyers RE, Cantley LC. Phosphoinositide kinase. Annu Rev Biochem 1998;67:481-507

[56] Bae SS, Cho H, Mu J, Birnbaum MJ. Isoform-specific regulation of insulin-dependent glucose uptake by Akt/protein kinase B. J Biol Chem 2003;278:49530-49536

[57] Farese RV. Function and dysfunction of a PKC isoforms for glucose transport in insulin-sensitive and insulin-resistant states. Am J Physiol Endocrinol Metab 2002;283:E1-E11

[58] Watson RT, Pessin JE. GLUT4 translocation: The last 200 nanometers. Cell Sign 2007;19,11:2209-2217

[59] Sano H, Roach WG, Peck GR, Fukuda M, Lienhard GE. Rab10 in insulin-stimulated GLUT4 translocation. Biochem J 2008;411:89-95

[60]   Larance M, Ramm G, James DE. The GLUT4 code. Mol Endocrinol 2008;22,2:226-233

[61]   Ishiki M, Klip A. Minireview: Recent developments in the regulation of glucose transporter-4 traffic: new signals, locations, and partners. Endocrinol 2005;146,2:5071-5078

[62]   Ver MR, Chen H, Quon MJ. Insulin signaling pathways regulating translocation of GLUT4. Curr Med Chem-Immun Endoc & Metab Agents 2005;5:159-165

[63]   Khan AH, Pessin JE. Insulin regulation of glucose uptake: a complex interplay of intracellular pathways. Diabetologia 2002;45:1475-1483

[64]   Ribon V, Printen JA, Hoffman NG, Kay BK, Saltiel AR. A novel, multifunctional c-Cbl binding protein in insulin signaling in 3T3-L1 adipocytes. Mol Cell Biol 1998;18:872-879

[65]   Cartee GD, Wojtaszewski JF. Role of Akt substrate of 160 kDa in insulin-stimulated and contraction stimulated glucose transport. Appl Physiol Nutr Metab 2007;32,3:557-566

[66]   Moodie SA, Alleman-Sposeto J, Gustafson TA. Identification of the APS protein as a novel insulin receptor substrate. J Biol Chem 1999;274:11186-11193

[67]Tanaka S, Morishita T, Hashimoto Y, *et al.* C3G, a guanine nucleotide-releasing protein expressed ubiquitously, binds to the SRC homology-3 domain of CRK and GRB2/ASH proteins. Proc Natl Acad Sci USA 1994;91:3443-3447

[68]   Baumann CA, Ribon V, Kanzaki M, *et al.* CAP defines a second signaling pathway required for insulin-stimulated glucose transport. Nature 2000;407:202-207

[69]   Chiang SH, Baumann CA, Kanzaki M, *et al.* Insulin-stimulated GLUT4 translocation requires the CAP-dependent activation of TC10. Nature 2001;410:944-948

[70]   Smart EJ, Graf GA, McNiven MA, *et al.* Caveolins, liquid-order domains, and signal transduction. Mol Cell Biol 1999;19:7289-7304

[71]   Watson RT, Shigematsu S, Chiang SH, *et al.* Lipid raft microdomain compartmentalization of TC10 is required for insulin signaling and GLUT4 translocation. J Cell Biol 2001;154:829-840

[72]   Chiang SH, Hwang J, Legendare M, Zhang M, Kimura A, Saltiel AR. TCGAP, a multidomain Rho GTPase-activating protein involved in insulin-stimulated glucose transport. EMBO J 2003;222679-2691

[73]   Chang L, Adams RD, Saltiel AR. The TC10-interacting protein CIP4/2 is required for insulin-stimulated Glut4 translocation in 3T3 adipocytes. Proc Natl Acad Sci USA 2002;99:12835-12840

[74]   Jiang ZY, Chawla A, Bose A, Way M, Czech MP. A phosphatidylinositol 3-kinase-independent insulin signaling pathway for N-WASP/Arp2/3/F-actin required for GLUT4 glucose transporter recycling. J Biol Chem 2002;277:509-515

[75]   JeBailey L, Rudich A, Huang X, Di Ciano-Oliveira C, Kapus A, Klip A. Skeletal muscle cells and adipocytes differ in their reliance on TC10 and Rac for insulin-induced actin remodeling. Mol Endocrinol 2004;18:359-372

[76]   Kanzaki M, Pessin JE. Insulin signaling: GLUT4 vesicles exit via the exocyst. Curr Biol 2003;13:R574-R576

[77]   Inoue M, Chang L, Hwang J, Chiang SH, Saltiel AR. The exocyst complex is required for targeting of Glut4 to the plasma membrane by insulin. Nature 2003;422:629-633

[78]   Lizunov VA, Lisinski I, Stenkula K, Zimmerberg J, Cushman SW. Insulin regulates fusion of GLUT4 vesicles independent of Exo70-mediated tethering. J Biol Chem 2009;284,12:7914-7919

[79]   Inoue M, Chiang S-H, Chang L, Chen X-W, Saltiel AR. Compartmentalization of the exocyst complex in lipid rafts controls Glut4 vesicle tethering. Mol Biol Cell 2006;17:2303-2311

[80]   Watson RT, Furukawa M, Chiang SH, *et al.* The exocytic trafficking of TC10 occurs through both classical and nonclassical secretory transport pathways in 3T3L1 adipocytes. Mol Cell Biol 2003;23:961-974

[81]   Bao Y, Lopez JA, James DE, Hunziker W. Snapin interacts with the Exo70 subunit of the exocyst and modulates GLUT4 trafficking. J Biol Chem 2008;283,1:324-331

[82]   Chang L, Chiang SH, Saltiel AR. TC10 alpha is required for insulin-stimulated glucose uptake in adipocytes. Endocrinol 2007;148,1:27-33

[83]   Saltiel AR, Pessin JE. Insulin signaling in microdomains of the plasma membrane. Traffic 2003;4:711-716

[84]   Longo N, Elsas LJ. Human glucose transporters. Adv Pediatr 1998;45:293-313

[85]   Blok J, Gibbs EM, Lienhard GE, *et al.* Insulin-induced translocation of glucose transporters from post-Golgi compartments to the plasma membrane of 3T3 L1 adipocytes. J Cell Biol 1998;106:69-76

[86]   Uemura E, Greenlee HW. Insulin regulates neuronal glucose uptake by promoting translocation of glucose transporter GLUT3. Exp Neurol 2006;198:48-53

[87]   Wilson CM, Mitsumoto Y, Maher F, Klip A. Regulation of cell surface GLUT1, GLUT3, GLUT4 by insulin and IGF-1 in L6 myotubes. FEBS Lett 1995;368:19-22

[88]   Kimball C, Murlin J. Aqueous extract of pancreas III. Some precipitation reactions of insulin. J Biol Chem 1923;58:337-348

[89]   Cryer PE. Hypoglycaemia: the limiting factor in the glycaemic management of Type I and Type II diabetes. Diabetologia 2002;45:937-948

[90]   Quesada I, Tudurí E, Ripoll C, Nadal Á. Physiology of the pancreatic α-cell and glucagon secretion: role in glucose homeostasis and diabetes. J Endocrinol 2008;199:5-19

[91]   Mojsov S, Heinrich G, Wilson IB, Ravazzola M, Orci L, Habener JF. Preproglucagon gene expression in pancreas and intestine diversifies at the level of post-translational processing. J BiolChem 1986;261:11880-11889

[92]   Dey A, Lipkind GM, Rouille Y, *et al.* Significance of prohormone convertase 2, PC2, mediated initial cleavage site, Lys 70-Arg 71, to generate glucagon. Endocrinol 2005;146:713-727

[93]   Gromada J, Bokvist K, Ding WG, *et al.* Adrenaline stimulates glucagon secretion in pancreatic A-cells by increasing the Ca^{2+} channels. J Gen Physiol 1997;110:217-228

[94]   Rorsman P, Salehi SA, Abdulkader F, Braun M, MacDonald PE. K_{ATP}-channels and glucose-regulated glucagon secretion. Trends Endocrinol Metab 2008;19,8:277-284

[95]   Göpel SO, Kanno T, Barg S, Rorsman P. Patch-clamp characterisation of somatostatin-secreting delta-cells in intact mouse pancreatic islets. J Physiol 2000;528(Pt3);497-507

[96]   Göpel SO, Kanno T, Barg S, Weng XG, Gromada J, Rorsman P. Regulation of glucose release in mouse-cells by K_{ATP} channels and inactivation of TTX-sensitive Na^+ channels. J Physiol 2000;528(Pt3):509-520

[97]   MacDonald PE, De Marinis YZ, Ramracheya R, *et al.* A K_{ATP} channel-dependent pathway within α cells regulates glucagon release from both rodent and human islets of Langerhans. PLoS Biology 2007;5,6:1236-1247

[98]   Kanno T, Göpel SO, Rorsman P, Wakui M. Cellular function in multicellular system for hormone secretion: electrophysiological aspect of studies on α-, β- and δ-cells of the pancreatic islet. Neurosc Res 2002;42:79-90

[99]   Nordlie RC, Bode AM, Foster JD. Recent advances in heaptic glucose-6-phosphatase regulation and function. Proc Soc Exp Biol Med 1993;203:274-285

[100]   Foster JD, Pederson BA, Nordlie RC. Glucose-6-phosphatase structure, regulation and function: an update. Proc Soc Exp Biol Med 1997;215:314-332

[101]   Herzig S, Long F, Jhala US, *et al.* CREB regulates hepatic gluconeogenesis through the coactivator PGC-1. Nature 2001;413:179-183

[102]   Yada T, Sakurada M, Ishihara H, *et al.* Pituitary adenylate cyclase-activating polypeptide (PACAP) in an islet substance serving as an intra-islet amplifier of glucose-induced insulin secretion in rats. J Physiol (London) 1997;505:319-328

[103]   Gromada H, Holst JJ, Rorsman P. Cellular regulation of islet hormone secreting by the incretin hormone glucagon-like peptide 1. Pflüg Arch 1998;435:583-594

[104]   Kanno T, Suga S, Nakano K, Kamimura N, Wakui M. Corticotropin-releasing factor modulation of Ca^{2+} in flux in rat pancreatic β-cells. Diabetes 1999;48:1741-1746

[105]   Mayo KE, Miller LJ, Batalie D, *et al.* The glucagon receptor family. Pharmacol Rev 2003;55:167-194

[106]   Slavin BG, Ong JM, Kern PA. Hormonal regulation of hormone-sensitive lipase activity and mRNA levels in isolated rat adipocytes. J Lipid Res 1994;35:1535-1541

[107]   Andersen B, Rassov A, Westergaard N, Lundgren K. Inhibition of glycogenolysis in primary rat hepatocytes by 1,4-dideoxy-1,4-imino-D-arabinitol. Biochem J 1999;342:545-550

[108]   Vons C, Pegorier JP, Giard J, Kohl C, Ivanov MA, Franco D. regulation of fatty-acid metabolism by pancreatic hormones in cultured human hepatocytes. Hepatology 1991;13:1126-1130

[109]   Brezeau P, Vale W, Burgus R, *et al.* Hypothalamic polypeptide that inhibits the secretion of immunoreactive pituitary growth hormone. Science 1973;179:77-79

[110]   Sakuri H, Dobbs R, Unger RH. Somatostatin-induced changes in insulin and glucagon secretion in normal and diabetic dogs. J Clin Invest 1974;54:1395-1401

[111]   Belenger A, Labrie F, Borgeat P, *et al.* Inhibition of growth hormone and thyrotropin release by growth hormone-release inhibiting hormone. Mol Cell Endocrinol 1974;1:329-333

[112]   Richardson UI, Schonbrunn A. Inhibition of adrenocorticotropin secretion by somatostatin in pituitary cells in culture. Endocrinol 1981;108:281-290

[113]   Epelbaum J, Enjalbert A, Krantic S, *et al.* Somatostatin receptors on pituitary somatotrophs, tyrotrophs, and lactotrophs: pharmacological evidence for loose coupling to adenylate cyclase. Endocrinol 1987;121:2177-2185

[114]   Zabel BU, Naylor SL, Sakaguchi AY, Bell GI, Shows TB. High resolution chromosomal location of human genes for amylase, proopiomelanocortin, somatostatin, and a DNA fragment (D3S1) by in situ hybrydyzation. Proc Natl Acad Sci USA 1983;80:6932-6936

[115]   Patel YC. Somatostatin and its receptor family. Front Neuroendocrinol 1999;20,3:157-198

[116]   Stangner JL, Samols E. The vascular order of islet cellular perfusion in the human pancreas. Diabetes 1992;41:93-97

[117] Efendic S, Nylen A, Roovete A, Uvnas-Wallenstein K. Effects of glucose and arginine on the release of immunoreactive somatostatin from the isolated perfused rat pancreas. FEBS Lett 1978;92:33-35

[118] Hermansen K, Christensen SE, Orskov H. Characterization of somatostatin release from the pancrease: the role of potassium. Scand J Clin Lab Invest 1979;39:717-722

[119] Levine AS, Morley JE. Peripheral administered somatostatin reduces feeding by a vagal mediated mechanism. Pharmacol Biochem Behav 1982;16:897-902

[120] Lotter EC, Krinsky R, McKay JM, Treneer CM, Porte Jr D, Woods SC. Somatostatin decreases food intake of rats and baboons. J Comp Physiol Psychol 1981;95:278-287

[121] Woods SC, Lutz TA, Geary N, Langhans W. Pancreatic signals controlling food intake; insulin, glucagon and amylin. Phil Trans R Soc B 2006;361:1219-1235

[122] Cherrington AD, Caldewell MD, Diets MR, Exton JH, Crofford DB. The effects of somatostatin on glucose uptake and production by rat tissues in vitro. Diabetes 1977;26:740-748

[123] Cherrington AD, Lacy WW, Chiasson JL. Effect of glucagon on glucose production during insulin deficiency in the dog. J Clin Invest 1978;62:664-667

[124] Ogihara M, Ui M. Effects of somatostatin on liver glycogen and fat metabolism in vivo. Japan J Pharmacol 1984;34:313-318

[125] Ensick JW, Vogel RE, Laschansky EC, et al. Endogenous somatostatin-28 modulates postprandial insulin secretion. J Clin Invest 1997;100,9:2295-2302

[126] Brown MJ, Rivier J, Vale W. Somatostatin-28: selective action of the pancreatic β-cell and brain. Endocrinol 1981;108:2391-2393

[127] Schuit FC, Derde M-P, Pipeleers DG. Sensitivity of rat pancreatic A and B cells to somatostatin. Diabetologia 1989;32:207-212

[128] Reubi J-C, Rivier J, Perrin M, Brown M, Vale W. Specific high affinity binding sites for somatostatin-28 on pancreatic β-cells: differences with brain somatostatin receptors. Endocrinol 1982;82:1049-1051

[129] Amherdt M, Patel YC, Orci L. Selective binding of somatostatin-14 and somatostatin-28 to islet cells revealed by quantitative electron microscopic autoradiography. J Clin Invest 1987;80:1455-1458

[130] Mandarino L, Stenner D, Blanchard W, et al. Selective effects of somatostatin-15, -25 and -28 on *in vitro* insulin and glucagon secretion. Nature 1981;291:76-77

[131] Lahlou H, Guillermet J, Hortala M, et al. Molecular signaling of somatostatin receptors. An N Y Acad Sci 2004;1014:121-131

[132] De Lecea L, Criada JR, Prospero-Garcia O, et al. A cortical neuropeptid with neuronal depressant and sleep-modulating properties. Nature 1996;381:242-245

[133] Strowski MZ, Kohler M, Chen HY, et al. Somatostatin receptor subtype 5 regulates insulin secretion and glucose homeostasis. Mol Endocrinol 2003;17,1:93-106

[134] Ribalet B, Eddlestone GT. Characterization of the G protein coupling to a somatostatin receptor of the K^+_{ATP} channel in insulin secreting mammalian HIT and RIN cell lines. J Physiol 1995;485,1:73-86

[135] Strowski MZ, Parmar RM, Blake AD, Schaeffer JM. Somatostatin inhibits insulin and glucagon secretion via two receptor subtypes: an *in vitro* study of pancreatic islets from somatostatin receptor 2 knockout mice. Endocrinol 2000;141,1:111-117

[136] Kumar U, Sasi R, Suresh S, et al. Subtype-selective expression of the five somatostatin receptors (hSSTR1 – 5) in human pancreatic islet cells: a quantitative double-label immunohistochemical analysis. Diabetes 1999;48:77-85

[137] Vanetti M, Kouba M, Wang X, Vogt G, Hollt V. Cloning and expression of a novel mouse somatostatin receptor (SSTR2B). FEBS Lett 1992;311:290-294

[138] Vanetti M, Vogt G, Hollt V. The two isoforms of the mouse somatostatin receptor (mSSTR2A and mSSTR2B) differ in coupling efficiency to adenylate cyclase and in agonist-induced receptor desensitization. FEBS Lett 1993;331:260-266

[139] Cooper GJS, Willis AC, Clark A, et al. Purification and characterization of a peptide from amyloid-rich pancreas of the type 2 diabetic patients. Proc Natl Acad Sci USA 1987;84:8628-8632

[140] Young AA, Gedulin BR, Vine W, et al. Gastric emptying is accelerated in diabetic BB rats and is slowed by subcutaneous injection of amylin. Diabetologia 1995;38:642-648

[141] Lutz TA. Amylinergic control of food intake. Physiol Behav 2006;89,4:465-471

[142] Gedulin BR, Rink TJ, Young AA. Dose-response for glucagonostic effect of amylin in rats. Metabolism 1997;46:67-70

[143] Lutz TA, Moller A, Rushing PA, Riediger T, Scharrer E. The anorectic effect of a chronic peripheral infusion of amylin is abolished in area postrema/nucleus of the solitary tract (AP/NTS) lesioned rats. Int J Obes Relat Metab Disord 2001;25:1005-1011

[144] Riediger T, Zuend D, Becskei C, Lutz TA. The anorectic hormone amylin contributes to feeding related changes of neuronal activity in key structures of the gut-brain axis. Am J Physiol Regul Integr Comp Physiol 2004;286:R114-R122

[145] Karra E, Batterham RL. The role of gut hormones in the regulation of body weight and energy homeostasis. Mol Cell Endocrinol 2009, doi:10.1016/j.mce.2009.06.010

[146] Fischer JA, Muff R, Born W. Functional relevance of G-protein-coupled-receptor-associated proteins, exemplified by receptor-activity-modifying proteins (RAMPS). Biochem Soc Trans 2002;30:455-460

[147] Berglund MM, Hipskind PA, Gehlert DR. Recent development in our understanding of the physiological role of PP-fold peptide receptor subtypes. Exp Biol Med 2003;228:217-244

[148] Hort Y, Baker E, Sutherland GR, Shine J, Herzog H. Gene duplication of the human peptide YY gene (PYY) generated the pancreatic polypeptide gene (PPY) on chromosome 17q21.1. Genomics 1995;26:77-83

[149] Track NS, McLeod RS, Mee AV. Human pancreatic polypeptide studies of fasting and postprandial plasma concentrations. Can J Physiol Pharmacol 1980;58:1484-1489

[150] Hazelwood RL. The pancreatic polypeptide (PP-fold) family: Gastrointestinal, vascular, and feeding behavioral implications. Proc Soc Exp Biol Med 1993;202:44-63

[151] Feletou M, Nicolas JP, Rodriguez M, *et al.* NPY receptor subtype in the rabbit isolated ileum. Br J Pharmacol 1999;127:795-801

[152] Pheng LH, Perron A, Quirion R, *et al.* Neuropeptide Y-induced contraction is mediated by neuropeptide Y Y2 and Y4 receptors in the rat colon. Eur J Pharmacol 1999;374:85-91

[153] Gehlert DR. Multiple receptors for the pancreatic polypeptide (PP-fold) family: Physiological implications. Proc Soc Exp Biol Med 1998;218:7-22

[154] Trinh T, van Dumont Y, Quirion R. High levels of specific neuropeptide Y/pancreatic polypeptide receptors in the rat hypothalamus and brainstem. Eur J Pharmacol 1996;318:R1-R3

[155] Whitcomb DC, Puccio AM, Vigna SR, Taylor IL, Hoffman GE. Distribution of pancreatic polypeptide receptors in the rat brain. Brain Res 1997;760:137-149

[156] Larhammar D. Structural diversity of receptors for neuropeptide Y, peptide YY and pancreatic polypeptide. Regul Pept 1996;65:165-174

[157] Mullins DE, Zhang X, Hawes BE. Activation of extracellular signal regulated protein kinase by neuropeptide Y and pancreatic polypeptide in CHO cells expressing the NPY, Y1, Y2, Y4 and Y5 receptor subtypes. Regul Pept 2002;105:65-73

[158] Mannon PJ, Mele JM. Peptide YY Y1 receptor activates mitogen-activated protein kinase and proliferation in gut epithelial cells via the epidermal growth factor receptor. Biochem J 2000;350:655-661

[159] Bard JA, Walker MW, Branchek TA, Weinshank RL. Cloning and functional expression of a human Y4 subtype receptor for pancreatic polypeptide, neuropeptide Y, and peptide YY. J Biol Chem 1995;270:26762-26765

[160] Lundell I, Blomqvist AG, Berglund MM, *et al.* Cloning of a human receptor of the NPY receptor family with high affinity for pancreatic polypeptide and peptide YY. J Biol Chem 1995;270: 29123-29128

[161] Perley MJ, Kipnis DM. Plasma insulin responses to oral and intravenous glucose studies in normal and diabetic studies. J Clin Invest 1967;46:1954-1962

[162] Nauck MA, Homberger E, Siegel EG, *et al.* Incretin effects of increasing glucose loads in man calculated from venous insulin and C-peptide response. J Clin Endocrinol Metab 1986;119:833-840

[163] Holst JJ, Gromada J. Role of incretin hormones in the regulation of insulin secretion in diabetic and nondiabetic humans. Am J Physiol Endocrinol Metab 2004;287:E199-E206

[164] Ranganath LR. The entero-insular axis: implications for human metabolism. Clin Chem Lab Med 2008;46,1:43-56

[165] Bell GI, Sanchez-Pescador R, Laybourn PJ, Najarian RC. Exon duplication and divergence in the human preproglucagon gene. Nature 1983;304:368-371

[166] Drucker DJ. Glucagon-like peptides. Diabetes 1998;47:159-169

[167] Huda MSB, Wilding JPH, Pinkney JH. Gut peptides and the regulation of appetite. Obesity Rev 2006;7:163-182

[168]. Mojsov S, Kopczynski MG, Habener JF. Both amidated and nonamidated forms of glucagon-like peptide 1 are synthesized in the rat intestine and pancreas. J Biol. Chem 1990;265:8001-8008

[169] Wettergren A, Pridal L, Wojdemann M, Holst JJ. Amidated and non-amidated glucagon-like peptide-1 (GLP-1): non-pancreatic effects (cephalic phase acid secretion) and stability in plasma in humans. Regul Pept 1998;77:83-87

[170] Orskov C, Rabenhoi L, Wettergren A, Kofod H, Holst JJ. Tissue and plasma concentrations of amidate and glycine-extended glucagon-like peptide 1 in humans. Diabetes 1994;43:535-539

[171] Nauck MA. Is glucagon-like peptide 1 an incretin hormone? Diabetologia 1999;42:373-379

[172] Burcelin R, Cani PD, Knauf C. Glucagon-like peptide-1 and energy homeostasis. J Nutr 2007;137:2534S-2538S

[173] Elliott RM, Morgan LM, Tredger JA, Deacon S, Wright J, Marks V. Glucagon-like peptide-1 (7 – 36) amide and glucose-dependent insulinotropic polypeptide secretion in response to nutrient ingestion in man: acute post-prandial and 24-h secretion patterns. J Endocrinol 1993;138:159-166

[174] Kreymann B, Williams G, Ghatei MA, Bloom SR. Glucagon-like peptide-1 7-36: a physiological incretin in man. Lancet 1987;2:1300-1304

[175] Mojsov S, Weir GC, Habener JF. Insulinotropin: glucagon-like peptide 1 (7 – 37) co-encoded in the glucagon gene is a potent stimulator of insulin release in the perfused rat pancreas. J Clin Invest 1987;79:616-619

[176] Ritzel R, Orskov C, Holst JJ, et al. Pharmacokinetic, insulinotropic, and glucagonostatic properties of GLP-1 (7 – 36 amide) after subcutaneous injection in healthy volunteers. Dose-response-relationship. Diabetologia 1995;38:720-725

[177] Furton MD, O'Shea D, Gunn I, et al. A role for glucagon-like peptide-1 in the central regulation of feeding. Nature 1996;379:69-72

[178] Drucker DJ, Philippe J, Mojsov S, Chick WL, Habener JF. Glucagon-like peptide 1 stimulates insulin gene expression and increases cyclic AMP levels in a rat islet cell line. Proc Natl Acad Sci USA 1987;84:3434-3438

[179] Drucker DJ. The biology of incretin hormones. Cell Metab 2006;3:153-165

[180] Negi G, Kumar A, Sharma SS, Gulati A. Biological actions of GLP-1 analogues: Recent advancements and development. CRIPS 2008;9,4:73-76

[181] Thorens B, Deriaz N, Bosco D, et al. Protein kinase A dependent phosphorylation of GLUT2 in pancreatic B cells. J Biol Chem 1996;271:8075-8081

[182] Beguin P, Nagashima K, Nishimura M, et al. PKA-mediated phosphorylation of the human K_{ATP} channel: separate roles of Kir6.2 and SUR1 subunit phosphorylation. EMBO J 1999;18:4722-4732

[183] Leiser M, Fleischer N. cAMP-dependent phosphorylation of the cardiac-type a1 subunit of the voltage-dependent Ca^{2+} channel in a murine pancreatic b cell line. Diabetes 1996;45:1412-1418

[184] Kwan EP, Gaisano HY. Glucagon-like peptide 1 regulates sequential and compound exocytosis in pancreatic islet beta-cells. Diabetes 2005;54:2734-2743

[185] Buteau J, Roduit R, Susini S, Prentki M. Glucagon-like peptide-1 promotes DNA synthesis, activates phosphatidylinositol 3-kinase and increases transcription factor pancreatic and duodenal homeobox gene 1 (PDX-1) DNA binding activity in beta (INS-1)-cells. Diabetologia 1999;42:856-864

[186] Fehmann HC, Habener JF. Insulinotropic hormone glucagon-like peptide-1(7 – 37) stimulation of proinsulin gene expression and proinsulin biosynthesis in insulinoma beta TC-1 cells. Endocrinol 1992;130:159-166

[187] Dupre J, Ross SA, Watson D, Brown JC. Stimulation of insulin secretion by gastric inhibitory polypeptide in man. J Clin Endocrinol Metab 1973;37:826-828

[188] Inagaki N, Seino Y, Takeda J, et al. Gastric inhibitory peptide: structure and chromosomal localization of the human gene. Mol Endocrinol 1989;3,6:1014-1021

[189] Takeda J, Seino Y, Tanaka K, et al. Sequence of an intestinal cDNA encoding human gastric inhibitory polypeptide precursor. Proc Natl Acad Sci USA 1987;84:7005-7008

[190] Deacon CF, Nauck MA, Meier J, Hucking K, Holst JJ. Degradation of endogenous and exogenous gastric inhibitory polypeptide in healthy and in type 2 diabetic subjects as revealed using a new assay for the intact peptide. J Clin Endocrinol Metab 2000;85:3575-3581

[191] Murphy MC, Isherwood SG, Sethi S, et al. Postprandial responses to meals of varying fat contents: modulatory role of lipoprotein lipase? Eur J Clin Nutr 1995;49:578-588

[192] Stoffel M, Fernald AA, Le Beau MM, Bell GI. Assignment of the gastric inhibitory polypeptide receptor gene (GIPR) to chromosome bands 10q13.2-q13.3 by fluorescence in situ. Genomics 1995;28,3:607-609

[193] Jhala US, Gianluca Cannetieri RA, Screaton RN, et al. cAMP promotes pancreatic beta-cells survival via CREB-mediated induction of IRS2. Genes Dev 2003;17:1575-1580

[194] Elahi D, Maneilly GS, Minaker KL, et al. Regulation of hepatic glucose production by gastric inhibitory polypeptide in man. Can J Physiol Pharmacol (Abstract) 1986;65:18

[195] O'Harte FPM, Gray AM, Flatt PR. Gastric inhibitory polypeptide and effects of glycation on glucose transport and metabolism in isolated mouse abdominal muscle. J Endocrinol 1998;156:237-243

[196] Wheeler MB, Gelling RW, McIntosh CH, Georgiou J, Brown JC, Pederson RA. Functional expression of the rat pancreatic islet glucose-dependent insulinotropic polypeptide receptor; ligand binding and intracellular signaling properties. Endocrinol 1995;136:4629-4639

[197] Yip RGC, Wolfe MM. GIP biology and fat metabolism. Life Sciences 2000;66:91-103

[198] Trumper A, Trumper K, Trusheim H, Arnold R, Goke B, Horsch D. Glucose-dependent insulinotropic polypeptide is a growth factor for beta (INS-1) cells by pleiotropic signaling. Mol Endocrinol 2001;15:1559-1570

[199] Ehses JA, Pelech SL, Pederson RA, McIntosh CH. Glucose-dependent insulinotropic polypeptide activates the Raf-Mek1/2-ERK1/2 module via a cyclic AMP/cAMP-dependent protein kinase/Rap1-mediated pathway. J Biol Chem 2002;277:37088-37097

[200] Kojima M, Hosoda H, Date Y, Nakazato M, Matsuno H, Kangawa K. Ghrelin is a growth-hormone-releasing acetylated peptide from stomach. Nature 1999;402:656-660

[201] Pusztai P, Sarman B, Ruzicska E, *et al.* Ghrelin: a new peptide regulating the neurohormonal system, energy homeostasis and glucose metabolism. Diabetes Metab Res Rev 2008;24:343-352

[202] Seim I, Collet C, Herington AC, Chopin LK. Revised genomic structure of the human ghrelin gene and identification of novel exons, alternative splice variants and natural antisense transcripts. BMC Genomics 2007;8:298, doi:10.1186/1471-2164-8-298

[203] Kanamoto N, Akamizu T, Tagami T, *et al.* Genomic structure and characterization of the 5'-flanking region of the human ghrelin gene. Endocrinol 2005;145:4144-4153

[204] Hosoda H, Kojima M, Matsuo H, *et al.* Purification and characterization of rat des-Gn(14)-ghrelin, a second endogenous ligand for the growth hormone secretagogue receptor. J Biol Chem 2000;275:21995-22000

[205] Kojima M, Kangawa K. Ghrelin: structure and function. Physiol Rev 2005;85:495-522

[206] Nishi Y, Hiejima H, Hosoda H, *et al.* Ingested medium-chain fatty acids are directly utilized for the acyl modification of ghrelin. Endocrinol 2005;146:2255-2264

[207] Broglio F, Benso A, Gottero C, *et al.* Non-acylated ghrelin does not posses the pituitaric and pancreatic endocrine activity of acylated ghrelin in humans. J Endocrinol Invest 2003;26:192-196

[208] Wren AM, Bloom SR. Gut hormones and appetite control. Gastroenterology 2007;132:2116-2130

[209] Hosoda H, Kojima M, Kangawa K. Biological, physiological, and pharmacological aspects of ghrelin. J Pharmacol Sci 2006;100:398-410

[210] Fukushima N, Hanada R, Teranishi H, *et al.* Ghrelin directly regulates bone formation. J Bone Miner Res 2005;20:790-798

[211] Cowley MA, Smith RG, Diano S, *et al.* The distribution and mechanism of action of ghrelin in the CNS demonstrates a novel hypothalamic circuit regulating energy homeostasis. Neuron. 2003;37:649-661

[212] Lu S, Guan JL, Wang QP, *et al.* Immunocytochemical observation of ghrelin-containing neurons in the rat arcuate nucleus. Neurosci Lett 2002;321:157-160

[213] Wu JT, Kral JG. Ghrelin. Integrative neuroendocrine peptide in health and disease. Ann Surg 2004;239:464-474

[214] Tritos NA, Kokkotou EG. The physiology and potential clinical applications of ghrelin, a novel peptide hormone. Mayo Clin Proc 2006;81,5:653-660

[215] Tschop M, Wawarta R, Riepl RL, *et al.* Post-prandial decrease of circulating human ghrelin levels. J Endocrinol Invest 2001;24:RC19-RC21

[216] Overduin J, Frayo RS, Grill HJ,Kaplan JM, Cummings DE. Role of the duodenum and macronutrient type in ghrelin regulation. Endocrinol 2005;146:845-850

[217] Cummings DE, Purnell JQ, Frayo RS, Schmidova K, Wisse BE, Weigle DS. A preprandial rise in plasma ghrelin levels suggests a role in meal initiation in humans. Diabetes 2001;50:1714-1719

[218] McCowen KC, Maykel JA, Bistrian BR, Ling PR. Circulating ghrelin concentrations are lowered by intravenous glucose or hyperinsulinemic euglycemic conditions in rodents. J Endocrinol 2002;175:R7-R11

[219] Anderwald C, Brabant G, Bernoider E, et a. Insulin-dependent modulation of plasma ghrelin and leptin concentrations is less pronounced in type 2 diabetic patients. Diabetes 2003;52:1792-1798

[220] Mohling M, Spranger J, Otto B, Ristow M, Tschop M, Pfeiffer AF. Euglycemic hyperinsulinemia, but not lipid infusion, decreases circulating ghrelin levels in humans. J Endocrinol Invest 2002;25:RC36-RC38

[221] Arafat MA, Otto R, Rochlitz H, *et al.* Glucagon inhibits ghrelin secretion in humans. Eur J Endocrinol 2005;153:397-402

[222] Nakazato M, Murakami N, Date Y, *et al.* A role for ghrelin in the central regulation of feeding. Nature 2001;409:194-198

[223] Wren AM, Seal LJ, Cohen MA, *et al.* Ghrelin enhances appetite and increases food intake in humans. J Clin Endocrinol Metab 2001;86:5992-5996

[224] Date Y, Nakazato M, Hashiguchi S, *et al.* Ghrelin is present in pancreatic alpha-cells of humans and rats and stimulates insulin secretion. Diabetes 2002;51:124-129

[225] Lee HM, Wang E, Englander EW, *et al.* Ghrelin, a new gastrointestinal endocrine pancreatic peptide that stimulates insulin secretion: Enteric distribution, ontogeny, influence of endocrine and dietary manipulations. Endocrinol 2002;143:185-190

[226] Egido EM, Rodriguez-Gallardo J, Silvestre RA, *et al.* Inhibitory effect of ghrelin on insulin and pancreatic somatostatin secretion. Eur J Endocrinol 2002;146:241-244

[227] Reimer MK, Pacini G, Ahren B. Dose-dependent inhibition by ghrelin of insulin secretion in the mouse. Endocrinol 2003;144;916-921

[228] Murata M, Okimura Y, Iida K, *et al.* Ghrelin modulates the downstream molecules of insulin-signaling in hepatoma. J Biol Chem 2002;227:5667-5674

[229] Broglio F, Arvat E, Benson A, *et al.* Ghrelin a natural GH secretagogue produced by the stomach, induces hyperglycemia and reduces insulin secretion in humans. J Clin Endocrinol Metab 2001;86:5083-5086

[230] Schaller G, Schmidt A, Pleiner J, *et al.* Plasma ghrelin concentrations are not regulated by glucose or insulin: a double-blind, placebo-controlled crossover clamp study. Diabetes 2003;52:16-20

[231] Tole V, Bassant MH, Zizzarri P, *et al.* Ultradian rhytmicity of ghrelin secretion in relation with GH, feeding behaviour, and sleep-wake patterns in rats. Endocrinol 2002;143:1353-1361

[232] DeVriese C, Gregoire F, Lema-Kisoka R, *et al.* Ghrelin degradation by serum and tissue homogenates: identification of the cleavage sites. Endocrinol 2004;145:4997-5005

[233] Smith RG, Van der Ploeg LH, Howard AD, *et al.* Peptidomimetic regulation of growth hormone secretion. Endocrinol Rev 1997;18:621-645

[234] McKee KK, Palyha OC, Feighner SD, *et al.* Molecular analysis of rat pituitary and hypothalamic growth hormone secretagogue receptors. Mol Endocrinol 1997;11:415-423

[235] Smith RG, Leonard R, Bailey AR, *et al.* Growth hormone secretagogue receptor family members and ligands. Endocrine 2001;14:9-14

[236] Howard AD, Feighner SD, Cully DF, *et al.* A receptor in pituitary and hypothalamus that functions in growth hormone release. Science 1996;273:974-977

[237] Guan XM, Yu H, Palyha OC, *et al.* Distribution of mRNA encoding the growth hormone secretagogue receptor in brain and peripheral tissues. Brain Res Mol Brain Res 1997;48:23-29

[238] Gnanapavan S, Kola B, Bustin SA, *et al.* The tissue distribution of the mRNA of ghrelin and subtypes of its receptor, GHS-R, in humans. J Clin Endocrinol Metab 2002;87:2988-2991

[239] Papotti M, Ghe C, Cassoni P, *et al.* Growth hormone secretagogue binding sites in peripheral human tissues. J Clin Endocrinol Metab 2000;85:3803-3807

[240] Kojima M, Hosoda H, Matusuo H, *et al.* Ghrelin: discovery of the natural endogenous ligand for the growth hormone secretagogue receptor. Trends Endocrinol Metab 2001;12:118-121

[241] Casanueva FF, Dieguez C. Growth hormone secretagogues: physiological role and clinical utility. Trends Endocrinol Metab 1999;10:30-38

[242] Ivy AC, Oldberg E. A hormonal mechanism for gallbladder contraction and evacuation. Am J Physiol 1928;86:599-613

[243] Takahashi Y, Fukushige S, Murotsu T, Matsubara K. Structure of human cholecystokinin gene and its chromosomal location. Gene 1986;50:353-360

[244] Konturek PC, Konturek SJ, The history of gastrointestinal hormones and the Polish contribution to elucidation of their biology and relation to nervous system. J Physiol Pharmacol 2003;54:83-98

[245] Beinfeld MC, Meyer DK, Eskay RL, Jensen RT, Brownstein MJ. The distribution of cholecystokinin immunoreactivity in the central nervous system in the rat as determined by radioimmunoassay. Brain Res 1981;212:51-57

[246] Crawler JN, Corwin RL. Biological actions of cholecystokinin. Peptides 1994;15:731-755

[247] Liddle RA, Goldfine ID, Rosen MS, Taplitz RA, Williams JA. Cholecystokinin bioactivity in human plasma. Molecular form, responses to feeding, and relationship to gallbladder contraction. J Clin Invest 1985;75:1144-1152

[248] Konturek SJ, Konturek PC, Konturek JW, Cześnikiewicz-Guzik M, Brzozowski T, Sito E. Neuro-hormonal control of food intake; basic mechanisms and clinical implications. J Physiol Pharmacol 2005;56,Suppl 6:5-25

[249] Beinfeld MC. Biosynthesis and processing of pro CCK: recent progress and future challenges. Life Sci 2003;72:747-757

[250] Wang BJ, Cui ZJ. How does cholecystokinin stimulate exocrine pancreatic secretion? From birds, rodents, to humans. Am J Physiol Regul Integr Comp Physiol 2007;292:R666-R678

[251] Rehfeld JF, Bungaard JR, Friis-Hansen L, Goetz JP. On the tissue-specific processing of procholecystokinin in the brain and gut: a short review. J Physiol Pharmacol 2003;54:S73-S79

[252] Gibbs J, Young RC, Smith GP. Cholecystokinin decreases food intake in rats. J Comp Physiol Psychol 1973;84:488-495

[253] Rose C, Vargas F, Facchinetti P, *et al.* Characterization and inhibition of a cholecystokinin-inactivating serine peptidase. Nature 1996;380:403-409

[254] Inoue H, Iannotti CA, Welling CM, Veile R, Donis-Keller H, Permutt MA. Human cholecystokinin type A receptor gene: Cytogenetic localization, physical mapping, and identification of two missense variations in patients with obesity and non-insulin-dependent diabetes mellitus (NIDDM). Genomics 1997;42:331-335

[255] Pisegna JR, de Weerth A, Wank SA. Molecular cloning of the human brain and gastric cholecystokinin receptor: Structure, functional expression and chromosomal localization. Biochem Biophys Res Commun 1992;189:296-303

[256] Noble F, Wank SA, Crawley JN, *et al.* International Union of Pharmacology. XXI. Structure, distribution, and functions of cholecystokinin receptors. Pharmacol. Rev 1999;51,4:745-781

[257] Dohlman HG, Thorner J, Caron MG, Lefkowitz RJ. Model systems for the study of seven-transmembrane-segment receptors. Annu Rev Biochem 1991;60:653-680

[258] Jensen RT, Wank SA, Rowley WH, Sato S, Gardner JD. Interaction of CCK with pancreatic acinar cells. Trends Pharmacol 1989;10:418-423

[259] Gully D, Fréhel D, Marcy, *et al.* Peripheral biological activity of SR 27897: A new potent non-peptide antagonist of CCK-A receptors. Eur J Pharmacol 1993;232:13-19

[260] Sandvik AK, Waldum HL. CCK-B (gastrin) receptor regulates gastric histamine release and acid secretion. Am J Physiol 1991;260:G925-G928

[261] Ji B, Bi Y, Simeone D, Mortensen RM, Logsdon CD. Human pancreatic acinar cells lack functional response to cholecystokinin and gastrin. Gastroenterol 2001;121:1380-1390

[262] Smith GP, Jerome C, Cuskin BJ, Eterno R, Simansky KJ. Abdominal vagotomy blocks the satiety effect of cholecystokinin in the rat. Science 1981;213:1036-1037

[263] Rushakoff RA, Goldfine ID, Beccaria LJ, *et al.* Reduced postprandial cholecystokinin (CCK) secretion in patients with noninsulin-dependent diabetes mellitus: evidence for a role for CCK in regulating postprandial hyperglycemia. J Clin Endocrinol Metab 1993;76:489-493

[264] Funakoski A, Miyasaka K, Kanai S, *et al.* Pancreatic endocrine dysfunction in rats not expressing the cholecystokinin-A receptor. Pancreas 1996;12:230-236

[265] Ahren B, Holst JJ, Efendic S. Antidiabetogenic action of cholecystokinin-8 in type 2 diabetes. J Clin Endocrinol Metab 2000;85:1043-1048

[266] Morisset J. The gastrointestinal cholecystokinin receptors in health and diseases. Annales Academiae Medicae Bialostocensis 2005,50:21-36

[267] Bataille D, Coundray AM, Carlqvist M, Rosselin G, Mut V. Isolation of glucagon-37 (bioactive enteroglucagon/oxyntomodulin) from porcine jejuno-ileum. Isolation of the peptide. FEBS Lett 1982;146:73-78

[268] Dubrasquet M, Bataille D, Gespach C. Oxyntomodulin (glucagon-37 or bioactive enteroglucagon): a potent inhibitor of pentagastrin-stimulated acid secretion in rats. Biosci Rep 1982; 2:391-395

[269] Bataille D, Gespach C, Tatemoto K, *et al.* Bioactive enteroglucagon (oxyntomodulin): present knowledge on its chemical structure and its biological activities. Peptides 1981;2,Suppl 2:41-44

[270] Holst JJ. Glucagon-like peptide 1 (GLP-1): an intestinal hormone, signalling nutritional abundance, with an unusual therapeutic potential. Trends Endocrinol Metab 1999;10:229-235

[271] Baldissera FG, Holst JJ. Glucagon-related peptides in the human gastrointestinal mucosa. Diabetologia 1984;26:223-228

[272] Read NW, McFarlane A, Kinsman RI, *et al.* Effect of infusion of nutrient solutions into the ileum on gastrointestinal transit and plasma levels on neurotensin and enteroglucagon. Gastroenterol 1984;86:274-280

[273] Ghatei MA, Uttenthal LO, Christofides ND, Bryant MG, Bloom SR. Molecular forms of human enteroglucagon in tissue and plasma: plasma responses to nutrient stimuli in health and in disorders of the upper gastrointestinal tract. J Clin Endocrinol Metab 1983;57,3:488-495

[274] LeQuellec A, Kervan A, Blache P, Ciurana AJ, Bataille D. Oxyntomodulin-like immunoreactivity: diurnal profile of a new potential enterogastrone. J Clin Endocrinol Metab 1992;74,6:1405-1409

[275] Baggion LL, Huang Q, Brown TJ, Drucker DJ. Oxyntomodulin and glucagon-like peptide-1 differentially regulate murine food intake and energy expenditure. Gastroenterol 2004;127,2:546-558

[276] Fehmann HC, Jiang J, Schweinfurth J, Wheeler MB, Boyd AE III, Goke B. Stable expression of the rat GLP-1 receptor in CHO cells: activation and binding characteristics utilizing LP-1 (7 – 36)-amide, oxyntomodulin, extendin-4, and extendin (9 – 39). Peptides 1994;15:453-456

[277] Cohen MA, Ellis SM, Le Roux CW, *et al.* Oxyntomodulin suppresses appetite and reduces food intake in humans. J Clin Endocrinol Metab 2003;88:4696-4701

[278] Stanley S, Wynne K, Bloom S. Gastrointestinal satiety signals III. Glucagon-like peptide 1, oxyntomodulin, peptide YY, and pancreatic polypeptide. Am J Physiol Gastrointest Liver Physiol 2004;286:6693-6697

[279] Konturek SJ, Konturek JW, Pawlik T, Brzozowski T. Brain-gut axis ant its role in the control of food intake. J Physiol Pharmacol 2004;55,1:137-154

[280] Dezaki K, Hosoda H, Kakei M, *et al.* Endogenous ghrelin in pancreatic islets restricts insulin release by attenuating Ca^{2+} signaling in beta cells: implication in the glycemic control in rodents. Diabetes 2004;53:3142-3151

[281] Jarrousse C, Bataille D, Jeanrenaud B. A pure enteroglucagon, oxyntomodulin (glucagon 37), stimulates insulin release in perfused rat pancreas. Endocrinol 1984;115,1:102-105

[282] Druce M, Ghatei M. Oxyntomodulin. Curr Opin Endocrinol Diabetes 2006;13,1:49-55

[283] Tatemoto K, Mutt V. Isolation of two novel candidate hormones using a chemical method for finding naturally occurring polypeptides. Nature 1980;285:417-418

[284] Hort Y, Baker E, Sutherland GR, Shine J, Herzog H. Gene duplication of the human peptide YY gene (PYY) generated the pancreatic polypeptide gene (PPY) on chromosome 17q21.1. Genomics 1995;26,1:77-83

[285] Tatemoto K. Isolation and characterization of peptide YY (PYY), a candidate gut hormone that inhibits pancreatic exocrine secretion. Proc Natl Acad Sci USA 1982;79:2514-2518

[286] Grandt D, Schimiczek M, Beglinger C, et al. Two molecular forms of peptide YY (PYY) are abundant in human blood: characterization of a radioimmunoassay recognizing PYY1-36 and PYY3-36. Regul Pept 1994;51:151-159

[287] McIntosh CH, Demuth H, Pospisilik JA, Pederson R. Dipeptidyl peptidase IV inhibitors: how do they work as new antibiotic agents? Regul Pept 2005;15,1:159-165

[288] Karra E, Chandarana K, Batterham RL. The role of peptide YY in appetite regulation and obesity. J Physiol 2009;587,1:19-25

[289] Dumont Y, Fournier A, St Pierre S, Quinion R. Characterization of neuropeptide Y binding sites in rat brain membrane preparations using [125I][Leu31,Pro34]peptide YY and [125I]peptide YY3-36 as selective Y1 and Y2 radioligands. J Pharmacol Exp Ther 1995;272:673-680

[290] Murphy KG, Bloom SR. Gut hormones and the regulation of energy homeostasis. Nature 2006;444:854-859

[291] Adrian TE, Ferri GL, Bacarese-Hamilton AJ, Fuessel HS, Polak JM, Bloom SR. Human distribution and release of a putative new gut hormone, peptide YY. Gastroenterol 1985;89:1070-1077

[292] Lin HC, Chey WY. Cholecystokinin and peptide YY are released by fat in either proximal or distal small intestine in dogs. Regul Pept 2003;114:131-135

[293] McGowan BMC, Bloom SR. Peptide YY and appetite control. Curr Opinion Pharmacol 2004,4:583-588

[294] Le Roux CW, Batterham RL, Aylwin SJ, et al. Attenuated peptide YY release in obese subjects is associated with reduced satiety. Endocrinol 2006;147:3-8

[295] Larhammar D. Structural diversity of receptors for neuropeptide Y, peptide YY and pancreatic polypeptide. Regular Pept 1996;65:165-174

[296] Batterham RL, Cowley MA, Small CJ, et al. Gut hormone PYY (3-36) physiologically inhibits food intake. Nature 2002;418:650-654

[297] Clark JT, Sahu A, Kalra PS, Balasubramaniam A, Kalra SP. Neuropeptide Y (NPY)-induced feeding behavior in female rats: comparison with human NPY ([Met17]NPY), NPY analog ([norLeu4]NPY) and peptide YY. Regul Pept 1987;17:31-39

[298] Stanley BG, Daniel DR, Chin AS, Leibowitz SF. Paraventricular nucleus injections of peptide YY and neuropeptide Y preferentially enhance carbohydrate ingestion. Peptides 1985;6:1205-1211

[299] Hagan MM, Castaneda E, Sumaya IC, Fleming SM, Galloway J, Moss DE. The effect of hypothalamic peptide YY on hippocampal acetylcholine release in vivo: implications for limbic function in binge-eating behavior. Brain Res 1998;805:20-28

[300] Corp ES, McQuade J, Krasnicki S, Conze DB. Feeding after fourth ventricular administration of neuropeptide Y receptor agonists in rats. Peptides 2001;22:493-499

[301] Bottcher G, Ahren B, Lundquist I, Sundler F. Peptide YY: intrapancreatic localization and effects on insulin and glucagon secretion in the mouse. Pancreas 1989;4,3:282-288

[302] Nieuwenhuizen AG, Karlsson S, Fridolf T, Ahren B. Mechanisms underlying the insulinostatic effect of peptide YY in mouse pancreatic islets. Diabetologia 1994;37:871-878

[303] Bertrand G, Gross R, Rove M, Ahren B, Ribes G. Evidence for a direct inhibitory effect of PYY on insulin secretion in rats. Pancreas 1992;5,5:595-560

[304] Boey D, Sainsbury A, Herzog H. The role of peptide YY in regulating glucose homeostasis. Peptides 2007;28:390-395

[305] Yoshinaga K, Mochizuki T, Yanaihara N, et al. Structural requirements of peptide YY for biological activity at enteric sites. Am J Physiol 1992;26:G695-G701

[306] Burcelin R, Brunner H, Seydoux J, Thorens B, Pedrazzini T. Increased insulin concentrations and glucagon storage in neuropeptide YY1 receptor-deficient mice. Peptides 2001;22,3:421-427

[307] Cho YR, Kim CW. Neuropeptide Y promotes beta-cell replication via extracellular signal-regulated kinase activation. Biochem Biophys Res Commun 2004;314,3:773-780

[308] Matsuda H, Brumovsky PR, Kopp J, Pedrazzini T, Hokfelt T. Distribution of neuropeptide Y Y1 receptors in rodent peripheral tissues. J Comp Neurol 2002;449,4:390-404

[309] Lynch DR, Walker MW, Miller RJ, Snyder SH. Neuropeptide Y receptor binding sites in rat brain: differential autoradiographic localizations with 125I-peptid YY and 125I-neuropeptide Y imply receptor heterogeneity. J Neurosci 1989;9:2616-2619

[310] Greeley GH, Lluis F, Gomez G, Ishizuka J, Holland B, Thorens JC. Peptide YY antagonizes β-adrenergic-stimulated release of insulin in dogs. Am J Physiol 1988;254:E513-E517

[311] Pittner R, Moore C, Bhavsar S, *et al.* Effects of PYY[3-36] in rodent models of diabetes and obesity. Int J Obes 2004;28,8:963-971

[312] van den Hoek AM, Heijboer AC, Corssmit EPM, *et al.* PYY3-36 reinforces insulin action on glucose disposal in mice fed a high-fat diet. Diabetes 2004;53:1949-1952

[313] Tatemoto K, Carlquist M, Mutt V. Neuropeptide Y – a novel brain peptide with structural similarities to peptide YY and pancreatic polypeptide. Nature 1982;296:659-660

[314] Larhammar D. Evolution of neuropeptide Y, peptide YY and pancreatic polypeptide. Regul Pept 1996;62:1-11

[315] Gehlert DR. Introduction to the reviews on neuropeptide Y. Neuropeptides 2004;38:135-140

[316] Cerda-Reverter JM, Larhammar D. Neuropeptide Y family of peptides: structure, anatomical expression, function, and molecular evolution. Biochem Cell Biol 2000;78:371-392

[317] Gehlert DR. Subtypes of receptors for neuropeptide Y: implications for the targeting of therapeutics. Life Sci 1994;55,8:551-562

[318] Ganguly PK. Neuropeptide Y receptors: future therapeutic target in congestive heart failure. J Health Sci 2000;46,6:430-433

[319] Cavadas C, Ribeiro CA, Cotrim M, Mosimann F, Brunner HR, Grouzmann E. Catecholamine and neuropeptide Y secretion from human adrenal chromaffin cells: effect of nicotine and KCl. Ann NY Acad Sci 2002;971:332-334

[320] Strand FL. Neuropeptides: regulators of physiological functions. MIT Press, MA 2000

[321] Sundler F, Böttcher G, Ekblad E, Håkanson R. PP, PYY and NPY – occurrence and distribution in the periphery. In: Colmers WF, Wahlestedt C (Eds.), The biology of neuropeptide Y and related peptides. Human Press Totowa NJ 1993:157-183

[322] Heilig M, Widerlov E. Neurobiology and clinical aspects of neuropeptide Y. Critical Rev Neurobiol 1995;9:115-136

[323] Ding WG, Kimura H, Fujimura M, Fujimiya M. Neuropeptide Y and peptide YY immunoreactivities in the pancreas of various vertebrates. Peptides 1997;18:1523-1529

[324] Myrsen U, Ahren B, Sundler F. Neuropeptide Y is expressed in subpopulations of insulin– and non-insulin-producing islet cells in the rat after dexamethasone treatment a combined immunocytochemical and *in situ* hybrydisation study. Regul Pept 1996;45:1306-1316

[325] Kamiji MM, Inui A. Neuropeptide Y receptor selective ligands in the treatment of obesity. Endocrine Rev 2007;26,6:664-684

[326] Park JJ, Lee HK, Shin MW, *et al.* Short-term cold exposure may cause a local decrease of neuropeptide Y in the rat hypothalamus. Mol Cells 2007;23:88-93

[327] Kalra SP, Kalra PS. NPY – an endearing journey in search of a neurochemical on/off switch for appetite, sex and reproduction. Peptides 2004;25:465-471

[328] Carvajal C, Dumont Y, Quirion R. Neuropeptide Y: role in emotion and alcohol dependence. CNS Neural Disord Drug Targets 2006;5:181-195

[329] Jacques D, Abdel-Samad D. Neuropeptide Y (NPY) and NPY receptors in the cardiovascular system: implication in the regulation of intracellular calcium. Can J Physiol Pharmacol 2007;85:43-53

[330] Sindelar DK, Palmiter RD, Woods SC, Schwartz MW. Attenuated feeding responses to circadian and palatability cues in mice lacking neuropeptide Y. Peptides 2005;26:2597-2602

[331] Krysiak R, Obuchowicz E, Herman ZS. Interactions between the neuropeptide Y system and the hypothalamic-pituitary-adrenal axis. Eur J Endocrinol 1999;140:130-136

[332] Beck B. Neuropeptide Y in normal eating and in genetic and dietary-induced obesity. Phil Trans R Soc B 2006;361:1159-1185

[333] Stanley BG, Leibowitz SF. Neuropeptide Y: stimulation of feeding and drinking by injection into the paraventricular nucleus. Life Sci 1984;35:2635-2642

[334] Flood JF, Morley JE. Increased food intake by neuropeptide Y is due to an increased motivation to eat. Peptides 1991;12:1329-1332

[335] Jewet DC, Cleary J, Levine AS, Schaal DW, Thompson T. Effects of neuropeptide Y, insulin, a 2-deoxyglucose, and food deprivation on food motivated behavior. Psychopharmacology 1995;120:267-271

[336] Lynch WC, Grace M, Billington CJ, Levine AS. Effects of Neuropeptide-Y on ingestion of flavored solutions in nondeprived rats. Physiol Behav 1993;54:877-880

[337] Ding WG, Kimura H, Fujimura M, Fujimiya M. Neuropeptide Y and peptide YY immunoreactivities in the pancreas of various vertebrates. Peptides 1997;18:1523-1529

[338] Moltz JH, McDonald JK. Neuropeptide Y: direct and indirect action on insulin secretion in the rat. Peptides 1985;6:1155-1159

[339] Pettersson M, Ahren B, Lundquist I, Bottcher G, Sundler F. Neuropeptide Y: intrapancreatic neuronal localization and effects on insulin secretion in the mouse. Cell Tissue Res 1987;248:43-48

[340] Bennet WM, Wang ZL, Jones PM, *et al.* Presence of neuropeptide Y and its messenger ribonucleic acid in human islets: evidence for a possible paracrine role. J Clin Endocrinol Metab 1996;81:2117-2120

[341] Imai Y, Patel HR, Hawkins EJ, Doliba NM, Matschinsky FM, Ahima RS. Insulin secretion is increased in pancreatic islets of neuropeptide Y-deficient mice. Endocrinol 2007;148,12:5716-5723

[342] Lindner D, Stichel J, Beck-Sickinger AG. Molecular recognition of the NPY hormone family by their receptors. Nutrition 2008;24:907-917

[343] Michel MC, Beck-Sickinger A, Cox H, *et al.* XVI. International Union of Pharmacology recommendations for the nomenclature of neuropeptide Y, peptide YY and pancreatic polypeptide receptors. Pharmacol Rev 1998;50,1:143-150

[344] Gerich J. Cryer PE, Rizza R. Hormonal mechanisms in acute glucose counterregulation: the relative roles of glucagon, epinephrine, norepinephrine, growth hormone and cortisol. Metabol 1980;29:1164-1175

[345] Cryer PE. Glucose counterregulation in man. Diabetes 1981;30:261-264

[346] Tappy L. Basics in clinical nutrition: Carbohydrate metabolism. E-SPEN Europ. e-J Clin Nutr Metab 2008;3:e192-e195

[347] Yamashima T. Jokichi Takamine (1854-1922), the samurai chemist, and his work on adrenalin. J Med Biogr 2003;11,2:95-102

[348] Bennett MR. One hundred years of adrenaline: the discovery of autoreceptors. Clin Auton Res 1999;9,3:145-159

[349] Berecek KH, Brody MJ. Evidence for a neurotransmitter role for epinephrine derived from the adrenal medulla. Heart Circul Physiol 1982;242,4:H593-601

[350] Li G, Xu J, Wang P, *et al.* Catecholamines regulate the activity, secretion, and synthesis of renalase. Circulation 2008;117:1277-1282

[351] Xu J, Li G, Wang P, *et al.* Renalase is a novel, soluble monoamine oxidase that regulates cardiac function and blood pressure. J Clin Invest 2005;115:1275-1280

[352] Koshimizu T, Yamauchi J, Hirasawa A, Tanoue A, Tsujimoto G. Recent progress in α_1-adrenoreceptor pharmacology. Biol Pharm Bull 2002;25,4:401-408

[353] Chen Z, Minneman KP. Recent progress in α_1-adrenoreceptor research. Acta Pharmacol Sin 2005;26,11:1281-1287

[354] Watt MJ, Howlett KF, Febbraio MA, Spriet LL, Hargreaves M. Adrenaline increases skeletal muscle glycogenolysis, pyruvate dehydrogenase activation and carbohydrate oxidation during moderate exercise in humans. J Physiol 2001;534,1:269-278

[355] Spriet LL, Ren JM, Hultman E. Epinephrine infusion enhances muscle glycogenolysis during prolonged electrical stimulation. J Appl Physiol 1988;64:1439-1444

[356] Febbraio MA, Lambert DL, Starkie RL, Proeitto J, Hargreaves M. Effect of epinephrine on muscle glycogenolysis during exercise in trained man. J Appl Physiol 1998;84:465-470

[357] Gray DE, Lickley HL, Vranic M. Physiologic effects of epinephrine on glucose turnover and plasma free fatty acid concentrations mediated independently of glucagon. Diabetes 1980;29:600-608

[358] Howlett K, Febbraio M, Hargreaves M. Glucose production during strenuous exercise in humans: role of epinephrine. Am J Physiol 1999;276:E1130-E1135

[359] Rizza RA, Cryer PE, Haymond MW, Gerich JE. Adrenergic mechanisms for the effects of epinephrine on glucose production and clearance in man. J Clin Invest 1980;65:682-689

[360] Sacca L, Morrone G, Cicala M, Corso G, Ungaro B. Influence of epinephrine, norepinephrine, and isoproterenol on glucose homeostasis in normal man. J Clin Endocrinol Metab 1980;50:680-684

[361] Hunt DG, Ivy JL. Epinephrine inhibits insulin-stimulated muscle glucose transport. J Appl Physiol 2002;93:1638-1643

[362] Nonogaki K. New insights into sympathetic regulation of glucose and fat metabolism. Diabetologia 2000;43:533-549

[363] Han XX, Bonen A. Epinephrine translocates GLUT-4 but inhibits insulin-stimulated glucose transport in rat muscle. Am J Physiol 1998;274:E700-E707

[364] Aslesen R, Jensen J. Effects of epinephrine on glucose metabolism in contracting rat skeletal muscles. Am J Physiol 1998;275:E448-E456

[365] Kreisman SH, Halter JB, Vranic M, Marliss EB. Combined infusion of epinephrine and norepinephrine during moderate exercise reproduces the glucoregulatory response of intense exercise. Diabetes 2003;52:1347-1354

[366] Kreisman SH, Mew NA, Arsenault M, *et al.* Epinephrine infusion during moderate intensity exercise increases glucose production and uptake. Am J Physiol Endocrinol Metab 2000;278:E949-E957

[367] Howlett K, Galbo H, Lorentsen J, *et al.* Effect of adrenaline on glucose kinetics during exercise in adrenalectomised humans. J Physiol 1999;519,3:911-921

[368] Doenst T, Taegtmeyer H. α-adrenergic stimulation mediates glucose uptake through phosphatidylinositol 3-kinase in rat heart. Circ Res 1999;84:467-474

[369] Huang MT, Lee CF, Dobson GP. Epinephrine enhances glycogen turnover and depresses glucose uptake *in vivo* in rat heart. FASEB J 1997;11:973-980

[370] Gromada J, Bokvist K, Ding W-G, *et al.* Adrenaline stimulates glucagon secretion in pancreatic A-cells by increasing the Ca^{2+} current and the number of granules close to the L-type Ca^{2+} channels. J Gen Physiol 1997;110:217-228

[371] Ullrich S, Wollheim CB. GTP-dependent inhibition of insulin secretion by epinephrine in permeabilized RINm5F cells: lack of correlation between insulin secretion and cyclic AMP levels. J Biol Chem 1988;263:8615-8620

[372] Peterhoff M, Sieg A, Brede M, Chao C-M, Hein L, Ullrich S. Inhibition of insulin secretion via distinct signaling pathways in α$_2$-adrenoceptor knockout mice. Europ J Endocrinol 2003;149:343-350

[373] Renström E, Ding WG, Bokvist K, Rorsman P. Neurotransmitter-induced inhibition of exocytosis in insulin-secreting β cells by activation of calcineurin. Neuron 1996;17:513-522

[374] Chernogubova E, Cannon B, Bengtsson T. Norepinephrine increases glucose transport in brown adipocytes via β$_3$-adrenoceptors through a cAMP, PKA and PI3-kinase-dependent pathway stimulating conventional and novel PKCs. Endocrinol 2004;145:269-280

[375] Kanda Y, Watanabe Y. Adrenaline increases glucose transport via a Rap1-p38MAPK pathway in rat vascular smooth muscle cells. Br J Pharmacol 2007;151:476-482

[376] Mulder AH, Tack CJ, Olthaar AJ, Smits P, Sweep FCGJ, Bosch RR. Adrenergic receptor stimulation attenuates insulin-stimulated glucose uptake in 3T3-L1 adipocytes by inhibiting GLUT4 translocation. Am J Physiol Endocrinol Metab 2005;289:E627-E633

[377] Ferrer JC, Favre C, Gomiss RR, *et al.* Control of glycogen deposition. FEBS Lett 2003;546:127-132

[378] Snell K. Regulation of hepatic glucose metabolism by insulin and counter-regulatory hormones. Proc Nutr Soc 1991;50:567-575

[379] Girard JR, Cuendet GS, Marliss EB, Kervran A, Rieutort M, Assan R. Fuels, hormones, and liver metabolism at term and during the early postnatal period in the rat. J Clin Invest 1073;52:3190-3200

[380] Snell K, Walker DG. Glucose metabolism in the newborn rat: temporal studies in vivo. Biochem J 1973;132:739-752

[381] Sperling MA, Ganguli S, Leslie N, Landt K. Fetal-perinatal catecholamine secretion: role in perinatal glucose homeostasis. Am J Physiol 1984;247:E69-E74

[382] Kim K, Cho SC, Cova A, Jang IS, Park SC. Alterations of epinephrine-induced gluconeogenesis in aging. Exptl Mol Med 2009;41,5:334-340

[383] Blair JB, James ME, Foster JL. Adrenergic control of glucose output and adenosine 3',5'-monophosphate levels in hepatocytes from juvenile and adult rats. J Biol Chem 1979;254:7579-7584

[384] Burnol AF, Letarque A, Ferré P, Girard J. Glucose metabolism during lactation in the rat: quantitative and regulatory aspects. Am J Physiol 1983;245:7579-7584

[385] Baltrusch S, Tiedge M. Glucokinase regulatory network in pancreatic β-cells and liver. Diabetes 2006;55,Suppl.2:S55-S64

[386] Shimazu T, Fukuda A. Increased activities of glucogenolytic enzymes in liver after splanchnic-nerve stimulation. Science 1965;150:1607-1608

[387] Shimazu T. Glycogen synthetase activity in liver: regulation by the autonomic nerves. Science 1967;156:1256-1257

[388] Uyama N, Geerts A, Reynaert H. Neural connections between the hypothalamus and the liver. Anat Rec A Discov Mol Cell Evol Biol 2004;280,1:808-820

[389] Shimazu T. Reciprocal innervation of the liver: its significance in metabolic control. Adv Metab Disord 1983;10:355-384

[390] Shimazu T. Neuronal regulation of hepatic glucose metabolism in mammals. Diabetes Metab Rev 1987;3:185-206

[391] Shimazu T, Ogasawara S. Effects of hypothalamic stimulation on gluconeogenesis and glycolysis in rat liver. Am J Physiol 1975;228:1787-1793

[392] Shimazu T, Amakawa A. Regulation of glycogen metabolism in liver by the autonomic nervous system: VI, possible mechanism of phosphorylase activation by the splenchnic nerve. Biochim Biophys Acta 1075;385:242-256

[393] Sakaguchi T, Iwanaga M. Effects of D-glucose anomers on afferent discharge in the hepatic vagus nerve. Experientia 1982;38:475-476

[394] Torii K, Niijima A. Effect of lysine on afferent activity of the hepatic branch of the vagus nerve in normal and L-lysine-deficient rats. Physiol Behav 2001;72:685-690

[395] Randich A, Spraggins DS, Cox JE, Meller ST, Kelm GR. Jejunal or portal vein infusion of lipids increase hepatic vagal afferent activity. Neuroreport 2001;12:3101-3105

[396] Takahashi A, Ishimaru H, Ikarashi Y, Kishi E, Maruyama Y. Effects of hepatic nerve stimulation on blood glucose and glycogenolysis in rat liver: studies with *in vivo* microdialisis. J Auton Nerv Syst 1996;61:181-185

[397] Vatamaniuk MZ, Horyn OV, Vatamaniuk OK, Doliba NM. Acetylcholine affects rat liver metabolism via type 3 muscarinic receptors in hepatocytes. Life Sci 2003;72:1871-1882

[398] Laloux M, Stalmans W, Hers HG. On the mechanism by which glucocorticoids cause the activation of glycogen synthase in mouse and rat livers. Eur J Biochem 1983;136:175-181

[399] Livingston JN, Lockwood DH. Effect of glucocorticoids on the glucose transporter system of isolated fat cells. J Biol Chem 1975;250:8353-8360

[400] Smith OL, Wong CY, Gelfand RA. Influence of glucocorticoids on skeletal muscle proteolysis in normal and diabetic-adrenalectonized eviscerated rats. Metabolism 1990;39:641-646

[401] Muller MJ, Thomsen A, Sibrowski W, Seitz HJ. 3,5,3'-triiodothyronine-induced synthesis of rat liver phosphoenolpyruvate carboxykinase. Endocrinol 1982;111:1469-1475

[402] Arrondo JL, Artetxe J, Sancho MJ, Macarulla JM. Liver glycogen metabolism in chicken: activation prior to triiodothyronine-induced protein synthesis enhancement. Horm Metab Res 1981;13:92-94

[403] Shahen O, Morgan DW, Wilcox HG, Keyes WS, Heimberg M. Modulation by thyroid status of the actions of glucagon and dibutyryl adenosine 3',5'-monophosphate on metabolism of free fatty acids by the isolated perfused rat liver. Endocrinol 1982;110:1740-1748

[404] Muller MJ, Seitz HJ. Interaction of thyroid hormones and cyclic AMP in the stimulation of hepatic gluconeogenesis. Biochem Biophys Acta 1983;756:360-368

[405] Nebioglu S, Wathanaronchai P, Nebioglu D, Pruden EL, Gibson DM. Mechanisms underlying enhanced glycogenolysis in livers of 3,5,3'-triiodothyronine-treated rats. Am J Physiol 1990;258:E109-E116

[406] Beauville M, Harant I, Crampes F, et al. Effect of long-term rhGH administration in GH-deficient adults of fat cell epinephrine response. Am J Physiol 1992;263:E467-E472

[407] Yin D, Clarke SD, Peters JL, Etherton TD. Somatotropin-dependent decrease in fatty acid synthase mRNA abundance in 3T3-F442A adipocytes is the result of a decrease in both gene transcription and mRNA stability. Biochem J 1998;331,(Pt3):815-820

[408] Gerich JE, Meyer C, Waerle HJ, Stumvoll M. Renal gluconeogenesis: its importance in human glucose homeostasis. Diabetes Care 2001;24,2:382-391

[409] Schoolwerth A, Smith B, Culpepper R. Renal gluconeogenesis. Miner Electrolyte Metab 1988;14:347-361

[410] Wirthensohn G, Guder W. Renal substrate metabolism. Physiol Rev 1986;66:469-497

[411] Cahill G. Starvation in man. N Engl J Med 1970;282:668-675

[412] Cano N. Bench-to-bedside review: Glucose production from the kidney. Critical Care 2002;6:317-321

[413] Meyer C, Stumvoll M, Welle S, Kreider M, Nair S, Gerich J. Human kidney substrate utilization and gluconeogenesis. Diabetologia 1974;40,Suppl.1:A24

[414] Stumvoll M, Meyer C, Perriello G, Kreider M, Welle S, Gerich J. Human kidney and liver gluconeogenesis: evidence for organ substrate selectivity. Am J Physiol 1998;274:E817-E826

[415] Cersosimo E, Judd R, Miles J. Insulin regulation of renal glucose metabolism in conscious dogs. J Clin Invest 1994;93:2584-2589

[416] Cersosimo E, Garlick P, Ferretti J. Regulation of splenchnic and renal substrate supply by insulin in humans. Metabolism 2000;49:676-683

[417] McGuinness O, Fugiwara T, Muyrell S, et al. Impact of chronic stress hormone infusion on hepatic carbohydrate metabolism in the conscious dogs. Am J Physiol 1993;265:E314-E322

[418] Stumvoll M, Meyer C, Kreider M, Perriello G, Gerich J. Effects of glucagon on renal and hepatic glutamine gluconeogenesis in normal postabsorptive humans. Metabolism 1998;47:1227-1232

[419] Stumvoll M, Meyer C, Parriello G, Kreider M, Welle S, Gerich J. Human kidney and liver gluconeogenesis: evidence for organ substrate selectivity. Am J Physiol 1998;274:E817-E826

[420] Corbett SW, Kaufman LN, Keesey RE. Thermogenesis after lateral hypothalamic lesions: contributions of brown adipose tissue. Am J Physiol 1988;255:E708-E715

[421] Williams G, Bing C, Cai XJ, et al. The hypothalamus and the control of energy homeostasis: different circuits, different purposes. Physiol Behav 2001;74:683-701

[422] Nieuwenhuizen AG, Rutters F. The hypothalamic-pituitary-adrenal-axis in the regulation of energy balance. Physiol Behav 2008;94:169-177

[423] Walker CA, Clark AM, Hewison M, Reide JP, Stewart PM. Functional expression, characterization, and purification of the catalytic domain of human 11-β-hydroxysteroid dehydrogenase type 1. J Biol Chem 2001;276:21343-21350

[424] Draper N, Stewart PM. 11 β-hydroxysteroid dehydrogenase and the prereceptor regulation of corticosteroid hormone action. J Endocrinol 2005;186:251-257

[425] Kawai A, Kuzuya N. Effects of glucocorticoids on hormone-stimulated lipolysis and calcium uptake in the adipose cells. Horm Metab Res 1981;13:224-228

[426] Pilkis SJ, Granner DK. Molecular physiology of the regulation of hepatic gluconeogenesis and glycolysis. Annu Rev Physiol 1992;54:885-909

[427] Ruzzin J, Wagman AS, Jensen J. Glucocorticoid-induced insulin resistance in skeletal muscles: defects in insulin signalling and the effects of a selective glycogen synthase kinase-3 inhibitor. Diabetologia 2005;48:2119-2130

[428] Rooney DP, Neely RDG, Cullen C, Ennis CN, Sheridan B, Atkinson AB. The effect of cortisol on glucose/glucose-6-phosphate cycle activity and insulin action. J Clin Endocrinol Metab 1994;77:1180-1183

[429] Rizza RA, Mandarino LJ, Gerich J. Cortisol-induced insulin resistance in man: impaired suppression of glucose production and stimulation of glucose utilization due t a postreceptor defect of insulin action. J Clin Endocrinol Metab 1982;54:131-138

[430] Oda N, Nakai A, Mokuno T, *et al.* Dexamethasone-induced changes in glucose transporter 4 in rat heart muscle, skeletal muscle and adipocytes. Eur J Endocrinol 1995;133:121-126

[431] Coderre L, Vallega GA, Pilch PF, Chipkin SR. *In vivo* effects of dexamethasone and sucrose on glucose transport (GLUT-4) protein tissue distribution. Am J Physiol 1996;271:E643-E648

[432] Owen OE, Cahill Jr GF. Metabolic effects on exogenous glucocorticoids in fasted man. J Clin Invest 1973;52:2596-2605

[433] Weinstein SP, Paquin T, Pritsker A, Haber RS. Glucocorticoid-induced insulin resistance: dexamethasone inhibits the activation of glucose transport in rat skeletal muscle by both insulin- and non-insulin-related stimuli. Diabetes 1995;44:441-445

[434] Harris HJ, Kotelevtsev Y, Mullins JJ, Seckl JR, Holmes MC. Intracellular regeneration of glucocorticoids by 11 β-hydroxysteroid dehydrogenase (11 β-HSD)-1 plays a key role in the regulation of the hypothalamic-pituitary-adrenal axis: analysis of 11 β-HSD-1-deficient mice. Endocrinol 2001;142:114-120

[435] Seckl JR, Walker BR. Minireview: 11 β-hydroxysteroid dehydrogenase type 1 – a tissue specific amplifier of glucocorticoid action. Endocrinol 2001;142:1371-1376

[436] Ekstrand A, Saloranta C, Ahonen J, Gronhagen-Riska C, Groop LC. Reversal of steroid-induced insulin resistance by a nicotinic-acid derivative in man. Metabol 1992;41:692-697

[437] Guillaume-Gentil C, Assimacopoulos-Jeannet F, Jeanrenaud B. Involvement of non-esterified fatty acid oxidation in glucocorticoid-induced peripheral insulin resistance *in vivo* in rats. Diabetologia 1993;36:899-906

[438] Delaunay F, Khan A, Cintra A, *et al.* Pancreatic beta cells are important targets for the diabetogenic effects of glucocorticoids. J Clin Invest 1997; 100:2094-2098

[439] Lambillotte C, Gilon P, Henquin J-C. Direct glucocorticoid inhibition of insulin secretion: an *in vitro* study of dexamethasone effects in mouse islets. J Clin Invest 1997;99:414-423

[440] Stubbs M, York DA. Central glucocorticoid regulation of parasympathetic drive to pancreatic β-cells in obese fa/fa rats. Int J Obes 1991;15:547-553

[441] Andrews RC, Walker BR. Glucocorticoids and insulin resistance: old hormones, new targets. Clin Sci 1999;96:513-523

[442] Sainsbury A, Cooney GJ, Herzog H. Hypothalamic regulation pf energy homeostasis. Best Pract Res Clin Endocrinol Metab 2002;16,4:623-637

[443] Silva JE. The thermogenic effect of thyroid hormone and its clinical implications. Ann Intern Med 2003;139:205-213

[444] Lechan RM, Hollenberg A. Thyrotropin-releasing hormone (TRH). In: Henry HL, Norman AW ed. Encyclopedia of hormones. Academic Press 2003:510-524

[445] Persani L. Hypothalamic thyrotropin-releasing hormone and thyrotropin biological activity. Thyroid 1998;8:941-946

[446] Chin WW, Carr FE, Burnside J, Darling DS. Thyroid hormone regulation of thyrotropin gene expression. Recent Prog Horm Res 1993;48:393-414

[447] Lechan RM. Update on thyrotropin-releasing hormone. Thyroid Today 1993;16:1-12

[448] Freeman ME, Kanyicska B, Lerant A, Nagy G. Prolactin: structure, function, and regulation of secretion. Physiol Rev 2000;80:1523-1631

[449] Yu R, Ashworth R, Hinkle PM. Receptors for thyrotropin-releasing hormone on rat lactotropes and thyrotropes. Thyroid 1998;8:887-894

[450] Fekete C, Lechan RM. Neuroendocrine implications for the association between cocaine- and amphetamine regulated transcript (CART) and hypophysiotropic thyrotropin-releasing hormone (TRH). Peptides 2006;27:2012-2018

[451] Lechan RM, Fekete C. Role of melanocortin signaling in the regulation of the hypothalamic-pituitary-thyroid (HPT) axis. Peptides 2006;27:310-325

[452] Fliers E, Wiersinga WM, Swaab DF. Physiological and pathophysiological aspects of thyrotropin-releasing hormone gene expression in the human hypothalamus. Thyroid 1998;8:921-928

[453] Dahl GE, Evans NP, Thrun LA, Karsch FJ. A central negative feedback action of thyroid hormones on thyrotropin-releasing hormone secretion. Endocrinol 1994;135:2392-2397

[454] Lechan RM, Kakucska I. Feedback regulation of thyrotropin-releasing hormone gene expression by thyroid hormone in the hypothalamic paraventricular nucleus. Ciba Found Symp 1992;168:144-158

[455] Sawin CT, Hershman JM, Chopra IJ. The comparative effect of T4 and T3 on the TSH response to TRH in young adult men. J Clin Endocrinol Metab 1977;44:273-278

[456] Braverman LE, Ingbar SH, Sterling K. Conversion of thyroxine (T4) to triiodothyronine (T3) in athyreotic human subjects. J Clin Invest 1970;49:855-864

[457] Robbins J. Thyroxine transport and the free hormone hypothesis. Endocrinol 1992;131:546-547

[458] Oppenheimer JH, Koerner D, Schwartz HL, Surks MI. Specific nuclear triiodothyronine binding sites in rat liver and kidney. J Clin Endocrinol Metab 1972;35:330-333

[459] Brent GA. The molecular basis of thyroid hormone action. N Engl J Med 1994;331,13:847-853

[460] Lazar MA. Thyroid hormone action: a binding contract. J Clin Invest 2003;112:497-499

[461] Lazar MA. Thyroid hormone receptors: multiple forms, multiple possibilities. Endocr Rev 1993;14:184-193

[462] Thompson CC, Weinberger C, Lebo R, Evans RM. Identification of a novel thyroid hormone receptor expressed in the mammalian central nervous system. Science 1987;237:1610-1614

[[463] Lazar MA, Chin WW. Nuclear thyroid hormone receptors. J Clin Invest 1990;86:1777-1782

[464] Baig M, Azhar A, Zaidi P, Khan S. Serum leptin and pituitary thyroid axis in hyperthyroid male patients. Pak J Med Res 2006;45,3

[465] Iacobellis G, Ribaudo MC, Zappaterreno A, Iannucci CV, Leonetti F. Relationship of thyroid function with body mass index, leptin, insulin sensitivity and adiponectin in euthyroid obese women. Clin Endocrinol 2005;62:487-491

[466] Näslund E, Andersson I, Degerblad M, et al. Association of leptin, insulin resistance and thyroid function with long-term weight loss in dieting obese men. J Intern Med 2000;248:299-308

[467] Chidakel A, Mentuccia D, Celi FS. Peripheral metabolism of thyroid hormone and glucose homeostasis. Thyroid 2005;15:899-903

[468] Granner DK, Pilkis S. The genes of hepatic glucose metabolism. J Biol Chem 1990;265:10173-10182

[469] Groot LJ, Jameson JL. Mechanism of thyroid hormone action. In: Endocrinology. 3rd ed. Degroot LJ Ed. Philadelphia, WB Saunders 1995:583-601

[470] Kim SR, Talbott EA, Tull E, Vogt M, Andersen S, Kuller LH. Contribution of abnormalities of thyroid hormones to type 2 diabetes. Diabetes Care 2000;23,2:260-261

[471] Viguerie N, Millet L, Aizou S, Vidal H, Larrouy D, Langin D. Regulation of human adipocyte gene expression by thyroid hormone. J Clin Endocrinol Metab 2002;87:630-644

[472] Koritschoner NP, Alvarez-Dolado M, Kurz SM, et al. Thyroid hormone regulates the obesity gene tub. EMBO Rep 2001;2:499-504

[473] Torrance CJ, Devente JE, Jones JP, Dohm GL. Effects of thyroid hormone on GLUT4 glucose transporter gene expression and NIDDM in rats. Endocrinol 1997;138:1204-1214

[474] Casla A, Rovira A, Wells JA, Dohm GL. Increased glucose transporter (GLUT4) protein expression in hyperthyroidism. Biochem Biophys Res Commun 1990;171:182-188

[475] Weinstein SP, O'Boyle E, Haber RS. Thyroid hormone increases basal and insulin-stimulated glucose transport in skeletal muscle. Diabetes 1994;43:1185-1189

[476] Weinstein SP, Watts J, Haber R. Thyroid hormone increases muscle/fat glucose transporter gene expression in rat skeletal muscle. Endocrinol 1991;129:455-464

[477] Klieverik LP, Janssen SF, van Riel A, et al. Thyroid hormone modulates glucose production via a sympathetic pathway from the hypothalamic paraventricular nucleus to the liver. PNAS 2009;106,14:5966-5971

[478] Chidakel A, Mentuccia D, Celi FS. Peripheral metabolism of thyroid hormone and glucose homeostasis. Thyroid 2005;15,8:899-903

[479] Comte B, Vidal H, Laville M, Riou J-P. Influence of thyroid hormones on gluconeogenesis from glycerol in rat hepatocytes: A dose-response study. Metabol 1990;39,3:259-263

[480] Franklyn JA. Metabolic changes in thyrotoxicosis. The Thyroid: A Fundamental and Clinical Text, eds Braverman LE, Utiger RD (Lippincott Williams & Wilkins, Philadelphia), 8th Ed 2000:667-672

[481] Dimitriadis GD, Raptis SA. Thyroid hormone excess and glucose intolerance. Exp Clin Endocrinol Diabetes 2001;109,Suppl.2:S225-S239

[482] Galofré JC, Pujante P, Abreu C, et al. Relationship between thyroid-stimulating hormone and insulin in euthyroid obese man. Ann Nutr Metab 2008;53:188-194

[483] Davidson MB. Effect of growth hormone on carbohydrate and lipid metabolism. Endocr Rev 1987;8:115-131

[484] Press M. Growth hormone and metabolism. Diabetes Metab Rev 1988;4:391-414

[485] Baumann G. Growth hormone heterogeneity: genes, isohormones, variants, and binding proteins. Endocr Rev 1991;12:424-449

[486] Baumann G. Growth hormone binding protein. The soluble growth hormone receptor. Minerva Endocrinol 2002;27:265-276

[487] Frantz AG, Rabkin MT. Effects of estrogen and sex difference on secretion of human growth hormone. J Clin Endocrinol 1965;25,11:1470-1480

[488] Plotnick LP, Thompson RC, Kowarski A, De Lacerda L, Migeon CJ, Blizzard RM. Circadian variation of integrated concentration of growth hormone in children and adults. J Clin Endocrinol Metab 1975;402:240-247

[489] Veldhuis JD, Roemmich JN, Richmond EJ, Bowers CY. Somatotropic and gonadotropic axes linkages in infancy, childhood, and the puberty-adult transition. Endocr Rev 2006;27:101-140

[490] Emerson MR. The central endocrine glands: interwining physiology and pharmacy. Am J Pharm Edu 2007;71,5:1-8

[491] Ross RJM. Growth hormone secretion: its regulation and the influence of nutritional factors. Nutr Res Rev 1990;3:143-162

[492] Frohman LA, Jansson JO. Growth hormone-releasing hormone. Endocr Rev 1986;7:223-253

[493] Barinaga M, Bilezikjian LM, Vale WW, Rosenfeld MG, Evans RM. Independent effects of growth hormone releasing factor on growth hormone release and gene transcription. Nature 1985;314:279-281

[494] Clemmons DR, Underwood LE. Nutritional regulation of IGF-I and IGF binding proteins. Annu Rev Nutr 1991;11:393-412

[495] Molitch ME. Neuroendocrinology. In: Feling P, Baxter JD, Frohman LA eds. Endocrinology and Metabolism. New York: McGraw-Hill 1995:221-288

[496] Holt RIG, Simpson HL, Sönksen PH. The role of the growth hormone-insulin-like growth factor axis in glucose homeostasis. Diabet Med 2003;20:3-15

[497] O'Sullivan LA, Liongue C, Lewis RS, Stephenson SE, Ward AC. Cytokine receptor signaling through the Jak-Stat-Socs pathway in disease. Mol Immunol 2007;44:2497-2506

[498] Kelly PA, Djiane J, Postel-Vinay MC, Edery M. The prolactin/growth hormone receptor family. Endocr Rev 1991;12:235-251

[499] Møller N, Jørgensen JOL. Effects of growth hormone on glucose, lipid, and protein metabolism in human subjects. Endocr Rev 2009;30,2:152-177

[500] Lanning NJ, Carter-Su C. Recent advances in growth hormone signaling. Rev Endocr Metab Disord 2006;7:225-235

[501] Wormald S, Hilton DJ. Inhibitors of cytokine signal transduction. J Biol Chem 2004;279:821-824

[502] Møller N, Vendelbo MH, Kapmann U, *et al.* Growth hormone and protein metabolism. Clin Nutr 2009;28:597-603

[503] Bak JF, Møller N, Schmitz O. Effects of growth hormone on fuel utilization and muscle glycogen synthase activity in normal humans. Am J Physiol 1991;260:E736-E742

[504] Press M, Tamborlane WV, Sherwin RS. Importance of raised growth hormone levels in mediating the metabolic derangements of diabetes. N Engl J Med 1984;310:810-815

[505] Fowelin J, Attval S, von Schenck H, Smith U, Lager I. Characterization of the insulin-antagonistic effect of growth hormone in insulin-dependent diabetes mellitus. Diabet Med 1995;12:990-996

[506] Fowelin J, Attval S, von Schenck H, Smith U, Lager I. Characterization of the insulin-antagonistic effect of growth hormone in man. Diabetologia 1991;34:500-506

[507] Randle PJ, Hales CN, Garland PB, Newsholme EA. The glucose fatty acid cycle. Its role in insulin sensitivity and the metabolic disturbance of diabetes mellitus. Lancet 1963;1:785-789

[508] Ferrannini E, Barrett EJ, Bevilacqua S, DeFronzo RA. Effect of fatty acids on glucose production and utilization in man. J Clin Invest 1983;72:1737-1747

[509] Busiquina S, Argente J, Garcia-Segura LM, Chowen JA. Anatomically specific changes in the expression of somatostatin, growth hormone-releasing hormone and growth hormone receptor mRNA in diabetic rats. J Neuroendocrinol 2000;12,1:29-39

[510] Gonzalez C, Jolin T. Effect of streptozotocin diabetes and insulin replacement on growth hormone in rats. J Endocrinol Invest 1985;8:7-11

[511] Olchovsky D, Bruno JF, Wood TL, *et al.* Altered pituitary growth hormone (GH) regulation in streptozotocin-diabetic rats: a combined defect of hypothalamic somatostatin and GH-releasing factor. Endocrinol 1990;126,1:53-61

[512] Amiel SA, Sherwin RS, Hintz RL, Gertner JM, Press GM, Tamborlane WV. Effect of diabetes and its control on insulin-like growth factors in the young subjects with type 1 diabetes. Diabetes 1984;33:1175-1179

[513] Hansen AP, Johansen K. Diurnal patterns of blood glucose, serum free fatty acids, insulin, glucagon and growth hormone in normals and juvenile diabetics. Diabetologia 1970;6:27-33

[514] Johnston DG, Davies RR, Prescott RWG. Regulation of growth hormone secretion in man: a review. J Royal Soc Med 1985;78:319-327

[515] Serné EH, de Jonhg RT, Eringa EC, Ijzerman RG, Stehouwer CDA. Microvascular dysfunction. A potential pathophysiological role in the metabolic syndrome. Hypertension 2007;50:204-211

[516] Jonk AM, Houben AJHM, de Jongh RT, Serné EH, Schaper NC, Stehouwer CDA. Microvascular dysfunction in obesity: a potential mechanism in the pathogenesis of obesity-associated insulin resistance and hypertension. Physiol 2007;22:252-260

[517] Verdant C, De Backer D. How monitoring of the microcirculation may help us at the bedside. Curr Opin Crit Care 2005;11:240-244

[518] DeFronzo RA, Ferrennini E, Sato Y, Felig P, Wahren J. Synergistic interaction between exercise and insulin on peripheral glucose uptake. J Clin Invest 1981;68:1468-1474

[519] Baron AD, Tarshoby M, Hook G et al. Interaction between insulin sensitivity and muscle perfusion on glucose uptake in human skeletal muscle. Evidence for capillary recruitment. Diabetes 2000;49:768-774

[520] Steinberg HO, Chaker H, Leaming R, Johnson A, Brechtel G, Baron AD. Obesity/insulin resistance is associated with endothelial dysfunction. Implications for the syndrome of insulin resistance. J Clin Invest 1996;97:2601-2610

[521] Baron A. Hemodynamic actions of insulin. Am J Physiol 1994;267:E187-E202

[522] Baron AD, Laakso M, Brechtel G, Edelman SV. Mechanism of insulin resistance in insulin-dependent diabetes mellitus: a major role for reduced skeletal muscle blood flow. J Clin Endocrinol Metab 1991;73:637-643

[523] Laakso M, Edelman SV, Brechtel G, Baron AD. Decreased effect of insulin to stimulate skeletal muscle blood flow in obese man. J Clin Invest 1990;85:1844-1852

[524] Laakso M, Edelman SV, Brechtel G, Baron AD. Impaired insulin-mediated skeletal muscle blood flow in patients with NIDDM. Diabetes 1992;41:1076-1083

[525] Yki-Jarvinen H, Utriainen T. Insulin-induced vasodilation: physiology or pharmacology? Diabetologia 1998;41:369-379

[526] Taddei S, Virdis A, Mattei P, Natali A, Ferrannini E, Salvetti A. Effect of insulin on acetylcholine-induced vasodilation in normotensive subjects and patients with essential hypertension. Circulation 1995;92:2911-2918

[527] Nuutila P, Raitakari M, Laine H, et al. Role of blood flow in regulating insulin-stimulated glucose uptake in humans: studies using bradykinin, [^{15}O] water, [^{18}F] fluoro-deoxyglucose and positron emission tomography. J Clin Invest 1996;97:1741-1747

[528] Zhang L, Vincent MA, Richards SM, et al. Insulin sensitivity of muscle capillary recruitment in vivo. Diabetes 2004;53:447-453

[529] Rattigan S, Clark MG, Barrett EJ. Hemodynamic actions of insulin in rat skeletal muscle: evidence for capillary recruitment. Diabetes 1997;46:1381-1388

[530] Clark MG, Wallis MG, Barret EJ, et al. Capillary recruitment and its role in metabolic regulation: a focus on insulin action in skeletal muscle. Am J Physiol 2003;284:E241-E258

[531] Grubb B, Snarr JF. Effect of flow rate on glucose concentration on glucose uptake rate by the rat limb. Proc Soc Exp Biol Med 1977;154:33-36

[532] Schultz TA, Lewis SB, Westbie DK, Gerich JE, Rushakoff RJ, Wallin JD. Glucose-delivery – a clarification of its role in regulating glucose uptake in rat skeletal muscle. Life Sci 1977;20:733-735

[533] Sobrevia L, Nadal A, Yudilevich DL, Mann GE. Activation of L-arginine transport (system y+) and nitric oxide synthase by elevated glucose and insulin in human endothelial cells. J Physiol 1996;490:775-781

[534] Zeng GY, Quon MJ. Insulin-stimulated production of nitric oxide is inhibited by wortmannin – directs measurement in vascular endothelial cells. J Clin Invest 1996;98:894-898

[535] Scherrer U, Randin D, Vollenweider L, Nicod P. Nitric oxide release accounts for insulin's vascular effects in humans. J Clin Invest 1994;94:2511-2515

[536] Vincent MA, Dawson D, Clark AD, et al. Skeletal muscle microvascular recruitment by physiological hyperinsulinemia precedes increases in total blood flow. Diabetes 1002;51:42-48

[537] Baron AD, Brechtel-Hook G, Johnson A, Cronin J, Leaming R, Steinberg HO. Effect of perfusion rate on the time course of insulin-mediated skeletal muscle glucose uptake. Am J Physiol 1996;271:E1067-E1072

[538] Steinberg HO, Brechtel G, Johnson A, Fineberg N, Baron AD. Insulin-mediated skeletal muscle vasodilation is nitric oxide dependent. A novel action of insulin to increase nitric oxide release. J Clin Invest 1994;94:1172-1179

[539] Kobzik L, Reid M, Bredt D, Stamler J. Nitric oxide in skeletal muscle. Nature 1994;372:546-548

[540] Silvagno F, Xia H, Bredt D. Neuronal nitric-oxide synthase-mu, an alternatively spliced isoform expressed in differentiated skeletal muscle. J Biol Chem 1996;271:11204-11208

[541] Segal SS, Brett SE, Sessa WC. Codistribution of NOS and caveolin throughout peripheral vasculature and skeletal muscle in hamsters. Am J Physiol 1999;277:H1167-H1177

[542] Vincent MA, Clerk LH, Lindner JR, *et al.* Microvascular recruitment is an early insulin effect that regulates skeletal muscle glucose uptake in vivo. Diabetes 2004;53:1418-1423

[543] Vincent MA, Barrett EJ, Lindner JR, Clark MG, Rattigan S. Inhibiting NOS blocks microvascular recruitment and blunts muscle glucose uptake in response to insulin. Am J Physiol 2003;285:E123-E129

[544] Kim JA, Montagnani M, Koh KK, Quon MJ. Reciprocal relationship between insulin resistance and endothelial dysfunction: molecular and pathophysiological mechanisms. Circulation 2006;113:1888-1904

[545] Clark MG, Wallis MG, Barrett EJ, *et al.* Blood flow and muscle metabolism: a focus on insulin action. Am J Physiol Endocrinol Metab 2003;284:E241-E258

[546] Caballero AE, Arora S, Saouaf R, *et al.* Microvascular and macrovascular reactivity is reduced in subjects at risk for type 2 diabetes. Diabetes 1999;48:1856-1862

[547] Clark MG. Impaired microvascular perfusion: a consequence of vascular dysfunction and a potential cause of insulin resistance in muscle. Am J Physiol Endocrinol Metab 2008;295:E732-E750

[548] King KD, Jones JD, Warthen J. Microvascular and macrovascular complications in diabetes. Am J Pharm Edu 2005;69,5,Art87:1-10

[549] Iin SM, Noh CI, Yang SW, *et al.* Endothelial dysfunction and microvascular complications in type 1 diabetes mellitus. J Korean Med Sci 2008;23:77-82

[550] Arrais RF, Dib SA. The hypothalamus-pituitary-ovary axis and type 1 diabetes mellitus: a minireview. Human Reprod 2006;21,2:327-337

[551] Godsland IF. Oestrogens and insulin secretion. Diabetologia 2005;48:2213-2220

[552] Wynn V, Doar J. Some effects of oral contraceptives on carbohydrate metabolism. Lancet 1966;7624:715-719

[553] Wynn V, Adams P, Godsland I, *et al.* Comparison of the effects of different combined oral-contraceptive formulations on carbohydrate and lipid metabolism. Lancet 1979;8125:1045-1049

[554] Fraenkel-Conrat HL, Herrig VV, Simpson ME, Evans HM. Mechanism of action of estrogens on insulin content of the rat's pancreas. Proc Soc Exp Biol Med 1941;48:333-337

[555] Houssay BA, Foglia VG, Rodriguez RR. Production and prevention of some types of experimental diabetes by oestrogens or corticosteroids. Acta Endocrinol 1954;17:146-164

[556] Tesone M, Chazenbalk G, Ballejos G. Estrogen receptor in rat pancreatic islets. J Steroid Biochem 1979;11:1309-1314

[557] Sutter-Dub M-T. Preliminary report: effects of female sex hormones on insulin secretion by the perfused rat pancreas. J Physiol (Paris) 1976;72:795-800

[558] Djursing H, Hagen C, Christensen F, Nickelsen C. Bromocriptine and estrogen modulation of gonadotropin release in normo and hyperprolactinemic patients with amenorrhea. Clin Endocrinol 1981;15:125-132

[559] Rosenfeld RL. Puberty in the female and its disorders. In: Sperling MA (ed) Pediatric Endocrinol 2nd ed. Philadelphia: WB Saunders 2002: 455-518

[560] Durando B, Deriso L, Krug E. Prevalence of menstrual abnormalities and androgen excess in women with type 1 and type 2 diabetes mellitus. Diabetes 2003;52,Suppl A:497-501

[561] Strotmeyer ES, Steenkiste AR, Foley TP, Berga SL, Dorman JS. Menstrual cycle differences between women with type 1 diabetes and women without diabetes. Diabetes Care 2003;26:1016-1021

[562] Nadal A, Alonso-Magdalena P, Soriano S, Quesada I, Ropero AB. The pancreatic β-cell as a target of estrogens and xenoestrogens: Implications for blood glucose homeostasis and diabetes. Mol Cell Endocrinol 2009;304:63-68

[563] Shi J, Simpkins JW. 17 beta-Estradiol modulation of glucose transporter1 expression in blood-brain barrier. Am J Physiol 1997;272:E1016-E1022

[564] Cheng CM, Cohen M, Wang J, Bondy CA. Estrogen augments glucose transporter and IGF 1 expression in primate cerebral cortex. Faseb J 2001;15:907-915

[565] Brinton RD. Estrogen regulation of glucose metabolism and mitochondrial function: Therapeutic implications for prevention of Alzheimer's disease. Adv Drug Del Rev 2008;60:1504-1511

[566] Konstanyan A, Nazaryan K. Rat brain glycolysis regulation by estradiol-17 beta. Biochim Biophys Acta 1992;1133:301-306

[567] Nilsen J, Irwin RW, Gallaher TK, Brinton RD. Estradiol *in vivo* regulation of brain mitochondrial proteome. J Neurosci 2007;27:14069-14077

[568] Thomas J. Modification of glucagon-induced hyperglycaemia by various steroidal agents. Metabol 1963;12:207-212

[569] Burghen GA, Givens JR, Kitabchi AE. Correlation of hyperandrogenism with hyperinsulinism in polycystic ovarian disease. J Clin Endocrinol Metab 1980;50:113-116

[570] Diamanti-Kandarakis E, Mitrakou A, Hennes MM, *et al.* Insulin sensitivity and antiandrogenic therapy in women with polycystic ovary syndrome. Metabol 1995;44:525-531

[571] Dunaif A, Green G, Futterweit W, Dobrjansky A. Suppression of hyperandrogenism does not improve peripheral or hepatic insulin resistance in the polycystic ovary syndrome. J Clin Endocrinol Metab 1990;70:699-704

[572] Lasco A, Cucinotta D, Gigante A, *et al.* No changes of peripheral insulin resistance in polycystic ovary syndrome after long-term reduction of endogenous androgens with leuprolide. Eur J Endocrinol 1995;133:718-722

[573] Volpi E, Liberman SA, Ferrer DM, *et al.* The relationships between testosterone, body composition, and insulin resistance. A lesson from a case of extreme hyperandrogenism. Diabetes Care 2005;28,2:429-432

[574] Yialamas MA, Dwyer AA, Hanley E, Lee H, Pittloud N, Hayes FJ. Acute sex steroid withdrawal reduces insulin sensitivity in healthy men with idiopathic hypogonadotropic hypogonadism. J Clin Endocrinol Metab 2007;92:4254-4259

[575] Yannucci J, Manola J, Garnick MB, Bhat G, Bubley GJ. The effect of androgen deprivation therapy on fasting serum lipid and glucose parameters. J Urol 200;176:520-525

[576] Marin P. Testosterone and regional fat distribution. Obes Res 1995;3,Suppl 4:S609-S612

[577] Pagotto U, Gambineri A, Pelusi C, *et al.* Testosterone replacement therapy restores normal ghrelin in hypogonadal men. J Clin Endocrinol Metab 2003;88:4139-4143

[578] Morimoto S, Mendoza-Rodriguez CA, Hiriart M, Larrieta ME, Vital P, Cerbón MA. Protective effect of testosterone on early apoptotic damage induced by streptozotocin in rat pancreas. J Endocrinol 2005;187:217-224

[579] Traish AM, Saad F, Guay A. The dark side of testosterone deficiency: II. Type 2 diabetes and insulin resistance. J Androl 2009;30,1:23-32

[580] Sato K, Iemitsu M, Aizawa K, Ajisaka R. Testosterone and DHEA activate the glucose metabolism-related signaling pathway in skeletal muscle. Am J Physiol Endocrinol Metab 2008;294:E961-E968

[581] Malkin CJ, Jones TH, Channer KS. The effect of testosterone on insulin sensitivity in men with heart failure. Eur J Heart Fail 2007;9:44-55

[582] Corbould A. Chronic testosterone treatment induces selective insulin resistance in subcutaneous adipocytes of women. J Endocrinol 2007;192:585-594

[583] Bandyopadhyay G, Sajan MP, Kanah Y, *et al.* PKC-ζ mediated insulin effects on glucose transport in cultured preadipocyte-derived human adipocytes. J Clin Endocrinol Metab 2002;87:716-723

[584] Kapoor D, Malkin CJ, Channer KS, Jones TH. Androgens, insulin resistance and vascular disease in men. Clin Endocrinol (Oxf) 2005;63,3:239-250

CHAPTER 4

Insulin Resistance and Disturbance of Glucose Metabolism

Abstract: Insulin resistance is an early and major feature in the development of type 2 diabetes mellitus (non-insulin-dependent diabetes mellitus), but it is also associated with hyperlipidemia, hypertension, obesity, cardiovascular disease, nonalcoholic fatty liver disease, and various monogenic disorders such as Rabson-Mendenhall syndrome, leprechaunism, type A insulin resistance, and CFTDM syndrome (congenital muscle fiber type disproportion myopathy). Moreover, disturbances in sleep (sleep apnoea) and ovarian dysfunction are also characterized by insulin resistance. It is a major problem that is increasing rapidly worldwide. A number of factors increase the risk for insulin resistance, including genetic predisposition, obesity and inactivity, aging, medications, polycystic ovary syndrome, and rare disorders such as partial lipodystrophy. Diets high in saturated fats and carbohydrates are associated with glucose intolerance, obesity, coronary heart disease, and type 2 diabetes mellitus. Glucotoxicity, lipotoxicity, and glucolipotoxicity are secondary phenomena that are proposed to play a role in all forms of type 2 diabetes. Insulin resistance typically reflects multiple defects of insulin receptor and post-receptor signaling that impair a diverse range of metabolic and vascular actions.

INTRODUCTION

The term first came into use to describe occasional diabetic patients who required increasingly large doses of insulin to control hyperglycemia. Most of these patients developed insulin resistance secondary to antibodies directed against the therapeutic insulin [1]. The words "insulin resistance" were earlier often used to designate a condition, where a patient with diabetes was treated with more than 200 units of insulin per day [2]. "Insulin resistance" has also been used to describe situations where genetic abnormalities of insulin itself, pro-insulin and insulin receptor, prevent the response generated by the insulin molecule interacting with its receptor [2]. Antibodies against the insulin or against insulin receptor are also described as causes of insulin resistance [3]. Recent "insulin resistance" defines a state in which a given concentration of insulin produces a less-than-expected biological effect.

In these situations, circulating insulin levels may be extremely high or patients with high blood glucose levels may be resistant to treatment with high doses (hundreds or thousand of units) of insulin per day [4]. When the fasting plasma glucose concentrations exceeds about 140 mg/dL, the β-cell can no longer maintain its elevated rate of insulin secretion [5]. The fasting insulin concentration declines progressively, resulting in impaired glucose tolerance (IGT) and/or type 2 diabetes mellitus [6, 7]. Patients with insulin resistance have hyperinsulinemia together with normoglycemia or hyperglycemia. On the other hand, impaired glucose tolerance (IGT) is defined as hyperglycemia during an oral glucose tolerance test which is insufficient for the diagnosis of diabetes mellitus. Impaired glucose tolerance is often a transition stage in the progression from normal glucose tolerance to non-insulin dependent diabetes [16].

Insulin resistance is highly heterogeneous in its presentation and progression,reflecting the involvement of genetic and environmental components [8 – 10, and 17]. It is determined by impaired sensitivity of insulin to its main target organs, i.e. adipose tissue, liver and muscle.

RISK FACTORS FOR INSULIN RESISTANCE

A number of apparent risk factors have been identified. Insulin resistance risk factors include, for example, genetic factors, obesity, diet, etc.

Genetic Factors

Many studies suggest that genetic factors influence insulin resistance. Most forms of insulin resistance involve defects of insulin receptor and post-receptor signaling [8 – 10]. Insulin binding to its receptor induces complex signaling cascades. Tyrosine phosphorylation of insulin receptor substrate (IRS) leads to the activation of two major pathways. The phosphatidylinositol 3-kinase (PI 3-kinase) is responsible for insulin action on glucose uptake and suppression of gluconeogenesis, and the mitogen-activated protein kinase (MAPK) pathway regulates gene expression. MAPK pathway interacts with PI 3-kinase pathway to control cell growth and differentiation [13].

Many mutations in the insulin receptor gene are known that affect receptor function [11]. Mutations of the insulin receptor gene are the best characterized causes of insulin resistance that have been identified to date [14, 15]. Impairment of intrinsic tyrosine kinase activity in the insulin receptor has been reported not only in patients with type 2 diabetes but also in non-obese normoglycemic patients with insulin resistance [14, 16]. The mutations in the insulin receptor gene impair insulin receptor biosynthesis and posttranslational modification of the receptor. Some of these mutations impair the binding of insulin to its receptor, the activation of the receptor tyrosine kinase, and receptor degradation [12]. These mutations typically behave in a recessive manner.

Insulin-resistant patients with type 2 diabetes have been demonstrated to have decreased insulin-receptor numbers, insulin-activated receptor tyrosine kinase activity, insulin receptor substrate-1 (IRS-1) activation, glycogen synthesis, activation of pyruvate dehydrogenase, muscle glucose uptake etc [18].

Mice that lack insulin receptors specifically in the liver exhibit insulin resistance, glucose intolerance, and failure of insulin in the regulation of hepatic glucose production [19]. A similar phenotype was demonstrated for mice in which phosphatidylinositol 3-kinase was inhibited [20]. These observations suggest that insulin resistance contributes to the pathogenesis of type 2 diabetes, based on results obtained with cultured cells [21].

A number of studies have estimated the heritability of insulin resistance. Insulin resistance occurs more commonly in the offspring of insulin resistant parents [11].

For more details see particular diseases due to insulin resistance.

Obesity

Obesity is now a considerable public health problem in most economically advanced countries. Obesity, specifically visceral abdominal obesity, is associated with a reduction in life expectancy of ~ 8 years, as well as with an increased risk of several major diseases, including type 2 diabetes, coronary heart disease and certain cancers [22 – 24]. By Zeyda and Stulnig [13] in the UK, rates of obese have increased by 30% in women, 40% in men, and 50% in children within the last decade resulting in 23% of adults being obese in 2007 and a prognosis of 50% for 2050.

Obesity is clinically defined as a body mass index (BMI) of ≥ 30 kg/m^2. A BMI of 30 represents an overweight of approximately 14 kg for any given high [25]. However, the relationship between standard indices of obesity, such as BMI, and insulin resistance is only moderate.

The prevalence of abdominal obesity (waist circumference > 102 cm for men and > 88 cm for women) is also high and growing [26]. A growing database of clinical evidence suggests that abdominal obesity is a stronger predictor of adverse cardiovascular outcomes than BMI [26]. The mechanism by which central abdominal fat generates insulin resistance is still not completely understood. It is suggested that release of fatty acids from visceral compartment into the portal vein increases gluconeogenesis and hepatic glucose output [4]. Visceral adipose tissue, by secreting adipocytokines, promotes the development of lipotoxicity in peripheral tissues [27]. The increasing prevalence of the cardiometabolic syndrome has been paralleled by a rise in the prevalence of obesity. Free fatty acids contribute to impaired glucose tolerance by accumulation in nonadipose tissues [28].

Visceral adipose tissue accumulation is an important predictive factor of lipid and glucose disturbances, while location of adipose tissue in the lower part of the body is not associated with increased alterations at the metabolic level [35]. There are several differences between visceral and subcutaneous tissue, including the expression of different genes involved in insulin resistance and different patterns of the expression, production and secretion of the adipokines [3, 37]. Wagenknecht and colleagues found a strong independent relationship between both visceral and subcutaneous adiposity and insulin resistance. Increased levels of fat were associated with lower insulin sensitivity. Visceral adipose tissue was a more potent predictor of insulin resistance than subcutaneous adipose tissue [38]. Visceral fataccumulation decreases peripheral insulin sensitivity, enhances hepatic gluconeogenesis [39] and the accumulation of fat within the liver and muscle leadsto insulin resistance in these tissues [40]. On the other hand, subcutaneous fat accumulation is more strongly correlated with insulin resistance than visceral fat accumulation in male diabetic patients [41].

Adipocytes are the only cells that are specialized and adapted to store lipids. They have the enzymes necessary to synthesize fatty acids and to store triacylglycerols during periods of abundant energy supply. Adipose tissue is composed of adipocytes and in addition to adipocytes, adipose tissue contains a matrix of conjunctive tissues (collagen and reticular fibers), nerve fibers, vascular stroma, lymph nodes and various cell types, such as immune cells (leukocytes, macrophages), fibroblasts and preadipocytes [65]. In mammals, there are two types of adipose tissue: white adipose tissue and brown adipose tissue. Their adipocytes exhibit important differences. Brown adipose tissue is specialized in thermogenesis and is practically absent in adult humans. It is found in fetuses and newborn infants [29]. Adipose tissue is the body's largest energy reservoir. Most energy reserves in the human body are stored in the fat cells as triacylglycerols [30].

White adipose tissue is a major secretory organ, particularly through the release of fatty acids during fasting, cholesterol, retinol, steroid hormones, and prostaglandins [31]. Adipose tissue is a complex and high active metabolic tissue that secretes multiple metabolically important proteins known as "adipokines" and other adipose specific molecules [32 – 35]. Some of these factors are implicated in the pathologies associated with obesity, particularly insulin resistance [34]. It is well known that white adipose tissue mass increases greatly in obesity. Several studies have shown that adipokines production is altered in obesity, type 2 diabetes and metabolic syndrome. Adipocyte enlargement is associated with dysfunctional fat cells which over-express and secrete excessive amounts of leptin IL-6, TNF-α, resistin. Altered secretion of these adipocytokines has been implicated in the development of insulin resistance in obesity [42].

Adipose Tissue as an Endocrine Organ

Role in Insulin Resistance

Leptin

Leptin is a peptide hormone, identified in 1994 as a product of the *ob* gene that had been described in mice [29]. The hormone, which consists of 167 amino acid residues [43], (molecular weight of 16 kDa) [29], is produced almost exclusively in adipose tissue. The human gene is located on chromosome 7q31.3 [29]. Many types of tissues express leptin, such as placenta, adeno-pituitary, gastric fundus mucosa, skeletal muscle etc, but subcutaneous fat is responsible of 80% of total leptin production [36].

Leptin has an important role in the regulation of energy balance and food intake [44, 45]. It is also necessary for reproduction, because deficiencies of or insensitivity to leptin are associated with hypothalamic hypogonadism both in humans and inrodents [29]. Leptin increases cytokine production, macrophage adhesion and phagocytosis, besides proliferation of T cells [46]. Leptin plays an important role inmodulating blood pressure mainly through its vascular, renal and sympathetic actions. Although depressor and pressor actions of leptin have been reported, the pressor effects of leptin appear to predominate [47]. It has been shown to promote NO (nitric oxide) release by the vascular endothelium that could potentially decrease blood pressure [48]. Independent of these effects, leptin improves peripheral, hepatic and skeletal muscle, insulin sensitivity and modulates pancreatic β-cell function [49].

Leptin receptors, OB-R, belong to the class I cytokine receptor family, which includes several interleukins (IL2 – IL7), growth hormone, prolactin and erythropoietin. Leptin receptor gene is mapped to the short arm of human chromosome 1 (1p31) [50]. The short leptin receptor isoform, OB-Ra, is expressed in the brain, with the highest levels in the choroid plexus and in microvessels [50]. The long form, OB-Rb, is highly expressed in selected nuclear groups in the rodent and human brain [43]. Hypothalamic as well as brain stem nuclei play a critical role in integrating the information on absorbed food, on the amount of energy stored in the form of fat, etc. Leptin receptor activation at these sites leads to repression of orexigenic pathways and induction of anorexigenic pathways. Leptin binding to the long isoform of the leptin receptor, results in activation of Janus kinase (JAK), which in turn phosphorylates OB-Rb, resulting in the recruitment and tyrosine phosphorylation of the transcription signal transducer, and activation of activators of transcription-3 (STAT3) [51]. Leptin binding to the leptin receptor also activates the IRS/phosphoinositide 3-kinase pathway [52]. Leptin receptor-mediated JAK-STAT signaling is essential for regulation of food intake and body weight. Leptin-stimulated PI 3-K signaling appears to be important for regulation of glucose metabolism. Leptin was shown to inhibit insulin secretion in lean animals. As body weight increases, leptin signaling protected the β-cell from adverse effects of overnutrition [56]. Insulin stimulates both leptin biosynthesis and secretion from adipose tissue [57]. It is an endocrine adipo-insular feedback loop, so called "adipo-insular axis" [57].

Obesity is known to be associated with hyperleptinemia, reflecting resistance to leptin. Obese subjects remain overweight despite the high circulating levels of leptin [53]. Both leptin deficient and leptin resistant obese rodents exhibit severe insulin resistance. This condition is rapidly ameliorated by leptin administration indeficient mice, even before reducing body weight [54]. Leptin administration to obese patients causes only modest effects on body weight [55]. In the majority of cases of obesity, leptin fails to induce weight loss. This diminished response to the anorexigenic and insulin-sensitizing effect of leptin is called "leptin resistance" [49]. The fact that leptin biosynthesis in adipose tissue is increased in obese individuals, except in leptin-deficient subjects led to the concept of leptin resistance.

In summary, "leptin resistance defines a situation when increased adipose biosynthesis is observed in the majority of obese individuals without adequate leptin-mediated end-organ response" [58].

The mechanisms underlying leptin resistance are currently under intense investigation. The inability of leptin to activate intracellular signaling pathways is associated with impairment of leptin transport across the blood-brain-barrier, reduction of leptin-mediated JAK-STAT signaling, and reduction of suppressor of cytokine signaling-3 [58], and appears to be restricted to the arcuate nucleus of the hypothalamus [47]. Therefore, it is very likely that leptin resistance is due to the inability of leptin to activate downstream signaling pathways in the arcuate nucleus.

Leptin promotes fatty acid oxidation. Impaired leptin action causes accumulation of triglycerides in skeletal muscle and pancreas. Accumulation of triglycerides and long-chain free fatty aids in these organs causes apoptosis. Lipotoxicity developing in skeletal muscle causes insulin resistance and in pancreas, causes β-cell dysfunction. It could be responsible for the development of type 2 diabetes. It has been demonstrated that decreased leptin actions partly underlie the development of type 2 diabetes in human lipodystrophy [59, 60]. Lipotoxicity may set the pathologic ground for the development of type 2 diabetes in metabolic syndrome subjects with impaired leptin actions due to obesity-related leptin resistance [47, 61].

TUMOR NECROSIS FACTOR-A (TNF-α)

A major step forward in the recognition of the secretory of white adipose tissue occurred in the early 1990s with the discovery that the proinflammatory cytokine tumor necrosis factor-α is synthesized and released by adipocytes [62]. TNF-α was the first adipose secreted product proposed to represent a molecular link between obesity and insulin resistance [63, 64]. This cytokine acts by two types of membrane receptors: TNFR I and TNFR II, which mediate transduction of the signal triggered by TNF-α [29].

Tumor necrosis factor-α is a proinflammatory cytokine produced by numerous cells, but mainly macrophages and lymphocytes. TNF-α is produced also by adipocytes in rodents, and in low quantities in humans. It has been described as a factor that induces cachexia in animals and inhibits lipogenesis and stimulates lipolysis. It is involved in inflammation, apoptosis, cytotoxicity and production of interleukin-1 and interleukin-6. It plays an important role in adipocyte metabolism; TNF-α acts directly in insulin dependent processes, including homeostasis of carbohydrate and lipid metabolism [66 – 68]. TNF-α was shown to have extensive metabolic effectsin adipose tissue, also including the stimulation of apoptosis [69].

In humans, adipose tissue TNF-α expression correlated with body mass index (BMI), percentage of body fat, and hyperinsulinemia. Its expression and secretion are increased in obesity, whereas weight loss decreased TNF-α level [70]. Tumor necrosis factor-α has been proposed as a link between adiposity and development resistance, because the majority of type 2 diabetic patients are obese [71].

A number of studies have demonstrated that TNF-α alters insulin signaling in cultured cells [72] and in vivo. It alters insulin sensitivity and induces insulin resistance. Neutralizing TNF-α in obese rats improves insulin resistance [62]. On the other hand, infusion of TNF-α-neutralizing antibodies to obese, insulin-resistant subjects, or type 2 diabetic patients, did not improve insulin sensitivity [73, 74]. Rather than acting systematically, TNF-α seems to act locally at the site of white adipose tissue through autocrine or paracrine mechanisms or both, having effects on insulin resistance [75].

One of the possible mechanisms by which this cytokine interferes with insulin sensitivity is through abnormal phosphorylation of insulin receptor substrate-1. The mechanisms affecting IRS-1 involve proteasome-mediated degradation, phosphatase-mediated dephosphorylation, and serine phosphorylation of IRS-1, which converts IRS-1 to a form that inhibits insulin receptor tyrosine kinase activity [76 – 78]. Abnormal phosphorylation of IRS-1 causes reduced phosphorylation of phosphatidylinositol 3-kinase and reduced synthesis and translocation of the glucose transporter GLUT 4 to the plasma membrane [79].

ADIPONECTIN

An adipose-secreted protein with homology with the complement factor C1q was cloned independently by different groups. It has been attributed several different names: in mice – Arcp30 (adipocyte complement-related protein of 30 kDa), adipoQ, GBP28 (gelatin-binding protein 28), and in humans – apM1 (adipose most abundant gene transcript 1) or adiponectin [80, 81]. Adiponectin is a 30 kDa protein and the human gene for adiponectin was first described in 1995 and is located at chromosome 3q27 [29]. Adiponectin consists of a collagenous tail and a globular head, which form trimer-dimers and high molecular weight complexes in the circulation [54].

Adiponectin effects are mediated through two distinct receptors named adiponectin receptor 1 (AdipoR1) and adiponectin receptor 2 (AdipoR2). The genes of human adiponectin receptors are located on chromosomes 1q32 and 12p13, respectively [29, 82]. Adiponectin receptors contain seven transmembrane domains, but differ both structurally and functionally from G protein-coupled receptors and do not seem to be coupled with G-protein [82]. AdipoR1 is expressed ubiquitously (primarily in muscle), whereas AdipoR2 is expressed most abundant in the liver [82]. Expression of both receptors is decreased in mouse models of obesity and insulin resistance [83, 84].

Adiponectin is a protein highly expressed in adipose cells. The expression of adiponectin mRNA is dependent on the adipose tissue. It is lower in visceral adipose tissue than in subcutaneous adipose tissue [85]. Plasma levels of adiponectin, which constitutes 0,01% of plasma proteins, are between 5 to 30 mg/L in lean control subjects.

Adiponectin enhances insulin sensitivity through activation of AMP-activated protein kinase (AMPK), which is known to regulate cellular malonyl-CoA concentrations by inhibiting CoA carboxylase [86]. The inhibition of CoA carboxylase results in a decreased level of intracellular malonyl CoA and a subsequent decreased lipogenesis associated with increased mitochondrial β-oxidation. Adiponectin is also able to regulate hepatic glucose production by lowering mRNA expression of two essential gluconeogenesis enzymes: phosphoenolpyruvate carboxykinase and glucose-6-phosphatase [80]. Adiponectin may have a protective effect on the vascular wall by acting early at several steps of the atherogenesis process, modulating TNF-α-induced inflammatory response, since it has been shown that adiponectin reduces TNF-α secretion of macrophages [87].

In contrast to other adipokines, a negative correlation has been demonstrated between the degree of obesity and levels of adiponectin in circulation. Adiponectin is unexpressed in obese patients with insulin resistance, with type 2 diabetes and in patients with coronary heart disease [36]. In animals (rhesus monkeys), plasma adiponectin decreases along with the development of insulin resistance associated with obesity and aging [88]. The studies in humans suggest that individuals with high adiponectin concentrations are less likely to develop type 2 diabetes than those with low concentrations [89, 90]. By Rabe and colleagues [49] upregulation of adiponectin or adiponectin receptors or enhancing adiponectin receptor function may represent a therapeutic strategy for obesity-linked insulin resistance.

INTERLEUKIN-6

Interleukin-6 (IL-6) is produced by many cell types (fibroblasts, endothelial cells, monocytes), and many tissues. Human white adipose tissue produces substantial amounts of IL-6 and this secretion, in the absence of an acute inflammatory process, might represent approximately 15 – 30% of circulating levels [91]. However, adipose tissue is composed of numerous cells other than adipocytes. The greater proportion of interleukin-6 is not produced by mature adipocytes but rather by cells of the stroma vascular fraction including preadipocytes, endothelial cells and monocyte/macrophages [92, 93]. Secretion of interleukin-6 is three times higher in visceral adipose than in subcutaneous adipose tissue [92, 93].

Interleukin-6 is a multifunctional cytokine acting on many cell types and several tissues. One of the main effects of interleukin-6, is the induction of hepatic C-reactive protein (CRP) production. There is a positive relationship between IL-6 levels in adipose tissue and circulating levels both interleukin-6 and CRP [94]. CRP is known to be an independent, major risk marker of cardiovascular complications [95]. Interleukin-6 has been proposed to play an important role in the link between obesity, inflammation, and coronary heart disease [96].

The interleukin-6 receptor belongs to the cytokine class I receptor family. In the presence of IL-6 the receptor activates intracellular signaling pathway, which uses Janus kinase (JAK) and signal transducers and activators of transcription (STATs).

Conflicting data exist regarding the role of interleukin-6 in insulin resistance [97, 98]. Plasma IL-6 is highly correlated with body mass and inversely related to insulin sensitivity [99, 100]. Circulating interleukin-6 levels are increased in obese and insulin resistant subjects [101, 102]. An interaction is now clearly established between interleukin-6 and insulin signaling pathways leading to an impaired biological effect of insulin. The exact mechanism has not yet been clearly elucidated, but there is evidence to suggest that interleukin-6 modulate insulin resistance through several distinct mechanism, including c-Jun N-terminal kinase 1 (JNK1)-mediated serine phosphorylation of IRS-1, JκB kinase (IKK)-mediated nuclear factor κB (NF-κB) activation and an interaction between suppressor of cytokine signaling-3 (SOCS-3) proteins and insulin receptor, which inhibits insulin-dependent receptor autophosphorylation [103 – 108].

Interleukin-6 reduces insulin-dependent hepatic glycogen synthesis [109, 110], glucose uptake in adipocytes [111] and enhances insulin-dependent glycogen synthesis and glucose uptake in myotubes [112, 113]. The effect of interleukin-6 on the hepatic glucose production is still under debate [114, 115]. On the other hand, interleukin-6 deficient mice developed mature-onset obesity, glucose intolerance [116] and intracerebroventricular administration of IL-6 decreasing body fat in rats [117]. These observations suggest that interleukin-6 might act at multiple levels, both centrally and on peripheral tissues [54].

RESISTIN

Resistin, also known as ADSF (adipocyte secreted factor) or FIZZ3 (found in inflammatory zones) was described in 2001 [118, 119]. Resistin has a molecular weight of 12,5 kDa [29]. The human resistin gene is located on chromosome 19 [29]. This adipokine is a member of the family proteins known as resistin-like molecules (RELM). These proteins are characterized by the consistent presence of a segment rich in cysteine (11 cysteines) at the C-terminal end.

The adipocyte is not the major cell type producing resistin in humans. Resistin is expressed more in preadipocytes than in mature adipocytes [29], and rather is produced by circulating monocytes and macrophages [120].

In animals, resistin studies have produced findings that absence of resistin activated AMPK and reduced gene expression encoding for hepatic gluconeogenesis enzymes [36]. These studies suggest that resistin could exert effects opposite to those of adiponectin. Infusion of resistin in the rat induced severe hepatic insulin resistance [121]. Although in rodents, resistin is expressed and secreted in lean individuals, circulating levels of resistin are increased in obesity [122]. In cultured adipocytes, resistin reduced insulin-stimulated glucose transport and inhibited adipocyte differentiation [119]. These studies suggest that resistin could be a link between adipose tissue, obesity, and insulin resistance.

There is considerable controversy about the role of resistin in humans. Studies reported contradictory findings with regards to a physiological role for resistin in glucose metabolism. Most of the studies found no correlation between plasma resistin levels, body mass index, and insulin resistance, although some studies reported an increase of resistinaemia in obesity and type 2 diabetes in humans.

As with TNF-α and interleukin-6, resistin has a role in inflammatory processes. Its expression in human peripheral-blood mononuclear cells is upregulated by TNF-α and IL-6 [123]. This adipokine was shown to be associated with disease activity in patients with inflammatory disease [124] and to be associated with coronary artery disease [125].

RETINOL BINDING PROTEIN 4 (RBP4)

Yang and colleagues [126] reported that retinol binding protein 4 was elevated in insulin-resistant adipose specific GLUT 4 knockout mice and in obese or type 2diabetic humans. They suggested a link between RBP4 and type 2 diabetes. Retinol binding protein 4 serum concentrations were elevated in insulin-resistant obese humans, impaired glucose tolerance and type 2 diabetes. RBP4 serum levels are elevated also in nonobese, normoglycemic subjects with a strong family history of type 2 diabetes [127].

By Rabe and colleagues [49] retinol binding protein 4 may act by two mechanisms: through retinol-dependent (via retinoic acid receptors {RARs} and retinoic acid-X receptors {RXRs} to regulate gene transcription) and retinol-independent mechanism (via cell surface receptors such as Megalin/gp320).

Several groups suggested RBP4 levels to be associated with insulin resistance [128, 129], type 2 diabetes [130, 131] and the metabolic syndrome [132]. An association was reported of RBP4 single nucleotide polymorphisms and insulin resistance, impaired insulin secretion and type 2 diabetes [133, 134]. However, other groups failed to identify changes in RBP4 levels in association with insulin resistance [135, 136], type 2 diabetes [136], and the metabolic syndrome [137].

In summary, the role of RBP4 in glucose metabolism in humans remains uncertain [49].

VASPIN

Vaspin is an adipokine identified in visceral adipose tissue of rats. It was identified as a member of the serine protease-inhibitor family [138]. It is strongly expressed in visceral adipose tissue, however human vaspin mRNA was reported to be expressed also in subcutaneous adipose tissue. In humans, it was shown to be associated with obesity and insulin resistance [139]. On the other hand, type 2 diabetes seemed to be abrogating this correlation [140]. Vaspin may represent an insulin-sensitizing adipokine, because vaspin injected into obese mice improves insulin resistance and glucose tolerance [138]. In the presence of insulin its tissue expression and plasma levels are normalized [141]. Vaspin expression decreases with worsening of diabetes and body weight loss [49].

VISFATIN

Visfatin is an adipokine identified by Shimomura and colleagues that is mainly synthesized and secreted in visceral fat [142]. It was originally identified as a pre-B-cell colony-enhancing factor (PBEF) that enhances the maturation of B cell precursor [148].

Plasma concentrations of visfatin were correlated with the amount of visceral fat in humans, type 2 diabetes and the presence of the metabolic syndrome [143 – 145]. It was reported to exert insulin-mimetic effects in cultured cells and to lower plasma glucose levels in mice [142]. It is to note that other studies did not confirm an association of visfatin and visceral adipose tissue or insulin sensitivity in humans [139, 146, and 147].

The hypoglycemic effect of visfatin has been seen both *in vivo* and *in vitro*. Intravenous infusion of visfatin leads to an acute fall of glucose in mice, and *in vitro*, visfatin enhanced glucose uptake by myocytes and adipocytes and inhibited hepatocyte glucose release [142].

Visfatin binds to the insulin receptor and induces IRS-1 and IRS-2 phosphorylation, and activation of phosphatidylinositol 3-kinase, protein kinase B and MAP kinase [36]. Other studies suggest that visfatin could be primarily regarded as an inflammatory mediator involved in several pathological processes [36].

By Antuna-Puente and colleagues [36] and by Lopez-Bermejo and colleagues [149], it is too early to consider visfatin in the development of hypoglycemic drugs.

OMENTIN

Omentin is strongly expressed in visceral adipose tissue, but poorly in subcutaneous fat. It is synthesized by visceral stromal vascular cells, but not mature fat cells, adipocytes [36, 49]. Human omentin is a protein of 313 amino acids. It increases insulin-stimulated glucose uptake and Akt phosphorylation in both omental and subcutaneous adipocytes [150]. These results suggest that omentin may improve insulin sensitivity.

Plasma omentin levels were correlated inversely with obesity, leptin levels and insulin resistance as determined by HOMA-R, and positively correlated with adiponectin and HDL levels [151]. Lean subjects have higher plasma omentin levels than do obese and overweight patients [151] and omentin gene expression is decreased with obesity [36]. The physiological role of omentin in glucose metabolism still needs to be determined.

CHEMERIN

Chemerin is an adipokine expressed in liver and white adipose tissue [152 – 154]. It modulates the expression of adipocyte genes involved in glucose and lipid metabolism, such as *SLC2A4*, fatty acid synthase, and adiponectin via its own receptor [152, 153]. In 3T3-L1 adipocytes, chemerin enhances insulin-stimulated glucose uptake and IRS-1 tyrosine phosphorylation. These results suggest that chemerin may increase insulin sensitivity in adipose tissue [155].

In rodents, data regarding the association of chemerin with obesity and diabetes were divergent. In humans, chemerin levels did not differ significantly between patients with type 2 diabetes and healthy subjects. On the other hand, in healthy subjects, chemerin levels were associated with body mass index, triglycerides and blood pressure [153].

SERUM AMYLOID A (SAA)

Serum amyloid A is an acute phase protein, which was previously believed only to be expressed in the liver in response to inflammation. SAA is expressed in adipose tissue. Subcutaneous adipose tissue displays higher levels of serum amyloid A expression than omental adipose tissue [164, 165]. Enlarged adipocytes have increased expression of SAA [165]. Plasma serum amyloid A levels are correlated with insulin resistance in obese subjects and type 2 diabetes [156]. Its expression in adipose tissue is largely increased in obesity and diabetes [157, 158]. Correlations were found between SAA levels and levels of C-reactive protein, interleukin-6, leptin, insulin, HbA$_{1C}$, and HOMA-IR. A majority of the correlations were strongest in women, and women had higher serum levels of SAA than men [166].

Serum amyloid A is an acute-phase reactant like C-reactive protein, used as a predictor for coronary artery disease and cardiovascular outcome [159]. The increase in acute phase serum amyloid A may affect lipid metabolism and thus contribute to the dyslipidemia associated with diabetes [160]. SAA displaces apolipoprotein A$_1$ from HDL-cholesterol, increasing HDL binding to macrophages, thus reducing their cardiovascular-protective effect [157].

Serum amyloid A consists of two closely related isoforms, SAA1 and SAA2 [161]. Additional members of the SAA family are SAA3 and SAA4 [162]. SAA3 is expressed in mammals, but not in humans [163] and SAA4 is a constitutively expressed member of the family [161]. SAA acts by the cell surface receptor selenoprotein S [167] and is also a ligand of the toll-like receptor-2 [168]. By Sjöholm and colleagues [166] SAA is a possible link between type 2 diabetes, atherosclerosis and inflammation.

ACYLATION-STIMULATING PROTEIN (ASP)

A substantial amount of acylation-stimulating protein is released by white adipose tissue [169]. ASP is a protein derived from the interaction of complement C3, factor B and adipsin [170]. It is an 8,9 kDa hormone [173]. ASP appears to be inactive as an immune modulator [54]. At the cellular level, acylation-stimulating protein stimulates glucose transport, enhances fatty acid re-estrification thus promoting triglyceride storage in adipose cells and inhibits glycolysis [171, 172]. In humans, plasma levels increased in obese subjects, but it is not known whether increased circulating levels of acylation-stimulating protein reflect increased activity or resistance to ASP [54]. Plasma levels of ASP are reduced in fasting [174] and in postobese women [175]. Resistance to ASP could preferentially channel fatty acid toward the liver [170].

A role of ASP was reported in the regulation of glucose homeostasis. ASP-deficient mice exhibit reduced fasting insulin levels and impaired glucose tolerance [176]. This result suggests that ASP reduces insulin sensitivity. ASP has effects on pancreatic islet function. It stimulates insulin secretion through a direct action on the β-cells [173]. By Ahrén and colleagues this effect depends on glucose phosphorylation, calcium uptake and protein kinase C (PKC). They also found that intravenous administration of acylation-stimulating protein in combination with glucose during the intravenous glucose tolerance test potentiated glucose-stimulated insulin secretion [173].

PLASMINOGEN ACTIVATOR INHIBITOR-1 (PAI-1)

Plasminogen activator inhibitor-1 is secreted by hepatocytes, endothelial cells and adipose tissue, where adipocyte participation in PAI-1 production is significant [177]. Cells of stromal vascular fraction and preadipocytes contribute PAI-1 production by human white adipose tissue [178]. It appears that visceral adipose tissue expresses more PAI-1 than does subcutaneous tissue.

Plasminogen activator inhibitor-1 controls the regulation of the fibrinolytic system in blood by inhibiting both urokinase-type and tissue-type plasminogen activators [179]. It provokes formation of thrombi and rupture of unstable atherogenic plaques. PAI-1 has been shown to influence cell migration and angiogenesis.

White adipose tissue is the main tissue source of elevated plasma PAI-1 in obesity, with the major participation of visceral fat [180, 1811]. Increased circulating levels of PAI-1 are found in patients with central obesity [182, 183]. Enhanced levels of PAI-1 are also found in patients with type 2 diabetes which is associated with a disturbance in glucose and lipid metabolism [179]. A defective insulin response in the liver contributes to the development of hyperglycemia, dyslipidemia and peripheral insulin resistance [179]. Several studies have appeared demonstrating a correlation in obese individuals between elevated levels of PAI-1 and hyperglycemia, hyperinsulinemia, fasting hypertriglyceridemia and high concentrations of LDL-cholesterol [184, 185]. As a result of increased circulating levels of PAI-1 is a decreased fibrinolytic capacity. It is to note that impairment of the fibrinolytic system is considered a cardiovascular risk factor [182]. The results obtained by Suzuki and colleagues suggest that glucose at high concentrations induces PAI-1 expression in vascular smooth muscle cells at least partially via MAPK and PKC activation [186]. Authors suggest that effect of glucose might have implications for the elevated plasma PAI-1 and atherosclerosis that are associated with diabetes.

Other Adipokines

White adipose tissue is an active endocrine and paracrine organ that releases a large number of cytokines and bioactive mediators that influence not only insulin resistance and diabetes but also inflammation, coagulation, fibrynolysis, atherosclerosis, and some forms of cancer [160, 187 and 188]. Obese white adipose tissue in infiltrated by macrophages, which may be a major source of locally produced proinflammatory cytokines. Weight loss is associated with a reduction in the macrophage infiltration of white adipose tissue [35].

Angiotensinogen decreases nitric oxide (NO) availability [189] and angiogenesis [190, 191], on the other hand, stimulating nuclear factor-κB (NF-κB), intracellular adhesion molecule-1 (ACM-1), vascular cell adhesion molecule-1 (VCAM-1), monocyte chemoattractant protein 1 (MCP-1) and monocyte colony-stimulating factor (M-CSF) [189]. It increases development of hypertension [65]. By Fonseca-Alaniz and colleagues [29] secreted by WAT tissue factor initiates coagulation cascade, and vascular endothelial growth factor (VEGF) stimulates angiogenesis in white adipose tissue. Monobutyrin, a non-protein substance, acts as vasodilator and inducer of vascular neoformation; transforming growth factor-B (TGF-B) regulates proliferation of preadipocytes and differentiation, development and apoptosis of adipocytes. Insulin-like growth factor-1 (IGF-1) and hepatocyte growth factor (HGF) stimulate proliferation, differentiation and development of adipocytes. White adipose tissue also releases macrophage migration inhibitory factor (MIF), lipoprotein lipase (LLP), cholesterol ester transfer protein (CEPT), prostaglandins, estrogens, glucocorticoids, and apelin.

INFLAMMATION

Many years ago, it was suggested that inflammation could be involved in insulin resistance and/or in the pathophysiology of type 2 diabetes [192]. On the other hand, inflammation is strongly associated with obesity. The molecular mechanisms involved are not clearly understood. Pro-inflammatory effects of cytokines were suggested. In obese patients, a chronic low-grade inflammation occurs as determined by increased plasma levels of inflammatory cytokines such as tumor necrosis factor-α (TNF-α), interleukin- and -8 (IL-6, IL-8), and monocyte chemoattractant protein-1 (MCP-1) [13]. Proinflammatory cytokines are able to alter insulin signaling. Reactive oxygen species and free fatty acids in obesity are also involved in insulin resistance.

Many kinases are involved in the inhibition of the specific intracellular signaling pathways, involving the nuclear factor-κB (NF-κB), IκB kinase, I-kappa-β kinase (I-KKβ), activating protein (AP-1) and c-Jun NH$_2$-terminal kinase (JNK) signaling molecules [13, 35 and 36]. All these pathways could interact with insulin signaling via inhibitory phosphorylation insulin receptor substrate [35]. TNF-α could also affect insulin sensitivity by altering the expression of the genes for insulin receptor, IRS-1, GLUT 4, adiponectin, PPARγ [13]. Interleukin-6 blocks IRS-mediated insulin signaling in liver and muscle via suppressor of cytokine signaling (SOCS) proteins [193].

Mechanisms of obesity-induced inflammation are not yet fully understood. It is suggested that endoplasmic reticulum stress plays a potential role in this process. Nutritional deficiency, viral infection or hypoxia can lead to impairment of endoplasmic reticulum function. Over-nutrition and obesity cause endoplasmic reticulum stress in liver and adipose tissue. It is due to an excessive lipid accumulation, disturbed energy metabolism, and changes in adipose tissue structural organization [194]. Endoplasmic reticulum stress triggers a stress response signaling network known as "unfolded protein response" (UPR). The UPR activates protective and apoptotic reactions. It also induces an inflammatory signal-transduction system by activating IKK, MAP kinases, JNK and NF-κB. Induction of endoplasmic reticulum stress with obesity leads to increase IRS-1 serine residue phosphorylation and inhibition of insulin signaling. Furthermore, endoplasmic reticulum stress downregulates the expression of GLUT 4 in adipocytes [195].

Summarizing, endoplasmic reticulum stress directly affects insulin signaling in insulin target cells by inducing inflammatory signal [13].

DIET

By Dedoussis and colleagues [196] in industrialized countries, a rapid increase in fat, saturated fatty acid and energy intake accompanies a decrease in physical activity, in the consumption of dietary fiber and diets with low glycemic index. The Westernization of diets, with an increase in availability of high calorie foods certainly contributes to the epidemic of insulin resistance. Diets high in saturated fats and carbohydrates are associated with glucose intolerance, obesity, coronary heart disease, and type 2 diabetes [197 – 200]. Diet and obesity are the main factors affecting the prevalence as well as the development and severity of type 2 diabetes. Nutrition represents a lifestyle element that can directly influence health.

In contrast to current Western diet, the traditional diets of many preagricultural people were low in carbohydrate [201 – 203]. There is evidence that the type of carbohydrate may influence insulin sensitivity and associated metabolic features. The findings in some studies that increasing the proportions of carbohydrate in relation to fat in the range of usually consumed quanties will influence insulin resistance may be explained further by the type of carbohydrate than the amount [204].

Over the past few decades, fructose consumption has dramatically increased. In 1970, individual consumption of fructose was only 0,5 lb/year, and in 1997, individual consumption of fructose was 62,4 lb/year. The consumption of fructose has increased largely because of an increased consumption of soft drinks and prepared desserts sweetened with sucrose and high fructose corn syrup, which contains between 55 – 90% fructose [206]. High fructose corn syrup is commonly found in soft drinks and juice beverages.

Fructose, compared with glucose, is preferentially metabolized to lipid in liver. In rodents, a high fructose diet induces accumulation of intrahepatocellular and intramyocellular lipids together with hepatic and muscle insulin resistance [208]. In humans, fructose ingestion results in increased rates of *de vovo* lipogenesis [209]. Thus, fructose is more lipogenic than is glucose. High-fructose diet increases fasting plasma triglycerides, very low-density lipoprotein (VLDL)-triglycerides, and glucose [210, 211]. A 7-d high fructose diet increased ectopic lipid deposition in liver and muscle and fasting VLDL-triglycerides and decreased hepatic insulin sensitivity [215]. On the other hand, the fructose diet had no significant effects of fasting plasma cholesterol, HDL-cholesterol, or LDL-cholesterol [206]. Fructose, unlike glucose, does not stimulate the secretion of insulin from pancreatic β-cells [212, 213] and leptin [206]. The lack of stimulation by fructose is likely due to the low concentrations of the GLUT 5 in pancreatic β-cells [206, 214].

The expression of genes was altered by high-fructose diet in skeletal muscle of healthy men. It was observed that high-fructose diet affected (significantly decreased) expression of genes, such as GLUT 4, acetyl-CoA decarboxylase-2, and proliferator-activated receptor-γ-coactivator-1α. On the other hand, fructose significantly increased expression of stearoyl-CoA desaturases-1 [216].

Many published experiments have shown that high-fructose diet induces hypertension in animals [217, 218]. The mechanism of fructose-induced hypertension is not well understood, but different factors have been implicated [219 – 221]. Surprisingly, in mice, addition of fructose to the diet did not result in an increase of brain GLUT 5 density and did not lead to increased weight and impaired glucose tolerance. High-fructose diet in mice, contrary to what has been observed in hamster, does not have same effect [222].

Interestingly, small catalytic quantities of fructose can have positive effects, and actually decrease the glycemic response to glucose loads, and improve glucose tolerance [223].

Fatty acids are an important source of energy for many tissues, including skeletal muscle. Skeletal muscle is the main site of manifestation of insulin resistance. Fatty acids elevated concentration in the serum is considered to be one of the important risk factors for development of insulin resistance [228], type 2 diabetes [224], glucose intolerance, obesity, and coronary heart disease [225, 226]. High-fat feeding has been presumed to be a cause of insulin resistance for at least twenty years [227]. A meta-analysis suggests that among overweight individuals, a total fat intake of < 30% total energy facilitates weight loss [229]. Thus, high-fat diets may promote insulin resistance via their obesogenic potential [204]. A number of studies have found that diets high in saturated fat result in increased weight and obesity. Mice placed on a 11-week high fat diet gained significantly more weight and had higher blood glucose levels than those fed on a low-fat diet [230]. The elevated free fatty acid serum levels were observed in the serum of subjects at high risk of type 2 diabetes (obesity, lipodystrophy) and acute elevation of fatty acids levels in healthy volunteers can also result in whole body and muscle insulin resistance [231]. In general, the high-fat diets significantly increased weight gain and insulin resistance, impaired glucose tolerance [232].

Mice with a β-cell overexpression of the cAMP-degrading enzyme phosphodiesterase 3B, early and rapidly develop glucose intolerance and insulin resistance as compared control animals, after 2 months of high-fat feeding. *In vitro* experiments revealed that the insulin secretory response to glucagon-like peptide-1 stimulation was markedly reduced in islets [233].

The data obtained by Randle and colleagues [234] and by Shulman [235] suggest that increases in plasma fatty acid concentration induce insulin resistance and reduce glucose transport. The reduction in insulin-activated glucose transport due to elevated plasma fatty acid concentration was observed in healthy volunteers and in patients with type 2 diabetes [236 – 238]. It is to note that high saturated fat content of the membrane makes for rigid, unresponsive membranes, whereas increased desaturation makes for improved membrane fluidity and responsiveness [239].

A number of studies have found an association between insulin sensitivity and various fatty acids. Several studies compared the effects of saturated and unsaturated fatty acids on insulin sensitivity in healthy subjects and those with type 2 diabetes [240 – 243]. There is a consistent positive association between the intake of saturated fatty acids (as for example for linoleic acid), and negative associations for palmitic, palmitoleic, and di-homo-γ-linolenic acids [247]. The observed association appears to be independent of adiposity [204].

Animal studies have established the connection between dietary lipids, membrane lipid profiles and insulin resistance [248, 249]. Results obtained by Storlien and colleagues showed that only by replacing sunflower oil (omega(n)-6), with fish oil (n-3) in rats fed on a high sucrose and high fat diet, the development of insulin resistance was attenuated [250]. In humans, insulin sensitivity was reduced by 10% on the diet high in saturated fatty acids [251]. The obesity and type 2 diabetes-prone Pima population proved to have 40% lower n-3 levels in their muscle membrane lipids than Australians [252].

The mechanism by which the nature of dietary fat might influence insulin sensitivity is not clearly understood. It is suggested that a change in the fatty acid composition of cell membranes influences insulin receptor binding or activity as well as ion permeability and cell signaling [252]. Another suggestion is that polyunsaturated fatty acids can act as ligands of PPAR γ [253, 254] or can modulate its expression, thus increasing transcription of *SLC2A4* [255, 256] and synthesis and improving insulin resistance.

LIFESTYLE

Data from throughout the world show that obesity, associated insulin resistance, and type 2 diabetes have dramatically increased in locations where lifestyle have recently been "westernized" [257 – 260]. The term "westernization" indicates an energy-dense diet and reduced physical activity [257].

Sedentary lifestyle increases the risk of developing cardiovascular diseases, diabetes [261, 262], and insulin resistance [263]. The pathways leading from a sedentary lifestyle to insulin resistance are incompletely understood. Studies have shown that moderate amounts of daily physical activity are able to ameliorate insulin sensitivity in diabetic patients or obese subjects [264, 265].

Hwu and colleagues reported an effect of physical inactivity, cigarette smoking and alcohol intake on insulin resistance in hypertensive patients [266]. Obtained results showed that sedentary hypertensive patients were more insulin resistant than the non-sedentary hypertensive. On the other hand, there were no differences in insulin sensitivity in subjects with different smoking status. Neither smoking nor alcohol intake was persistently associated with insulin resistance in the study. According to authors, physical inactivity is an important lifestyle determinant of insulin resistance in hypertensive patients and influences of smoking and alcohol intake on insulin resistance are less significant than physical inactivity in hypertensive patients [266]. Amati and colleagues [269] compared insulin sensitivity in athletes (younger and older), normal weight (younger and older), and obese (younger and older) subjects using a glucose clamp. It is to note that the non-athletes were sedentary. Results suggest that insulin resistance may not be characteristic of aging, but rather associated with obesity and physical inactivity. Blanc and colleagues [267] investigated the consequences of physical inactivity on fuel homeostasis during 7 days of head-down bed rest, a model mimicking weightlessness. Surprisingly, obtained results suggest gender different response to sedentary lifestyle. Increased age, overweight and physical inactivity are as strong risk factors for LADA (Latent autoimmune diabetes) as for type 2 diabetes [269]. Regular exercise may protect against the development of insulin resistance and normalize of glucose tolerance by means of short-term effects of exercise in some individuals with abnormal glucose tolerance [270].

A number of studies have demonstrated that short periods of inactivity lad to insulin resistance in humans [271 – 273]. Physical inactivity, during 5 days of bed rest, was associated with the development of insulin resistance, dyslipidemia (increased total cholesterol and triglycerides), increased blood pressure, and impaired microvascular function in healthy volunteers [274]. These studies suggest that the vasculature is highly sensitive to the metabolic changes associated with physical inactivity. Another study [275] demonstrated that high-saturated fat intake associated with physical inactivity after a period as short as 60 h is sufficient to significantly impair insulin sensitivity in healthy subjects. On the other hand, physical activity with a high-saturated fat diet did not significantly impair insulin sensitivity. These results suggest that even mild physical activity may confer protection against the deterious effects of a high fat diet.

HORMONAL FACTORS AND DRUGS

The term "glucocorticoid" represents both secreted hormones and anti-inflammatory and immunosuppressive agents [276]. As a family of therapeutic drugs, glucocorticoids have widespread use in nonendocrine and endocrine diseases [277]. Glucocorticoids are used in anti-inflammatory and immunosuppressive therapies such as allergic and hematological disorders and renal, intestinal, liver eye, and skin diseases. These drugs are also used in rheumatic diseases, bronchial asthma and in organ transplantation surgery [276, 278].

Glucocorticoids are steroid hormones released from the adrenal cortex. In humans, the main endogenous glucocorticoid is cortisol. Glucocorticoid hormones constitute an integral component of the response to stress; in times of stress, cortisol release is increased up to 10-fold of the basal value [279]. Synthesis and release of these hormones are regulated by the pituitary and hypothalamus, and this regulatory system is termed the hypothalamo-pituitary-adrenal (HPA) axis [279]. Endogenous and exogenous glucocorticoids readily cross the cellular membranes and act on intracellular receptors to influence the transcription of target genes [280, 281]. Glucocorticoid hormones play a key role in cellular growth and development. They have multi-systemic effects that are essential for survival in times of stress, influencing the regulation of salt and water homeostasis, blood pressure, immune function and cellular energy metabolism [280, 282].

The importance of glucocorticoids is exemplified in clinical syndrome deficiency (Addison's diseases or hypopituitarism). Cortisol deficiency is characterized by postural hypotension, weight loss and hypoglycemia. On the other hand, glucocorticoids have been reported to induce Cushing's syndrome [277]. Cortisol excess is characterized by central obesity, hypertension, glucose intolerance, osteoporosis and impaired response to infection.

The effects of glucocorticoids on glucose metabolism are well characterized [282]. For many genes involved in glucose metabolism, glucocorticoid effects oppose those of insulin. As a result, these hormones induce a state of insulin resistance. The effect of glucocorticoids *in vivo* appears to include impaired insulin-dependent glucose uptake in the periphery, enhanced gluconeogenesis in the liver [283, 284] and reduced central appetite [285]. Glucocorticoid hormones inhibit insulin secretion from pancreatic β-cells [286 – 288], and the central action of these hormones may enhance vagal stimulation of insulin secretion [289]. Glucocorticoid-induced whole body insulin resistance is highly correlated to its metabolic effects in individual organs.

The expression of GLUT 4 at the plasma membrane is even increased, or remains normal, by glucocorticoids in skeletal muscle and adipose tissue [290 – 292]. Glucocorticoids decrease glucose transport in skeletal muscle through a lowering of translocation of GLUT 4 to the cell surface in response to insulin and to other stimuli [290, 292 – 294]. Recent studies have indicated that peroxisome proliferator-activated receptor-α also contributes toward development of insulin resistance.

Glucose utilization in adipose tissue also affects whole body glucose disposal. Dexamethasone, a synthetic glucocorticoid, significantly inhibits total mRNA and tyrosine phosphorylation of insulin substrate-1 in 3T3-L1 adipocytes [295, 296]. Similar to the skeletal muscle, glucocorticoids decrease glucose transport in adipose tissue through inhibition of GLUT 4 translocation to the cell surface [295].

The liver is also the metabolic target of glucocorticoid action. A positive relationship has been observed between glucocorticoid effects in the liver and whole body insulin resistance [276]. Altered hepatic glucose metabolism due to glucocorticoids involves the enhancement of glucose output and reduction of glucose utilization [297]. It is to note, that dexamethasone treatment does not change insulin receptor and insulin substrate-1 [298], but it decreases PI 3-kinase activity in the liver [276]. For details see Chapter 3, part "Role of the hypothalamic-pituitary axis in the carbohydrate homeostasis".

Growth hormone has marked effects on energy metabolism, influencing all major pathways of substrate metabolism. It is an important regulator of glucose metabolism and insulin sensitivity in healthy subjects and in patients with acromegaly [299, 300]. Growth hormone hypersecretion is a known cause of insulin resistance and carbohydrate intolerance [301, 302]. Patients with acromegaly have elevated fasting insulin concentrations and some have impaired glucose tolerance [303, 304].

Many studies have been performed to establish the effect of growth hormone on glucose metabolism. Unfortunately, the results have been quite divergent. On the other hand, these effects appear to be independent of changes in body fat [306].

Prolonged growth hormone exposure is associated with insulin resistance and in particular by inhibition of insulin-stimulated glucose uptake in skeletal muscle [307]. The inhibition of glucose uptake is accompanied by unaltered insulin binding and reduced glucose oxidation [308], reduced glycogen synthase activity [308, 309], and increased intracellular glucose levels [309]. High-dose growth hormone treatment for 6 weeks resulted in reduced insulin sensitivity, but after 6 months of treatment, insulin sensitivity returned to pretreatment levels [310]. Study of Hwu and colleagues [311] did not observe any untoward effects on insulin sensitivity after 12 months of treatment. On the other hand, persistent decreased insulin sensitivity was reported after 6 months of treatment with a physiological growth hormone dose [312]. Short-term (1 week) and long-term (6 months) growth hormone therapy resulted in impaired insulin-stimulated glucose uptake, which deterioration of glucose tolerance. The decrease in glucose uptake was associated with an increase in lipid oxidation and a concomitant decrease in glucose oxidation [305].

The molecular mechanisms underlying these effects of growth hormone are not fully understood. According to Rose and Clemmons [306] the change in insulin sensitivity is believed to be mediated directly by growth hormone, binding to its receptor. Growth hormone activation of its receptor with subsequent activation of its intracellular signaling pathways leads to alterations in insulin sensitivity, but localization of the point within the insulin signaling pathway that is impaired has not been determined [306]. For details see Chapter 3, part "Role of the hypothalamic-pituitary axis in the carbohydrate homeostasis".

The impairment of glucose metabolism correlates strongly with an increased rate of lipid oxidation and intramyocellular triglyceride and free fatty acids content. The cytosolic mechanisms linking free fatty acids to insulin resistance remain unclear. Several studies have demonstrated that free fatty acids interfere with insulin signaling and in particular may blunt insulin substrate-1-associated PI 3-kinase activity [313]. In animals study, Dominici and colleagues [314] showed that insulin receptor number was reduced in the liver of growth hormone overexpressing animals and that induction of receptor phosphorylation and PI 3-kinase activation by insulin in the liver was attenuated. Therefore, according authors, hepatic sensitivity to insulin was impaired.

The association between thyroid hormones, insulin resistance and metabolic syndrome was observed. Kumar and colleagues [315, 316] reported that total triiodothyronine and thyroid-stimulating hormone showed positive correlation with insulin and HOMA-IR. Total triiodothyronine and thyroid-stimulating hormone correlated more with variables of metabolic syndrome than free triiodothyronine and thyroxine. Thyroid-stimulating hormone is also significant associated with insulin resistance in women with polycystic ovary syndrome. The association appeared to be independent of age and BMI [317]. For details see Chapter 3, part "Role of the hypothalamic-pituitary axis in the carbohydrate homeostasis".

Interaction of sex hormones and insulin has been described extensively in women [318] and men [319]. Hormone replacement therapy improves insulin resistance in women with type 2 diabetes [320]. It is known that hyperandrogenicity correlates with insulin resistance in women with polycystic ovary syndrome and in healthy women with abdominal obesity [319].

Testosterone is an important regulator of insulin sensitivity in men. Hormone levels are low in men with diabetes and metabolic syndrome. Short-term testosterone replacement therapy produces an improvement in insulin sensitivity in men [319]. By Kapoor and colleagues [319] hypotestosteronemia may have a role in the pathogenesis of insulin-resistance states. It is to note, that in children normal puberty is associated with a reduction in insulin-stimulated glucose uptake in peripheral tissues [321]. Elevated levels of androgens and estrogens could contribute to the insulin resistance observed [319]. Animal studies have demonstrated that also short-term moderate increases of testosterone concentration are followed by a marked decrease in whole-body insulin sensitivity [322]; however, the mechanisms involved are uncertain [319]. For details see Chapter 3, part "Role of the hypothalamic-pituitary axis in the carbohydrate homeostasis".

Anti-adrenergic therapy with β-blockers has been widely accepted as an important therapeutic intervention in patients with chronic heart failure. Various anti-adrenergic drugs may carry differential effects on insulin sensitivity [327]. Anti-adrenergic drug may increase myocardial glucose uptake, and may blunt actions of norepinephrine and glucagon. An increase in glycosylated hemoglobin was observed [329]. Treatment with these drugs may impair glucose disposal to skeletal muscle and blocking the sympathetic beta-stimulation of glucose production may have theoretical adverse consequences [327].

DISEASES

Insulin resistance also has other factors that contribute to its presence in the body. A numerous diseases are also associated with insulin resistance and patients with various diseases show insulin resistance. By Krentz [16] insulin resistance is associated with – for example: thyrotoxicosis, polycystic ovary syndrome, acromegaly, phaeochromocytoma, Cushing's syndrome, insulinoma, glucagonoma syndrome, congestive cardiac failure, atheromatous disease microvascular angina, hepatic cirrhosis, chronic renal failure, myotonic dystrophy, Prader-Willi syndrome, Alström's syndrome, Laurence-Moon-Biedl syndrome, Werner syndrome and Friedreich's ataxia. There are also syndromes associated with extreme insulin resistance [16]: leprechaunism, Rabson-Mendenhall syndrome, type A insulin resistance, type B insulin resistance, type C insulin resistance, and lipodystrophic diabetes syndromes.

For example, glucose abnormalities in patients with heart failure are common and often associated with worsening symptomatic status [323]. Up to 43% of patients with left ventricular dysfunction have documented glucose abnormalities [324, 325]. Patients with heart failure have up to a 4 times higher risk of developing diabetes mellitus [326]. The mechanism of insulin resistance in dysfunctional myocardium is currently unknown [327]. On the other hand, the relationship between heightened sympathetic activation and the development of myocardial and peripheral insulin resistance is observed [328].

Glucotoxicity

Glucotoxicity and lipotoxicity are secondary phenomena that are proposed to play a role in all forms of type 2 diabetes [330]. The concept of "glucotoxicity" and "lipotoxicity" has been advanced to explain the pathogenesis of type 2 diabetes mellitus [331, 337].Unger and Grundy first introduced the concept of glucotoxicity [332].

As long as insulin resistance and the resulting mild hyperglycemia persist, the pancreas is forced to constantly over-secrete insulin, a condition termed "allostatic load" [331]. Normal glucose tolerant individuals with a high pancreatic allostatic load have an increased risk of developing type 2 diabetes compared to individuals with a low pancreatic allostatic load [333]. One of the possible ways that an increased allostatic load can eventually load to failure of the endocrine pancreas is through the direct detrimental affect of hyperglycemia on the β-cell. It is commonly referred to as glucotoxicity [334]. Mechanisms of glucotoxicity include decrease in expression of relevant genes, β-cell de-differentiation and increased apoptosis [335, 336]. Multiple biochemical pathways and mechanisms of action for glucose toxicity have been suggested, such as glucose autoxidation, protein kinase C activation, methylglyoxal formation and glycation, hexosamine metabolism, sorbitol formation, and oxidative phosphorylation [339]. It is suggested that chronic hyperglycemia *per se* can worsen insulin resistance [6].

Glucose is the major nutrient regulator of pancreatic β-cell function. It controls all steps of insulin gene expression, insulin biosynthesis and insulin secretion [340]. Glucose metabolism regulates hepatic gene expression. Glucose disposal issufficient to activate the transcription of key genes of the glycolysis, pentose phosphate, and lipogenesis pathways [346].

The term "glucose toxicity" was originally coined to describe the adverse effects of chronic exposure of pancreatic β-cells to high concentrations of glucose [6, 338]. On the other hand, the term "glucose toxicity" can be, and is currently used more broadly, to describe the pathogenic role of high glucose on multiple organ systems.

Poitout and Robertson observed the decreased levels of insulin mRNA, insulin content, and insulin release in β-cell lines (HIT-T15) cultured in media containing high concentrations of glucose [330]. It is to note, that insulin gene expression, insulin content and glucose-induced insulin secretion were progressively and drastically comprised over time when the higher glucose concentration was used in the media [341]. Exposure of β-cells to elevated glucose levels for several weeks impaired insulin gene expression [342]. This is associated with detoriation in insulin promoter activity as well as pancreas-duodenum homeobox-1 (PDX-1) and mammalian homologue of avian MafA/L-Maf (MafA) [343 – 345].

It has been proposed that the β-cells response to increased insulin demand and hyperglycemia can be classified into 4 phases of adaptation [336]. Phase 1 is characterized by successful adaptation to increased demand which appears to be mediated by increasing the residual β-cell mass by hypertrophy. β-cell function otherwise remains normal. Phase 2 is classified as mild decompensation in which glucose-stimulated insulin secretion is impaired. This phase is observed at minimally elevated glucose, i.e. before the development of overt diabetes. The defect in insulin secretion is at the level of secretion, and not at the level of insulin gene expression. Phase 3 occurs in response to a longer duration of high glucose exposure and is termed severe decompensation. At this stage glucose stimulated insulin secretion is impaired and responses to non-glucose stimuli are also decreased. β-cell insulin mRNA then decreases. In 4th phase, β-cell decompensation is accompanied by structural damage.

Patients with type 2 diabetes are subjected to chronic oxidative stress [347 – 350]. Oxidative stress is associated with molecular mechanism of the decreased insulin biosynthesis and secretion [351].

Pancreatic β-cells have very low levels of antioxidant enzymes compared with other tissues. These observations suggest that β-cell is particularly at risk for oxidative stress [352 – 355].

Metabolic reactions continuously produce reactive oxygen species (ROS), such as superoxides (O_2^-), hydroxyl radicals (OH^-), peroxyl radicals (ROO^-) or nitric oxide (NO). ROS are involved in inflammation, carcinogenesis, aging, and atherosclerosis [351]. On the other hand, several antioxidant enzymes, such as Cu/Zn superoxide dismutase, Mn superoxide dismutase, catalase, and glutathione peroxidase, help to maintain low levels of ROS. It is to note, that high glucose concentrations caused cellular stress in islets, but did not induce higher activities of the antioxidant enzymes [360].

Glucose-related pathways through which ROS can be formed include autoxidation, oxidative phosphorylation, glycosylation, and the glucosamine pathways [356 – 359]. Oxidative stress can damage cellular components, such as lipids, proteins or DNA [361], and oxidative stress can be a key event in diabetic complications [362, 363].

Various pathways are thought to be involved in the increase in oxidative stress in a hyperglycemic state. With the first pathway, more oxidative stress is caused by hyperglycemia because a non-enzymatic glycosylation reaction is enhanced in the hyperglycemic state. Another pathway involves the mitochondrial electron transfer system, which also becomes a source of oxidative stress [351]. This system is located in the mitochondrial inner membrane, where ATP is produced and water molecules are generated by deoxidation of four of the electrons of oxygen molecules. ROS is produced as an intermediate product in this process. Part of the oxygen is produced as superoxide anions, and their production increases in the hyperglycemic state [364]. The hexosamine pathway also becomes a source of oxidative stress [365]. In summary, at least six pathways are emphasized in the literature as being major contributors of ROS [339]: enolization and α-ketoaldehyde formation, protein kinase C (PKC) activation, dicarbonyl formation and glycation, sorbitol metabolism, hexosamine metabolism, and oxidative phosphorylation.

Glucotoxicity also participates in insulin resistance of insulin-sensitive tissues, such as liver, skeletal muscle, and adipose tissue. Oxidative stress is strongly suspected to be involved in chronic hyperglycemia-induced insulin resistance [366]. Exposure of primary adipocytes to chronic elevated glucose levels can induce oxidative stress [367] and oxidative stress induces insulin resistance in the 3T3-L1 adipocytes by inhibition the translocation of Glut 4 to the plasma membrane [368]. It is to note that oxidative stress can induce insulin resistance in intact rat muscle [369].

As mentioned above, the term "glucose toxicity" can be also used to describe the pathogenic role of high glucose on multiple organ systems, such as eyes (retinopathy) [370, 371], kidney (nephropathy) [372], nerves (neuropathy) [373], skin/mucous membranes (microvascular lesions, necrobiosis lipoidica diabeticorum, staphylococcus and streptococcus infections, fungal infections) [351], vascular system (atherosclerosis, endothelial cell dysfunction, restenosis) [374 – 377]. High glucose levels also act on the fetus (macrosomia, congenital anomalies, and shoulder dystonia).

Lipotoxicity

Not only plasma glucose levels are increased in uncontrolled type 2 diabetes increased plasma free fatty acids and increased storage of fatty acids in tissues including non-adipose tissue, such as muscle and liver, have long been recognized [378]. The focus of research towards type 2 diabetes has long been glucocentric rather than lipocentric. Accumulation of excess lipids in non-adipose tissue leads to cell dysfunction or cell death. Lipotoxicity may play an important role in the pathogenesis of diabetes and heart failure in humans [379]. The important role of fatty acids and lipid metabolism in the development of type 2 diabetes was outlined in the 1992 paper by McGarry [380]. Unger first introduced the concept of lipotoxicity [381].

Disorders of lipid metabolism were proposed to contribute to β-cell dysfunction in type 2 diabetes [381]. Exposure of isolated islets and insulin-secreting cells to elevated levels of fatty acids *in vitro* impairs insulin gene expression [382 – 386]. The mechanisms by which fatty acids impair β-cell function are largely unknown [337]. Possible mechanisms underlying the lipotoxic effect of free fatty acids on the β-cell include overproduction of NO [387], interleukin 1B [388], and ceramide [384, 389]. It is interesting, that ceramide synthesis does not appear to mediate fatty acid impairment of insulin secretion [390].

Ceramide activates c-jun N-terminal kinase. Therefore, Poitout and colleagues [340] hypothesize that ceramide-induced c-jun N-terminal kinase activation might inhibit insulin gene transcription via c-jun-dependent and – independent pathways. Alternatively, by these authors, ceramide might inhibit protein kinase B thereby allowing the transcription factor FoxO1 to translocate into the nucleus and repress its target genes.

The mechanisms of lipotoxicity in β-cells also involve the PDX-1 and MafA transcription factors. Hagman and colleagues showed in isolated rat islets that palmitate inhibits PDX-1 and MafA binding activity [383]. It is interesting that PDX-1 and MafA appear to be affected by palmitate through different mechanism; under lipotoxic conditions, PDX-1 is expressed but retained in the cytoplasm and MafA mRNA levels are decreased [340].

Prolonged exposure of β-cells to fatty acids *in vitro* increases basal insulin release and inhibits glucose-stimulated insulin secretion [391 – 394]. It has also been observed *in vivo* in rats [395] and in humans [396]. Poitout and Robertson pointed out that [330] these two effects have distinct mechanisms. The increase in basal insulin release involves enhanced low K_m glucose usage [397, 398]. Fatty acids decrease the activity of citrate synthase in culturing islets, resulting in lowered citrate levels and increased phosphofructokinase activity [398, 399]. This in turn reduces glucose-6-phosphate levels, disinhibits hexokinase, and increases glucose usage at low glucose concentrations [330]. It is to note, that *in vivo* fatty acids decrease sympathetic nervous system activity enhancing insulin secretion [400].

The mechanisms underlying the decrease in glucose-stimulated insulin secretion by fatty acids are less clear. Uncoupling protein-2 (UCP-2) is a ubiquitously expressed mitochondrial carrier that has been suggested to uncouple the respiratory chain from ATP synthesis [401]. Numerous evidences suggest that UCP-2 modulates insulin secretion and plays a role in lipotoxicity: increased UCP-2 expression in β-cells impairs insulin secretion [402, 403], UCP-2 KO animals have increased insulin levels and are protected from diabetes [401, 404], UCP-2 expression is increased in islets after high-fat feeding in rodents [403, 405], and very important observation – islets isolated from UCP-2 KO animals are protected from lipotoxicity [404]. In summary, fatty acids activate the expression of UCP-2 in β-cells, perhaps resulting in mitochondrial uncoupling, and such uncoupling is predicted to impair insulin secretion, because glucose-induced insulin secretion depends upon ATP generation from glucose metabolism [330].

Fatty acids can induce β-cell death by apoptosis in the presence of high glucose [406]. It is to note, that *in vitro*, saturated fatty acids induce β-cell apoptosis [407, 408], whereas unsaturated fatty acids are usually protective [406, 407]. Several mechanisms have been proposed to mediate fatty acid-induced apoptosis in β-cells, such as ceramide formation [409 – 411], altered lipid partitioning [406, 412 and 413] and the generation of oxidative stress [414 – 417]. Unfortunately, the effects of fatty acids on β-cell apoptosis *in vitro* are difficult to interpret, because [330]: significant differences exist between clonal cells and primary β-cells in their sensitivity to the cytotoxic effects of fatty, there are species-related differences in the ability of fatty acids to cause cell death, and the concentrations of fatty acids used *in vitro* vary among publications. There is also evidence that free fatty acids have effects on expression of PPARα, glucokinase, GLUT 2 and prepro-insulin [379].

In humans, the cardiac lipid overload that occurs with inherited defects in the mitochondrial fatty acid oxidation pathways is associated with heart failure and sudden death [418]. In animal models of obesity and diabetes, deposition of fat in cardiomyocytes is followed by evidence of apoptotic cardiomyocytes death [419]. In transgenic mice, cardiac restricted overexpression of acyl-CoA synthetase leads to increased cardiac myocyte free fatty acid uptake and intramyocyte accumulation of triglyceride and phospholipids; lipid accumulation is associated with early evidence of cardiomyocytes apoptosis, initial cardiac hypertrophy, decrease in systolic function and premature death [420]. In other animal models, in dependence on mutation, fatty acid metabolism disorders are associated with increased very low density lipoprotein (VLD) triglyceride, cardiac hypertrophy, increased mortality, cardiomyocytes accumulation of free fatty acids and cholesterol esters, poorcontractile function, ventricular hypertrophy and systolic ventricular dysfunction [379].

Adipose tissue progressively loses its ability to buffer excessive lipid fluxes as obesity develops. This disorder is associated with an increase in free fatty acid flux to the muscle of obese subject [421]. Increased plasma free fatty acids lead to intramyocellular lipid accumulation in humans. The skeletal muscle lipid overload has been proposed to play a critical role in the genesis of insulin resistance and type 2 diabetes [17]. Some possible mechanisms have been proposed, including the effect of free fatty acids on cellular membrane fluidity [422] and activation of the hexosamine pathway [423]. Intramyocellular lipid accumulation is associated with activation of serine/threonine kinase cascade that ultimately results in reduced IRS-1 tyrosine phosphorylation, reduced insulin receptor substrate-1-associated phosphatidylinositol 3-kinase activity and failure to promote translocation of the GLUT 4 to the plasma membrane in response to insulin stimulation [424, 425]. These studies indicate that acute elevations of plasma free fatty acids result in intramyocellular increases of insulin desensitizing lipid moieties.

Recent data suggest that intramyocellular lipids are specifically harmful when combined with reduced mitochondrial function, both conditions that characterize type 2 diabetes. The reduction in the transcription factor PPARγ co-activator-1α, which is involved in mitochondrial biogenesis, may be a result of consumption of high-fat diets and high plasma fatty acid levels. Thus, muscular lipotoxicity may impair mitochondrial function and may be central to insulin resistance and type 2 diabetes mellitus [426, 427].

Lipid overload in the liver leads to dysregulated liver function. Evidence is found in animal models and in human disease. In a mouse model of impaired β-oxidation, lipid accumulation in the liver may lead to cell dysfunction, manifest as failure to approximately carry out gluconeogenesis [428] and neonatal hypoglycemia contributes to rather early mortality. In humans, triglyceride and free fatty acid accumulation in the liver is associated with non-alcoholic steatohepatitis [429]. The effect of long chain fatty acids on glycogen synthase has been proposed as a possible mechanism [430, 431].

There are also studies suggest that free fatty acids carried by filtered albumin in the setting of proteinuria play a role in the genesis of tubulointerstitial injury [432].

Metabolic Syndrome

Reports of clustering of metabolic risk factors are not new and date back to the early 1920s [433]. Metabolic syndrome was initially observed in 1923 by Kylin. He described the clustering of hypertension, hyperglycemia and gout as the syndrome [434]. However, there was little interest in this phenomenon until 1988. In 1988 Reaven coined the term "syndrome X" to describe a disorder consisting of insulin resistance, glucose intolerance, increased triglyceride and decreased high-density cholesterol levels and hypertension [23]. The syndrome has given several names including the insulin resistance syndrome, the cardiovascular metabolic syndrome, the plurimetabolic syndrome, the deadly quartet, the dysmetabolic syndrome [435 – 439, and 442]. Reaven postulated that the common feature was insulin resistance and that all the other changes were likely to be secondary to this basic abnormality and that the more obese and sedentary an individual, the greater the degree of insulin resistance [440]. The World Health Organization (WHO) first defined the syndrome in 1998 [441]. In 1998, WHO proposed a unifying definition for the syndrome and chose to call it the "metabolic syndrome" rather than the "insulin resistance syndrome" [441], a term that had been used by Zimmet in 1991 [443]. This name was chosen primarily because it was the cause of all components of the syndrome [444]. As per The World Health Organization's criteria the metabolic syndrome required the presence of diabetes mellitus, impaired fasting glucose, impaired glucose tolerance, or insulin resistance plus 2 additional factors. In 1999, the European Group for the Study of Insulin Resistance suggested that a more appropriate term would be the "insulin resistance syndrome" and modified the criteria to require fasting hyperinsulinemia plus 2 other factors using different outpoints than those used by the WHO [440, 445].

Although there are divergent criteria for the identification of the metabolic syndrome, they all tend to agree that the metabolic syndrome core components include obesity, insulin resistance, dyslipidemia and hypertension [450].

Criteria for diagnosis of the metabolic syndrome by WHO (World Health Organization, 1985) is based on [441]: *insulin resistance* {impaired glucose tolerance (IGT), impaired fasting glucose (IFG), type 2 diabetes mellitus or lowered sensitivity}, and two of the following – *obesity* {waist-hip-ration (WHR) in men ≥ 0.9, in women ≥ 0.85, and/or body mass index (BMI) ≥ 30 kg/m^2, waist circumference (WC) > 96 cm}, *dyslipidemia* {triglycerides ≥ 150 mg/dL = ≥ 2.0 mmol/liter, and/or HDL-C (high density lipoprotein cholesterol) in men ≤ 35 mg/dL and ≤ 39 mg/dL in women}, *blood pressure* (BP) {$\geq 140/90$ mm Hg}, *glucose* {IGT, IFG or type 2 diabetes mellitus}, and *other* – microalbuminuria.

Criteria for diagnosis of the metabolic syndrome by EGIR (European Group for the Study of Insulin Resistance, 1999) is based on [445]: *insulin resistance* {plasma insulin > 75th percentile = top 25% of the fasting insulin values among nondiabetic individuals}, and two of the following – *obesity* {WC ≥ 94 cm for men, and ≥ 80 cm for women}, *dyslipidemia* {triglycerides ≥ 150 mg/dL, and/or HDL-C < 39 mg/dL in men or women}, *blood pressure* {$\geq 140/90$ mmHg or antihypertensive medication}, *glucose* {fasting plasma glucose (FPG) ≥ 110 mg/dL = ≥ 6.1 mmol/liter, IGT, IFG, but not diabetes}.

Criteria for diagnosis of the metabolic syndrome by NCEP:ATP III (National Cholesterol Education Program-Adult Treatment Panel III, 2001) is based on [446]: *insulin resistance* {none}, three or more of the following features – *obesity* {WC ≥ 102 cm in men, and ≥ 88 cm in women}, *dyslipidemia* {triglycerides ≥ 150 mg/dL, HDL-C ≤ 40 mg/dL in men, and ≤ 50 mg/dL in women}, *blood pressure* {$\geq 130/85$ mmHg}, *glucose* {fasting plasma glucose (FPG) ≥ 110 mg/dL = ≥ 6.1 mmol/liter, includes diabetes}.

Criteria for diagnosis of the metabolic syndrome by AACE (American Association of Clinical Endocrinology, 2003) is based on [447]: *insulin resistance* {IGT or IFT}, and two or more of the following – *obesity* {BMI ≥ 25 kg/m^2}, *dyslipidemia* {triglycerides ≥ 150 mg/dL, HDL-C < 40 mg/dL in men, and < 50 mg/dL in women}, *blood pressure* {$\geq 130/85$ mmHg}, *glucose* {IGT or IFG but not diabetes}, and *other* – other features of insulin resistance (includes family history of type 2 diabetes mellitus, polycystic ovary syndrome, sedentary lifestyle, advancing age, and ethnic groups susceptible to type 2 diabetes mellitus).

Criteria for diagnosis of the metabolic syndrome by IDF (International Diabetes Association, 2005) is based on [448]: *insulin resistance* {none}, *obesity* {central obesity as defined by ethnic/racial, specific WC}, and 2 of the following – *dyslipidemia* {triglycerides ≥ 150 mg/dL or on TG Rx, HDL-C ≤ 40 mg/dL in men, and ≤ 50 mg/dL in women or on HDL-C Rx}, *blood pressure* {$\geq 130/85$ mmHg}, *glucose* {FPG ≥ 100 mg/dL, includes diabetes}.

Criteria for diagnosis of the metabolic syndrome by AHA/NHLBI (American Heart Association/National Heart, Lung, and Blood Institute, 2005) is based on [449]: *insulin resistance* {none}, but three of following five features – *obesity* {WC in men ≥ 102 cm and ≥ 88 cm in women}, – *dyslipidemia* {triglycerides ≥ 150 mg/dL or on TG Rx, HDL-C ≤ 40 mg/dL in men, and ≤ 50 mg/dL in women or on HDL-C Rx}, *blood pressure* {$\geq 130/85$ mmHg or on hypertension Rx}, *glucose* {FPG ≥ 100 mg/dL, or on Rx for elevated glucose}.

The mechanisms underlying the metabolic syndrome are not fully known; however resistance to insulin stimulated glucose uptake seems to modify biochemical responses in a way that predisposes to metabolic risk factors [23, 435, and 451].

Data from the Third National Health and Nutrition Examination Survey suggested that about 20 – 30% of adults in developed countries have the metabolic syndrome. Its prevalence increases markedly among older people: in those aged 60 years or more, nearly 50% of people are estimated to have the metabolic syndrome [452].The metabolic syndrome is a proinflammatory and prothrombotic state with glucotoxicity and lipotoxicity contributing to the metabolic and vascular abnormalities [440]. The metabolic syndrome is characterized by a clustering of risk factors for cardiovascular disease that include insulin resistance, abdominal obesity, atherogenic dyslipidemia, hypertension and hyperuricemia. The metabolic syndrome is also characterized by a cluster of metabolic disorders that increase the risk of type 2 diabetes mellitus. Insulin resistance is believed to play a key role in the development of cardiometabolic syndrome [454]. During few years the prevalence of the cardiometabolic syndrome increased from 23,1% to 26,7% [455]. In the San Antonio Heart Study, the risk of cardiovascular disease was 1,7-fold and that of type 2 diabetes 5,8-fold increased in subjects with as compared with those without the metabolic syndrome [459].

As given above the mechanisms underlying the metabolic syndrome are not full known. Many studies have reported that resistance to insulin stimulated glucose uptake seems to modify biochemical responses in a way that predisposes to metabolic risk factors [435, 451].

The major pathogenic factor in the metabolic syndrome is central obesity [456, 457]. While abdominal obesity is determined by the accumulation of both subcutaneous adipose tissue and visceral adipose tissue, the excess accumulation of visceral adipose tissue appears to play a more significant pathogenic role [458]. It was found that visceral adipose tissue was nearly 50% higher in patients with metabolic syndrome in comparison with healthy subjects. Higher subcutaneous adipose tissue as well as higher intermuscular adipose tissue were significantly associated with metabolic syndrome in normal-weight and overweight, but not in obese subjects [460]. Visceral adipose tissue, by secreting adipocytokines, promotes the development of lipotoxicity in peripheral tissues [27]. Several adipokines have been implicated in the evolution of insulin resistance; for example: adiponectin, resistin, leptin, tumor necrosis factor-α, and interleukin 6 [461]. Adipose tissue is a source of metabolically active substances including elevated levels of free fatty acids, which affect parallel insulin-signaling pathway in the liver, skeletal muscle, and blood vessels, leading to hyperglycemia and endothelial dysfunction [440].

Metabolic syndrome is commonly associated with an abnormal lipoprotein phenotype characterized by elevated triglycerides, a low level of high-density lipoprotein cholesterol, and an accumulation of small, dense low-density lipoprotein particles (the so-called atherogenic dyslipidemic phenotype). It is to note that low-density lipoprotein cholesterol levels are often normal [468]. On the other hand, abnormal lipids were identified as the strongest risk for coronary heart disease in type 2 diabetes [469]. The presence of small, dense low-density lipoprotein particles is associated with an increased risk of ischemic heart disease [470] and isimplicated in the development of type 2 diabetes [471].

Adipose tissue insulin resistance appears to be important to the pathophysiology of the metabolic syndrome [472 – 473]. In the setting of insulin resistance and expanded adipose tissue triglyceride stores, the process of free fatty acid mobilization from stored adipose tissue triglyceride is accelerated [474], because insulin is unable to suppress lipolysis, resulting in relatively more free fatty acids being secreted into the plasma [472]. It is to note, that insulin resistance and hyperinsulinemia are strongly associated with decreased adipose triglyceride lipase and hormone-sensitive lipase mRNA and protein expression [475].

The increased risk of cardiovascular disease associated with the metabolic syndrome has many causes but dyslipidemia plays a prominent role [453]. Although the obesity is a major pathogenic factor in the metabolic syndrome, not all obese develop the syndrome and even lean individuals can be insulin resistant. Both lean and obese insulin resistant individuals have an excess of fat in the liver which is not attributable to alcohol or other known causes of liver disease. The fatty liver is insulin resistant [462, 463]. It overproduces both glucose [463] and VLDL [464, 465] leading to hyperglycemia, hypertriglyceridemia, and a low HDL cholesterol concentration. Overproduction of glucose, VLDL, CRP (C-reactive protein), and coagulation factors by the fatty liver could contribute to the excessive risk of cardiovascular disease associated with the metabolic syndrome [466].

Increases in free fatty acid flux have been shown to impair hepatic insulin action [476]. Insulin resistance in the liver increases hepatic glucose output, the synthesis of proinflammatory cytokines and changes of lipoprotein metabolism. In this state of insulin resistance, free fatty acid flux is high, triglyceride synthesis and storage are increased, and excess triglyceride is secreted as VLDL [477]. Dyslipidemia associated with insulin resistance is a direct consequence of increased VLDL secretion by the liver [478] and alterations in lipoprotein lipase have been associated with the metabolic syndrome.

Hepatic steatosis is related to insulin resistance and to the metabolic syndrome. By Jiang and Torok [479], this includes simple deposition of excessive hepatic fatty acids as triglycerides in the liver and nonalcoholic steatohepatitis.

The relationship between insulin resistance and hypertension has been established [480 – 482]. Insulin is a vasodilator and in the insulin resistant state, the vasodilatory effect of hormone can be lost [483]. On the other hand, in this state, insulin has an effect on sodium reabsorption in the kidney [484]. By Hanley and colleagues [485], insulin resistance contributes only modestly to the increased prevalence of hypertension in the metabolic syndrome.

Insulin resistance is known to activate the renin-angiotensin-aldosterone system (RAAS) [435]. Angiotensin II acting through its type 1 receptor (AT1) induces insulin resistance by inhibiting the actions of insulin in vascular and skeletal muscle tissue [486]. RAAS may also promote oxidative stress and endothelial dysfunction [487]. It is to note that activation of RAAS is associated with increased NADH and NADPH oxidase activity and increased reactive oxygen species such as superoxide anion and hydrogen peroxide [488]. These changes also result in hypertension, a major feature of the metabolic syndrome.

Metabolic syndrome is associated with an elevated inflammatory state [489]. Chronic, subclinical inflammation is part of metabolic syndrome. This is evidenced by the elevations of proinflammatory molecules including C-reactive protein, tumor necrosis factor-α, plasma resistin, interleukin 6, interleukin 18 [490 – 494], and inflammatory markers, including C-reactive protein, tumor necrosis factor-α, interleukin 18, and plasminogen activator inhibitor-1 activity showing an increase [495 – 499]. Individual inflammatory markers are also associated with singular components of the metabolic syndrome [450]. These factors are regulated by proinflammatory regulators such as nuclear factor κβ and the c-Jun NH_2-terminal signaling pathways to modulate the expression of genes that code for inflammatory proteins and to alter insulin signaling [500]. The result of these changes is an inflammatory state with increased risk for coagulation and decreased insulin sensitivity, both key features of the insulin resistance syndrome [461]. It is to note that levels of the antiinflammatory adipokine adiponectin are depressed in the metabolic syndrome [492, 501, and 502]. Adiponectin inhibits inflammation and promotes insulin sensitivity. In healthy subjects adiponectin decreases endothelial expression of adhesion molecules (intracellular adhesion molecule-1 {CAM-1}, vascular cell adhesion molecule-1 {VCAM-1}, and P-selectin) and decreases macrophage phagocytic activity [503]. Resistin, which is expressed primarily in macrophages, increases the expression of CAM-1 and VCAM-1 while enhancing that of monocyte chemoattractant protein-1 [504]. Both adiponectin and resistin interfere with monocyte adherence to vascular endothelium, promoting monocytic migration to the subendothelial space, one of the key events in the development of atherosclerosis [460]. It is to note, that macrophage and T cell infiltration is a major feature of atherosclerotic plaques, especially at sites of plaque rupture. Studies show positive association of systemic markers of inflammation with atherothrombotic disease [505 – 509]. It is now well known that inflammation and oxidation play key roles in the etiology and progression of cardiovascular disease [510].

Insulin resistance in the skeletal muscle due to decreased muscle glycogen synthesis promotes the development of atherogenic dyslipidemia, resulting in an increase in plasma triglyceride concentrations and a reduction in plasma HDL concentrations [467]. In muscle, increased plasma free fatty acid disrupts a glucose-fatty acid cycle [511, 512]. It has been hypothesized that triglyceride accumulation in skeletal muscle plays a direct role in the etiology of insulin resistance [473].

Insulin resistance tends to cluster in families and may be influenced by both genetic and environmental factors. The effect of genetics on insulin sensitivity is about 30% to 40% [513]. Familial aggregation is most evident for the individual components of metabolic syndrome. On the other hand, some studies suggest that specific genes, such as those that encode for 11β-hydroxysteroid dehydrogenase, adiponectin, and the β3-adrenergic receptor may predispose to the development of metabolic syndrome [514 – 516].

Several genes regulate insulin action at target organ level. It includes genes regulating insulin receptor function [517], intracellular insulin signaling [518], and nuclear receptors peroxisome proliferators activated receptor gamma (PPAR-γ). Significant evidence for linkage of insulin sensitivity, disposition index, and acute insulin response to glucose to different regions on chromosome 11 and 12 was observed. A most recent report focused on the endothelial nitric oxide synthase gene and its role in the metabolic syndrome. It was suggested that genetic variation at the endothelial nitric oxide synthase locus was associated with features of metabolic syndrome [519].

Type 1 Diabetes Mellitus

Type 1 diabetes (previously known as juvenile or insulin-dependent diabetes) results due to autoimmune progressive destruction of insulin-producing pancreatic β-cells by CD4+ and CD8+ T cells and macrophages infiltrating the islets [520]. Although, the etiology of the type 1 diabetes is believed to have a major genetic component, studies on the risk of developing type 1 diabetes suggest that environmental factors may be important etiological determinants. Evidence of an autoimmune etiology is found in about 95% of these cases and is classified as type 1 A (immune mediated). The remaining 5% lack defined markers of autoimmunity and therefore are classified as type 1 B, also termed idiopathic (non-immune mediated) [521].

Type 1 diabetes is observed in approximately 10% of patients with diabetes mellitus [522]. The incidence of type 1 diabetes varies regionally. In Finland the disease incidence is 40 per 100.000 children per year, 20.1 per 100.000 children in Kuwait, less than 2 per 100.000 in Japan, and 0,1 per 100.000 in Zunai region in China and in Venezuela [522 – 526]. Studies highlight the geographical differences in the incidence of type 1 diabetes, with the highest occurring in Caucasoid populations, mainly in Northern Europe and the lowest in Asia and South America. The incidence among boys is slightly higher than among girls [527]. The incidence of type 1 diabetes is projected to increase 40% between 1997 and 2010. The study suggest an annual, global increase of 3 – 4% with the highest increase expected in the 0 – 4 year age group [528, 529]. This rapid rise strongly suggests that the action of the environment of susceptibility genes contributes to the evolving epidemiology of type 1 diabetes [522].

Given the range of complications associated with type 1 diabetes such as nephropathy, retinopathy, neuropathy, coronary heart disease and peripheral vascular disease, improved understanding of the pathogenesis and identification of preventative therapies are the major aims of physicians. Bone mineral density appears to be reduced in patients with type 1 diabetes in most studies [532 – 536].

Type 1 diabetes is a complex polygenic dissorder. It cannot be classified strictly by dominant, recessive, or intermediate inheritance, making identification of disease susceptibility or resistant gene difficult [530, 531]. Genetic susceptibility is important in the development of type 1 diabetes. The lifetime of type 1 diabetes risk for a number of the general population is often quoted as 0,4%. Eight-five percent of cases of type 1 diabetes occur in individuals with no family of the disease. Differences in risk also depend on which parent has diabetes. The risk increases to 1 – 2% if the mother has diabetes and intriguingly to 3 – 7% if the father has type 1 diabetes [537, 538]. The sibling risk is 6% [539]. The classic indicator of the role of genetics in any disease is found by comparing concordance rates in monozygotic vs. dizygotic twins. Monozygotic twins have a concordance rate of 30 to 50%, whereas dizygotic twins have a concordance rate of 6 to 10% [537]. In Finland, with the highest incidence of type 1 diabetes, concordance rates of 27 for monozygotic twins and 3,8% for dizygotic twins were reported [540]. The study showed that 88% of the phenotypic variance was due to genetic factors, and the remaining variance is due to unshared environmental factors [540]. Over the last three decades, the study of type 1 diabetes has led the field in the identification of genes underlying complex multifunctional disease.

In both rodents and humans, the most important genetic link is the major histocompatibility complex (MHC). In humans, the MHC is known as the human leukocyte antigen (HLA) and contains over 200 genes [541]. It is located on chromosome 6p21.3 [542], encoding HLA class I, and class II molecules [543]. HLA class I and II genes are highly polymorphic and consist of many different alleles [550]. These genes encode cell surface proteins that are required for interaction with cells of immune system, and are involved in immune recognition and killing. Distinct loci within the HLA region determine risk [544, 545], though the HLA class II region appears to be most influential [546]. The HLA is considered to contribute about half of the familial basis of type 1 diabetes [547, 548]. Disease susceptibility is highly associated with inheritance of the HLA alleles DR3 and DR4 as well as the associated alleles DQ2 and DQ8. More than 90% of patients with type 1 diabetes express either DR3DQ2 or DR4DQ8. Heterozygous genotypes DR3/DR4 are most common in children diagnosed with type 1 diabetes prior to the age of 5 (50%) [530]. Individuals with the HLA haplotype DRB1*Q302-DQA1*0301, especially when combined with DRB*10201-DQA1*0501 are highly susceptible (10 – 20-fold increase) to type 1 diabetes. On the other hand, HLA class II haplotypes such as DR2DQ6 confer dominant protection [549]. Individuals with the haplotype DRB1*0602-DQA1*0102 rarely develop type 1 diabetes. The precise mechanism through which HLA-DQ determines disease susceptibility is still not clear [551].

Candidate genes studies also identified the insulin gene as the second most important genetic susceptibility factor, contributing 10% of genetic susceptibility to type 1 diabetes [552]. Over the last decade, whole genome screen has indicated that there are at least 15 other loci associated with type 1 diabetes [553 – 555], such as cytostatic T-lymphocyte antigen (CTLA-4) gene [557, 558], *PTPN22* [559], interleukin 2 receptor alpha (IL2RA) gene [560], interferon induced with helicase C domain 1 (IFIH1) gene [561], vitamin D receptor gene (VDR) [562], KIAAO350 (also known as CLEC 16A) gene [563], phosphotyrosine protein phosphatase, non-receptor 2 gene (PTPN2) [564], and others [565].

To date, no single gene is either necessary or sufficient to predict the development of type 1 diabetes. Although type 1 diabetes is likely a polygenic disorder, epidemiological pattern of type 1 diabetes suggests that environmental factors are involved [556].

Histological analysis of the pancreas from patients with type 1 diabetes shows that immunological activity is not present in a healthy or a type 2 diabetic pancreas [566]. This activity is limited to insulin-containing islets, including infiltration by activated lymphocytes, antibodies and components of the complement system. These histological findings are consistent with type 1 diabetes being an immune-mediated disease [546]. The autoimmune nature of type 1 diabetes is a fairly recent discovery. The initial evidence for autoimmunity in patients with type 1 diabetes came from immunofluorescence studies, which showed that a high percentage of sera from newly diagnosed type 1 patients reacted with pancreatic islets [543, 567, and 568]. Autoantibodies, called islet cell autoantibodies (ICA), are detected in individuals with type 1 diabetes. Over the years, the specificities of several islet cell autoantibodies have been clarified, although some still remain unidentified. Three major autoantibodies have now been identified.

The first is an isoform of glutamic acid decarboxylase (GAD65). GAD65 is a protein expressed in neuroendocrine cells, including pancreatic islets. The function of protein in the islets is not known. Between 60 and 80% of newly diagnosed type 1 diabetic patients have autoantibodies to GAD65.

The second major autoantigen is insulinoma associated antigen-2 (IA-2, also known as ICA512). It is a member of the transmembrane protein-tyrosine phosphatase family [570]. Experiments suggest that it may play a role in insulin secretion [571].

Between 60 and 70% of newly diagnosed patients with type 1 diabetes have autoantibodies against IA-2.

The third major autoantigen is insulin. Autoantibodies against insulin are among the first autoantibodies to appear in the prediabetic state and are usually found in very young children. Between 30 and 50% of young children with type 1 diabetes have autoantibodies against insulin [530]. Once insulin therapy begins, insulin antibodies may not be a useful marker since some patients develop antibodies to exogenous insulin. The frequency of autoantibodies against insulin is lower in individuals who develop type 1 diabetes at an older age. Other candidate autoantigens include carboxypeptidase, hSP 60, and ganglioside (GM2-1). It is estimated from animal studies that between 80 and 90% of the β-cells that must be destroyed are clinically apparent.

Epidemiological studies link viral infection to the acquisition of type 1 diabetes. The most popular candidates are viruses, with enteroviruses [572], rotaviruses [573] and rubella being suspects. Viral involvement is strongly supported in human type 1 diabetes acquired after congenital rubella. Approximately 20% of such children go on to develop type 1 diabetes [526]. It is to note, that more than 10 viruses have been reported to be associated with the development of type 1 diabetes-like syndromes in animals [574].

Type 1 diabetes is often associated with other well established autoimmune diseases such as chronic thyroiditis, non-destructive Addison's disease, celiac disease, and autoimmune polyendocrinopathy syndrome. Up to 25% of patients with type 1 diabetes will have evidence of thyroid disease, the commonest autoimmune disease associated with type 1 diabetes [575]. The prevalence of celiac disease is increased at 7% in patients with type 1 diabetes, but not other types of diabetes [576]. The prevalence of islet cell antibody has been reported to be as high as 6% in patients with Addison's disease [577].

By Neufeld and colleagues [578, 579], where multiple autoimmune endocrinopathies are present, they tend to segregate in definable groups. These are termed autoimmune polyglandular syndrome (ASP). Type 1 diabetes can occur in all of these, but is most frequent in APS 2, Schmidt's Syndrome [546]. It is characterized by the presence of Addison's disease with type 1 diabetes and/or autoimmune thyroiditis. Clustering of type 1 diabetes with other autoimmune diseases suggest that possible defects in immune regulation may contribute to the development of multiple autoimmune phenotypes [526].

Type 1 diabetes mellitus is recognized to include an element of insulin resistance. Insulin resistance is an independent risk factor for the development of macro- and microvascular complications of type 1 diabetes and may contribute to the development of the disease [937]. Insulin resistance plays a larger role in the type 1 diabetes disease process than is commonly recognized. The onset of type 1 diabetes is often heralded by an antecedent illness and/or the onset of puberty, both conditions associate with insulin resistance. Insulin resistance is a transient feature of normal puberty and peaks at Tanner stage 3 [938]. Despite evidence in the literature of insulin resistance in adults with type 1 diabetes mellitus [939 – 941] and in adolescent during metabolic decomposition [942, 943, and 947] and puberty [944, 945], insulin resistance is not routinely considered to contribute to type 1 diabetes mellitus pathophysiology.

The presence of insulin resistance in type 1 diabetes mellitus was probably first noted by Himsworth in 1936 [946]. Though Ginsberg reported on measurements of insulin sensitivity in patients with type 1 diabetes as early 1977 [952], the concept that changes in insulin sensitivity have a role in type 1 diabetes has only recently been gaining acceptance [953].

The mechanisms of insulin resistance in type 1 diabetes mellitus remain poorly defined. The phenotype of insulin resistance in type 1 diabetes mellitus youth is unique, suggesting a pathophysiology that is different from type 2 diabetes mellitus [948]. Insulin resistance is associated with a metabolic syndrome, phenotype of high triglycerides, triglyceride to high-density lipoprotein ratio, visceral fat, intramyocellular lipid, obesity, inflammation, and low high-density lipoprotein and adiponectin. Type 1 diabetic youth patients observed by Nadeau and colleagues [948] lacked these abnormalities. Single small studies individually found that adult patients with type 1 diabetes mellitus lacked central adiposity, hepatic steatosis, hypoadiponectinemia and low high-density lipoprotein [949, 950]. On the other hand, according to other authors, some mechanisms are likely to be similar to those already proposed for type 2 diabetes mellitus [951]. Insulin insensitive patients with type 1 and type 2 diabetes both have raised intramyocellular lipid [939] recognized to interfere with insulin signaling and glucose uptake by skeletal muscle [954]. Adipokines whose levels are influenced by insulin resistance in both type 1 and type 2 diabetes [955, 956], have modulatory effects on insulin signaling.

Mechanisms contributing to insulin resistance have been described in patients with type 1 diabetes [937]. Impaired insulin-stimulated vasodilatation can reduce blood flow and hence glucose delivery for extraction in skeletal tissues [957 – 959]. Patients with type 1 diabetes with insulin resistance express lower tissue levels of the insulin receptor [960] and GLUT 4 is reported to be expressed at a lower level in the skeletal muscle of obese patients with type 1 diabetes [961].

Insulin resistance is recognized to the aetiology of micro- (nephropathy, neuropathy and retinopathy) and macrovascular (coronary artery disease and peripheral vascular disease) disease in patients with type 1 diabetes mellitus [937, 948, and 959]. Studies demonstrate a clear association between clinical surrogates of insulin resistance with the development of vascular complications in type 1 diabetes [937]. There are yet no study examining the relationship between insulin resistance and cerebrovascular disease in type 1 diabetes mellitus [937].

The mechanism of association between insulin resistance and progression of type 1 diabetes is not clear [962, 963], but insulin resistance has a capacity to both disrupt β-cell physiology and alter autoimmunity in those at risk [937]. Thus many, but not all, studies demonstrate a role of insulin resistance in type 1 diabetes. One potential explanation for the development of insulin resistance in patients with type 1 diabetes is the role of counter-regulatory hormone. In particular, an inappropriate excess of growth hormone clearly contributes to the insulin resistance in type 1 diabetes [964, 965]. Another possibility is a direct role of impaired glucose metabolism since either hyperglycemia per se, or hyperinsulinemia or both could contribute directly to impaired insulin action [966]. According to suggestion by Pang and Narendran [937], immune cells express receptors for adipocytokines [967] and manipulating the levels of these cytokines influences the rate of development of type 1 diabetes [968]. Metabolically active β-cells synthesize and are more susceptible to the toxic effects of inflammatory cytokines [969]. They up-regulate islet self-antigens, which may make them more susceptible to autoimmune attack [970]. These processes, according to Pang and Norendran [937], may in part explain the association between insulin resistance and progression to type 1 diabetes mellitus.

LADA

Late autoimmune diabetes in adults (LADA), type 1.5 diabetes [581] or slow progressive insulin dependent diabetes mellitus (SPIDDM) [582] is a common form of diabetes [580]. The term "latent autoimmune diabetes in adults", abbreviated as LADA, was coined by Tuomi and colleagues [583] to describe patients with a slowly progressive form of autoimmune or type 1 diabetes who could be treated initially without insulin injections. Yet the risk factors are poorly characterized. Age, overweight and physical inactivity are important risk factors for type 2 diabetes by way of increasing insulin resistance. These findings suggest a role for insulin resistance in the pathogenesis of LADA [584].

LADA is defined by three features including: adult age at diagnosis, the presence of diabetes-associated autoantibodies, and delay from diagnosis in the need for insulin therapy to manage hyperglycemia. The first and last are not categorical traits, being dependent on the mode of ascertainment and decision making by physicians, the second feature lacks disease specificity because it is based on positivity for autoantibodies found in type 1 diabetes mellitus [585].

Latent autoimmune diabetes in adults is a disorder in which, despite the presence of islet antibodies at diagnosis of diabetes, the progression of autoimmune β-cell failure is slow. Patients with LADA are therefore not insulin dependent, at least during the first 6 months after diagnosis of diabetes. This clinical observation was intended to distinguish LADA from classic type 1 diabetes, where insulin is required from diagnosis, and from type 2 diabetes, where insulin is not required at all or at least until some years after diagnosis [580]. Individuals with slowly progressive type 1 diabetes had previously been identified by an immunofluorescence staining pattern to islet cell antibodies restricted to β-cells [586, 587]. Among patients with phenotypic type 2 diabetes, LADA occurs in 10% of individuals older than 35 years and in 25% below that age [588].

The concept of LADA is ambiguous [584]. The controversy primarily concerns that it can be viewed as a separate form of diabetes or a rather mild form of type 1 diabetes [589]. With regard to the etiological differences between type 1, type 2 diabetes, and LADA, Carlsson and colleagues [590] found that smoking is associated with a reduced risk of LADA and type 1 diabetes but an increased risk of type 2 diabetes. With regard to age, BMI, and physical inactivity, there is a similarity between LADA and type 2 diabetes [584].

Pathogenesis of LADA still remains unclear. By Bandurska-Stankiewicz and colleagues [591], there are several factors considered to be responsible for slow and/or partial progression of β-cells destruction, such as less extensive genetic predisposition to have type 1 diabetes could explain why LADA occurs in adult age, possible action of genes responsible for beta cells protection, partial regeneration of beta cells, immune tolerance after the onset of immune process against beta cells, and quantitative decrease of exposition for environmental factors damaging beta cells.

A subset of adults who present with type 2 diabetes has detectable ICA (about 6% of these patients) and GAD (about 10% of these patients) antibodies [592]. In the United Kingdom Prospective Diabetes Study, the level of antibodies was higher in a younger group of patients; in a group of patients aged 25 – 34 years, GAD antibodies level was detected positive in 34% and ICA – in 21% [593, 594].

All four islet autoantibodies – ICAs, GAD autoantibodies, IA-2 autoantibodies and insulin autoantibodies – are common in childhood type 1 diabetes. ICAs and GAD antibodies are also common in LADA, but both IA-2 autoantibodies and insulin autoantibodies are much less common in LADA than in type 1 diabetes [595]. Type 1 diabetic patients are very often positive for two or more autoantibodies, whereas single autoantibodies are common in LADA patients [596]. It is to note that glutamic acid decarboxylase (GAD) antibodies can be detected in 1 – 15,8% of healthy subjects with diabetic history in their family, but even then most of these individuals do not develop clinical symptoms of diabetes. It is possible that there are some factors protecting islets against destruction [591].

In type 1 diabetes, it is clearly established that HLA BR3, DR4 and DQB1*0201 and 0302 confer risk of type 1 diabetes. It is estimated that ~ 50% of the risk of type 1 diabetes can be attributed to HLA. Furthermore, other HLA alleles including DR2 and DQB1*0301 and 0602 confer protection against type 1 diabetes. Many groups have measured HLA in LADA patients, but unfortunately, many of the reports do not agree, and consequently there is still considerable controversy in this area [596]. Some genetic studies of the LADA patients suggest that occurrence of alleles DR3, DR4 and DQB1*0201 and 0302 is similar to the patients with type 1 diabetes and higher than in control group [594,597, and 598]. On the other hand, children with the diabetes-protective HLA DR2, DQB1*0602, are unlikely to develop diabetes [599], whereas in type 1 diabetes of adult-onset and LADA, the same alleles carry less protection [600, 601].

Allelic variations at several non-HLA loci have also been associated with increased risk for and protection from classic type 1 diabetes, although these effects are weaker than for HLA. Unfortunately, the significance of these genes in LADA has not been confirmed [602]. Only in one study, the TNF2 allele was significantly lower in LADA compared with type 1 diabetes or nondiabetic control subjects [600].

Non-genetic factors play a major role in causing type 1 diabetes. We know little of the current incidence of autoimmune diabetes in adults and LADA. The incidenceof a range of autoimmune diseases has increased over the last three decades [603]. The current low selection density and relative stability of HLA polymorphism indicate that this increasing incidence cannot be due to genetic selection pressures and is most likely the result of monogenetic factors [604, 605]. It is to note, that among some of LADA patients there are observed other autoimmune diseases, such as Graves disease, Hashimoto thyroiditis, Addison's disease, pernicious anaemia, and hypoparathyroidism [591].

Type 2 Diabetes Mellitus

Type 2 diabetes mellitus, previously called non-insulin-dependent diabetes mellitus, is a complex heterogeneous group of metabolic disorders including hyperglycemia and impaired insulin action and/or insulin secretion. Current theories of type 2 diabetes include a defect in insulin-mediated glucose uptake in muscle, a dysfunction of the pancreatic β-cells, a disruption of secretory function of adipocytes, and an impaired insulin action in liver [606]. In contrast to insulin resistance, the decline in β-cell function is considered a late event [607] and was shown to be, at least in part, caused by an irreversible loss of β-cell mass [608]. The etiology of human type 2 diabetes is multifactorial with genetic background and environmental factors of the modern world which favor the development of obesity. Overweight and obesity represent a major risk factor for type 2 diabetes [609 – 611]. However, some 10% of type 2 diabetic patients display normal weight, and many obese subjects never develop type 2 diabetes, indicating that type 2 diabetes is not exclusively caused by environmental factors [612] but pathogenesis of type 2 diabetes is not fully understood.

Type 2 diabetes clearly represents a multifunctional disease, and several findings indicate that genetics is an important contributing factor. It has been estimated that 30% – 70% of type 2 diabetes risk can be attributed to genetics [613]. The lifetime risk of type 2 diabetes is about 7% in a general population, about 40% in offspring of one parent with type 2 diabetes, and about 70% if both parents have type 2 diabetes [615]. Patterns of inheritance suggest that type 2 diabetes is both polygenic and heterogeneous – i.e. multiple genes are involved and different combinations of genes play a role in different subsets of individuals [614].

Genetic research efforts of the last decade have led to the identification of at least 27 (confirmed and potential) type 2 diabetes susceptibility genes [612] and most recent genome-wide association studies have identified 20 common genetic variants associated with type 2 diabetes [616]. Many loci appear to regulate the capacity of β-cells to increase insulin secretion in response to an increase in insulin resistance or obesity (*TCF7L2, KCNJ11, HHEX, SLC30A8, CDKAL1, CDKN2A/CDKN2B, IGF2BP2, KCNQ, MTNR1B, WFS1*), genes related to insulin sensitivity (*PPARG, ENPP1*), glucose transport (*CAPN10*), obesity (*MC4R, FTO*), and insulin secretion (*CDC123/CAMK1D, JA2F1, KCNO1, TSPAN8/LGR5*). Four other loci (*ADAMTS9, HFN1B, NOTCH2, THADA*) have unknown roles in type 2 diabetes [612, 616]. Most of the gene variants could be confirmed in many ethnicities (*TCF7L2, SLC30A8, HHEX, CDKAL1, CDKN2A/CDKN2B, IGF2BP2, FTO*), whereas other may have higher relevance for certain ethnic groups, e.g. *ENPP1* for African-Americans [617, 618]. Notably, no gender-specific differences in the known genes impact on the diabetes risk were observed [612].

An evolutionary theory regarding the genetics of this process was first proposed by Neel [619]. When humans were hunter-gatherers and did not know when the next meal was expected, some individuals developed "thrifty genes". Thrifty genes caused the body to become insulin resistant. Insulin resistance was due to mechanisms that allowed blood glucose to be transported into cells where it would be used for energy. Pancreas had to make more insulin. The excess insulin allowed cells to store fat for use during times of relative famine, leading to a much higher survival rate [619 – 621]. These genes may include uncoupling proteins, PPAR-γ, PPAR-α, CALPAIN10, and adrenergic receptor polymorphisms [622 – 624]. When agrarian societies began to develop, thrifty genes began to cause weight gain because food was more plentiful [619 – 621].

During puberty, resistance to the action of insulin increases, resulting in hyperinsulinemia [625]. In children who have a genetic predisposition and environmental risk exposures, the additional burden of insulin resistance at puberty may lead to uncompensated hyperinsulinemia and glucose intolerance [626].

In normoglycemic subjects, insulin displays rapid variations in blood concentrations. The insulin response to a meal normally occurs in a biphasic pattern, and the amount of insulin released is highly responsive to the prevailing glucose value [627]. Insulin is secreted with secretory peaks every 5 – 10 min, that are though necessary for normal regulation of hepatic glucose production, and larger oscillations every 60 – 120 min, especially after meals, to maximize the efficiency of nutrient clearance following meals [628 – 630]. In overt type 2 diabetic patients, a reduction or an absence of rapid secretory peaks is observed [631, 632]. An acute rise in glucose, that can be experimentally replicated with intravenous glucose, normally causes a large burst of insulin secretion that lasts 5 – 10 min (first phase) and is followed by a second insulin response that lasts as long as hyperglycemia (second phase). In type 2 diabetes, first phase insulin secretion is abolished [633 – 635]. As mentioned above, early phase insulin secretion is pivotal in the transition from fasting state to fed state, as it suppresses hepatic glucose production [636], and lipolysis [637], and crosses the endothelial barrier, preparing target cells for the action of insulin [638].

In healthy subjects, the pancreatic β-cell adapts its secretion rate to the level required by insulin sensitivity. If compensation is impaired, plasma glucose rises gradually. Part of the normal β-cell compensation to insulin resistance is an increase in the β-cell mass. A study of a large number of weight-matched subjects with type 2 diabetes and healthy subjects (controls) showed a 40 – 60% reduction of β-cell mass with this disease [639, 640]. Considerable current research is focused on trying to determine the pathogenic reason for the lowered β-cell mass in type 2 diabetes, with several proposed mechanisms. An observation first made, at the turn of the century was the occurrence of amyloid plaques in islets from patients with type 2 diabetes [641, 642]. Studies in the late 1980s showed the amyloid developed from a normal β-cell secreted protein that is co-packed with insulin in insulin granules, and is termed Islet Associated Polypeptide (IAPP) [643 – 645]. Studies in humans have demonstrated that islet amyloid is associated with loss of β-cell mass [646]. It has been proposed that very small developing intracellular amyloid fibrils cause the β-cell destruction in the early stages of the disease [647]. A significant loss of β-cells does not seem likely at the early phases of clinical hyperglycemia in type 2 diabetes [648]. This conclusion is supported by autopsy studies suggesting that at death perhaps ≤ 20 – 50% of the β-cells are lost after many ears of disease [649 – 651]. The reduction of β-cell mass is attributable to accelerated apoptosis. The major factors for progressive loss of β-cell function and mass are: glucotoxicity, lipotoxicity, oxidative stress, proinflammatory cytokines, and leptin [652 – 656].

Since skeletal muscle accounts for ~ 75% of whole body insulin-stimulated glucose uptake, defects in this tissue play a major role in glucose homeostasis in patients with type 2 diabetes [657]. Insulin resistance in skeletal muscle is among the earliest detectable defects in humans with type 2 diabetes [7, 568, and 659]. Insulin elicits its pleiotropic metabolic responses by binding to and activating a specific plasma membrane receptor with tyrosine kinase activity [660]. It activates a series of lipid and protein kinase enzymes linked to the translocation of glucose transporters (GLUT 4) to the cell surface, synthesis of glycogen, protein, mRNA, and nuclear DNA, which affect cell survival and proliferation [661]. In states of insulin resistance, one or more of the following molecular mechanisms to block insulin signaling are likely to be involved. Insulin receptor tyrosine phosphorylation appears to be normal or reduced in type 2 diabetic patients [662]. Type 2 diabetic patients have impaired insulin-stimulated tyrosine phosphorylation of IRS-1 in skeletal muscle. A similar impairment is observed at the level of PI 3-kinase in type 2 diabetic muscle [662].

The dysregulation of the insulin receptor or IRS constitutes a common feature of insulin resistance [606]. Mechanisms for this dysregulation might include TNF-α-mediated downregulation of mRNA transcription [663 – 665], kinase-mediated serine/threonine phosphorylation [666 – 669], proteasome-mediated degradation [670], and phosphatase-mediated dephosphorylation [671 – 674]. These signaling abnormalities could result in an impaired glucose transport. It is to note that insulin-stimulated glucose transport is reduced in the skeletal muscle of patients with type 2 diabetes [662].

Type 2 diabetic patients are characterized by a decreased fat oxidative capacity and high levels of circulating free fatty acids [675 – 677]. The latter is known to cause insulin resistance by reducing insulin stimulated glucose uptake, most likely via accumulation of lipid inside the muscle cell [678 – 679]. A reduced fat oxidative capacity and metabolic inflexibility are important components of skeletal muscle insulin resistance [680].

In type 2 diabetic patients, GLUT 4 expression is downregulated in adipose tissue [681]. The hyperglycemia associated with type 2 diabetes cannot be explained by the decreased uptake of glucose into adipocytes due to downregulation of GLUT 4 because skeletal muscle is the major site of glucose disposal [606]. The results obtained in animal studies by Zisman and colleagues [682] and Abel and colleagues [683] indicate that adipocyte Glut 4 deficiency may result in generation of circulating factors that are responsible for cross-organ communication. Adipocytes secrete factors which may alter systemic insulin action and hepatic glucose production, including adiponectin, resistin, leptin, interleukin 6, tumor necrosis factor-α, retinol-binding protein 4, and free fatty acids [682 – 684]. The inhibition of signaling downstream of the insulin receptor may be a primary mechanism through which this inflammatory state causes insulin resistance [606].

Impaired insulin sensitivity and deregulated insulin action in the liver contribute significantly to the pathogenesis of type 2 diabetes [685]. Dysfunction of IRS proteins in liver initially leads to postprandial hyperglycemia, increased hepatic glucose production, and deregulated lipid synthesis, and is considered as a major pathophysiological mechanism for the development of insulin resistance and type 2 diabetes [686 – 688].

Patients with diabetes are highly susceptible to infections [689], and develop remarkable changes in lymphocyte metabolism [690]. Infectious diseases were a major cause of death among diabetic patients before the advent of insulin therapy. Type 2 diabetic patients show reduced thymidine uptake by lymphocytes, a reduced percentage of interleukin-2 receptor-positive cells and increased plasma levels of tumor necrosis factor-α when compared with controls [691 – 693]. These patients show impaired intensity of deoxy-D-glucose transport into peripheral blood cells [694 – 697] and changed glucose transporters expression in these cells [698 – 701]. High and low glucose levels also affect these processes in lymphocytes [702].

Several mutations in mitochondrial DNA (mtDNA) have been found to be associated with enhanced risk for developing diabetes [703]. Most of them are rare [704]. For example, the A3243G mutation in the mtDNA-encoded tRNA^{Leu,UUR} gene is associated with the MIDD (maternally inherited diabetes and deafness) syndrome and accounts for 0,2 – 2% of the diabetic cases [705 – 707]. Highest frequencies are found in Japan [704]. The penetrance of this mutation is high, as > 85% of the carriers will develop diabetes during life [708]. Surprisingly, laughter regulates gene expression in patients with type 2 diabetes [709].

Gestational Diabetes Mellitus

Gestational diabetes mellitus (GDM) is defined as "carbohydrate intolerance with onset or first recognition during pregnancy" [710]. This definition includes pregnancies in which the following occur: insulin therapy is required, diabetes persists after delivery, and diabetes may have been present, but not recognized, prior to the pregnancy [711]. Gestational diabetes is one of the most common complications of pregnancy, occurring in 2,2% – 8,8% of each year, depending on the ethnic mix of the population and the criteria used for diagnosis [712]. It can have a much higher incidence in certain minority populations with a greater predisposition to diabetes. The incidence of gestational diabetes is increasing, in parallel to the increase in type 2 diabetes. Women at risk of type 2 diabetes are at risk of GDM [713].

During early pregnancy, glucose tolerance is normal or slightly improved and peripheral sensitivity to insulin and hepatic basal glucose production is normal [714 – 716]. Insulin responses to oral glucose are also greater in the first trimester than before pregnancy. The second phase of insulin response is not significantly different in early pregnancy from the pregravid state [717]. Studies of glucose tolerance during gestation show a progressive increase in nutrient-stimulated insulin responses despite an only minor deterioration in glucose tolerance, consistent with progressive insulin resistance [718]. Insulin action in late normal pregnancy is 50% – 70% lower that of nonpregnant women [714 – 716]. A progressive increase in basal and postprandial insulin concentrations is seen with advancing pregnancy, and by the third trimester, basal and 24-h mean insulin concentrations may double [719]. Thus there is a 50% – 70% reduction in insulin sensitivity in women with gestational diabetes compared with controls [726]. The first and second phases of insulin release are 3- to 3,5-fold greater in late pregnancy [714].

In early pregnancy, basal glucose and insulin concentrations do not differ significantly from nongravid values [715] and basal hepatic glucose production does not differ at 12 – 14 wk of gestation [717]. By the third trimester, basal glucose concentrations are lower and insulin is almost twice the concentration of nongravid women. Postprandial glucose concentrations are significantly elevated, glucose peak is prolonged [720] and increases production of hepatic glucose [721, 722]. Glucose production increases with maternal body weight [722]. Endogenous glucose production remains sensitive to increased insulin concentration through gestation in contrast with the progressive decrease in peripheral insulin sensitivity [717].

Gestational diabetes mellitus is a heterogeneous disorder in which age, obesity, and genetic background contribute to the severity of the disease. Risk factors for GDM include being overweight before pregnancy (BMI > 25kg/m^2), having a first-degree relative with diabetes, previous glucose intolerance, previous macrosomia or large-for-gestational-age baby, polycystic ovarian syndrome, age > 25 years, and being a member of an ethnic group with the high prevalence of GDM [723]. Low-risk ethnic groups are those other than Hispanic, African-American, Native American, South Asian, East Asian, Pacific Islander, and Indigenous Australian [724]. Multiparous women have a very high prevalence of gestational diabetes mellitus [725].

There has been relatively little research in the area of gestational diabetes genetics [727]. There are studies that have examined the familial clustering of gestational diabetes and type 1 and type 2 diabetes. Dorner and colleagues [728] reported increased familial aggregation of diabetes on the maternal side of offspring with type 1 diabetes whose mothers had gestational diabetes. Similarly, there is evidence for clustering of type 2 diabetes and impaired glucose tolerance in families with a GDM [729] and evidence for higher prevalence of type 2 diabetes in mothers of women with gestational diabetes [730].

Freinkel and colleagues [731] observed that HLA DR3 and DR4 antigens were uncommon overall, but nonetheless in higher frequency in women with gestational diabetes than in women with normal pregnancies. Similarly, Ober and colleagues [732] reported association between variation in the insulin receptor gene in Caucasian and African-American women with gestational diabetes. On the other hand, no associations between insulin receptor gene were observed in Hispanic women with gestational diabetes [732]. There have also been observed several reports of association between variations in glucokinase gene and gestational diabetes [733 – 736]. By Ellard and colleagues [736], the prevalence of glucokinase gene variants may be as high as 80% in a small subset of women with gestational diabetes selected by highly specific clinical criteria. There have also been reports of association between variation in the P2 promoter region of *HNF4A* and gestational diabetes [727]. Variation in *HFN4A* may contribute to the β-cell dysfunction observed in GDM [727].

The pathophysiology of gestational diabetes remains controversial; GDM may reflect a predisposition to type 2 diabetes under the metabolic conditions of pregnancy or it may represent the extreme manifestation of metabolic alterations that normally occur in pregnancy [717]. Only a 1,6% incidence of islet cell antibodies is found by using a specific monoclonal antibody in women with GDM[737]. As the increase in insulin resistance is greatest in the third trimester, GDM usually develops in this period [713]. The pathophysiology of gestational diabetes involves abnormalities of insulin-sensitive tissue. Beta cell sensing of glucose is also abnormal and is manifested as an inadequate insulin response for a given degree of glycemia [738]. Women with gestational diabetes have decreased insulin sensitivity in comparison with a weight-matched control groups. Ryan and colleagues [739] reported a 40% decrease in insulin sensitivity in women with gestational diabetes in comparison with a pregnant control groups in late pregnancy. Postpartum studies in women with gestational diabetes have demonstrated defects in insulin-secretory response [740]. Gestational diabetes induces a state of dyslipidemia consistent with insulin resistance.

During pregnancy, women with gestational diabetes do have higher serum triacylglycerol concentrations but lower LDL-cholesterol concentrations than do normal pregnant women [741]. Carr and colleagues [742] found that gestational diabetes increases the risk of cardiovascular disease in women with a family history of type 2 diabetes and these women were more likely to have experienced cardiovascular disease events at a younger age.

During pregnancy, gestational diabetes is associated with a number of complications for child. Because insulin does not cross the placenta, the fetus is exposed to the maternal hyperglycemia. At the 11th or 12th week of gestation, the fetal pancreas is capable of responding to this hyperglycemia [743]. The fetus thus becomes hyperinsulinemic, which in turn promotes growth and subsequent macrosomia [724]. Fetus born to mother with gestational diabetes has higher risk of developing macrosomia, neonatal hypoglycemia, hyperbilirubinemia, respiratory distress syndrome, polycythemia, hypertrophic cardiomyopathy, hypocalcemia, shoulder dystonia with its attendant risk of brachial plexus injury and clavicle fracture, jaundice [744 – 749]. These complications have been reported with varying frequency [750]. Additionally, there are some data that suggest an increase in fetal malformation and perinatal mortality [751 – 754]. Cesarean sections are also more common, and GDM is associated with a higher risk of pre-eclampsia [747 – 749].

Infants exposed to maternal diabetes in uterus have an increased risk of diabetes and obesity in childhood and adulthood [755]. Studies indicate that the magnitude of fetal-neonatal risks is proportional to the severity of maternal hyperglycemia [756].

MODY

Maturity onset diabetes of young (MODY) is a monogenic and autosomal dominant form of diabetes mellitus. MODY was described by Tattersall in 1974 – 1975 [757, 758] and since then newer gene mutations and subgroups of MODY have been identified. Tattersall and Fajans coined the acronym MODY for "individuals with a fasting hyperglycemia diagnosed under age 25 which could be treated without insulin for more than two years" [758]. Criteria used in genetic studies of MODY families are as follows [759]: 1) early onset diabetes before the age of 25 years in at least two family members MODY pedigrees show a phenomenon of anticipation, i.e. a progressive reduction in the age of diagnosis in succeeding generations; 2) non insulin dependent diabetes demonstrated by the absence of insulin treatment 5 years after diagnosis or by significant circulating C-peptide concentrations; 3) autosomal dominant inheritance; 4) absence of obesity (though obese people can get MODY), or other problems associated with type 2 diabetes or metabolic syndrome (e.g. hypertension, hyperlipidemia, and polycystic ovary syndrome). Of note, pancreatic autoantibodies, as for example GAD are not found. To distinguish MODY from type 1 diabetes tests need to be done to establish the absence of diabetes antibodies (anti-insulin, anti-islet, anti-GAD). In obese people, the absence of insulin resistance (which will be shown by a C-peptide test), will differentiate it from type 2 diabetes. MODY presents in children, adolescent or young adults and may account for up to 5% of diabetes cases [760]. The prevalence is 0,5% – 1% of all patients of NIDDM in most white European populations [759]. In France, MODY has been found in 13% of Caucasian NIDDM families [761]. There are reports that MODY could represent more than 18% of NIDDM population in India [762].

MODY patients have a strong family history of diabetes, suggestive of a primary genetic cause [763, 764]. MODY is caused by changes to a single gene and if either one of the parents carries this gene they have a 50% chance of passing it on to their child; this is known as autosomal dominant inheritance. So MODY can appear in several generations of a family. Whereas multiple acquired factors contribute to the pathophysiology of type 2 diabetes, disease progression in MODY is though to be largely independent of nongenetic factors other than time [760]. A primary physiological defect caused insulin release [763 – 765].

Nine genetic forms of MODY have been identified to date, and these have been termed MODY 1 – 9. These rare diabetic disorders are associated with heterozygosity for mutations in single genes, including 7 transcription factors and 2 metabolic enzymes. For each form of MODY, multiple specific mutations involving different amino acid substitutions have been discovered. In some cases, there are significant differences in the activity of the mutant gene product that contribute to variations in the clinical features of the diabetes.

MODY 1

MODY 1 is due to a loss-of-function mutation in the HNF4α gene on chromosome 20q12 [614] that codes for hepatocyte nuclear factor 4α. HNF4α is a nuclear transcription factor responsible for the regulation of hepatic and pancreatic β-cell gene expression [766, 767]. It controls function HNF1α (see MODY 3) and perhaps HNF1β (MODY 5) as well and plays a role in the early development of the pancreas, liver, and intestines. In the pancreas these genes influence expression of among others, the genes for insulin, GLUT 2 and several proteins involved in glucose and mitochondrial metabolism [760, 768, and 769]. MODY due to HNF4α mutations closely resembles classic type 2 diabetes. Several HNF4α mutations have been described [770 – 773], but this still remains a rare cause of MODY, accounting for 5% of UK MODY families [759, 771]. Presence of any one of these mutations prevents efficient stimulation of insulin gene transcription. Consequently, not enough insulin is produced in response to high blood glucose. Patients with HNF4α mutations have diabetes as a result of β-cell dysfunction rather than insulin resistance. Pancreatic polypeptide secretion is also impaired in patients with MODY 1. Liver effects are subtle and not clinically significant. These patients may have alteration in triglyceride, lipoprotein(s) and apolipoproteins AII and CIII. It was found that a common variant of HNF4α was associated with high serum lipids and metabolic syndrome [775]. Macrosomia and neonatal hypoglycemia have also been reported in MODY 1 [776]. The prevalence of microvascular and macrovascular complications is similar to IDDM [777].

MODY 2

MODY 2 is due to any of several mutations in the *GCK* gene on chromosome 7p15 [614] for glucokinase [778]. MODY 2 is one of the common forms of MODY [779]. Glucokinase serves as the glucose sensor for the β-cell, which catalyzes the first and rate-limiting step of glycolysis. Loss-of-function mutations in glucokinase result that is less sensitive or less responsive to rising levels of glucose [780 – 783]. The β-cells in MODY 2 have a normal ability to make and secrete insulin, but do so only above an abnormally high threshold. Gain-of-function mutations in glucokinase gene do not lead to diabetes, but to the "complementary" condition, congenital hyperinsulinism. Missense mutations fall into three main categories [759]: mutations of conserved active site residues (these have drastic effect on catalytic activity), mutations predicted to distort the enzyme structure (those show reduced activity), and mutations of surface residues that eliminate conserved interactions with other residues, and may reduce the stability of the structure (show small reduction in activity). Patients have remarkably similar phenotype despite the variety of mutations [784]. The pathophysiology involves chronic, mild hyperglycemia which is usually asymptomatic. Only 2% of patients require insulin therapy and diabetes associated complications are rare.

An affected mother will pass MODY 2 to 50% of her children. A small number of infants will have a new mutation not present in their mothers. If the mother is affected and the fetus is not, the maternal glucose will be somewhat high and the fetal pancreas will make lots of insulin, resulting in a large infant. If the fetus is affected but mother is not, glucose will be normal and fetal insulin production will be low, resulting in intrauterine growth retardation. Homozygous mutations result in permanent neonatal diabetes mellitus [785].

MODY 3

MODY 3 is the most common type of MODY in populations with European ancestry, accounting for about 70% of all cases in Europe. It is due to mutations in the *HNF-1α* gene on chromosome 12q24 [614, 786]. *HNF-1α* is expressed in the liver, kidney, pancreas and bowel. It is a transcription factor that is thought to control a regulatory network important for differentiation of β-cells. Mutations of this gene lead to reduced β-cell mass or impaired function. MODY 1 and MODY 3 diabetes are clinically similar, and clinical features are markedly different from *GCK* mutations [780]. Most subjects under the age of 10 years have a normal glucose tolerance and fasting blood glucose levels. The average age of manifestation is 22 – 26 years. Most patients exhibit pronounced polyuria when diagnosed. MODY 3 patients show considerable, progressive hyperglycemia, after 16 years of diabetes 50% have retinopathy, 15% – 20% show severe forms of pre-proliferative or proliferative macular edema, and 20% of cases have nephropathy [769, 786, and 787].

MODY 4

MODY 4 arises from mutations of the insulin promoter factor-1 (IPF-1) homeobox gene on chromosome 13q12 [614]. IPF-1 is a transcription factor vital to the development of the embryonic pancreas and in adult, it continues to play a role in the regulation and expression of genes for insulin, GLUT 2, glucokinase, and somatostatin. IPF-1 has been described as a master switch for both endocrine and exocrine function of pancreas [768]. It plays a key role in the regulation of insulin secretion [759]. It is suggested that homozygosity for the mutation is associated with agenesis of pancreas and neonatal diabetes and heterozygosity with MODY [763, 788].

MODY 4 is so rare that only a single family has been well-studied. A number of older relatives who were heterozygous had mild hyperglycemia or diabetes.

MODY 5

MODY 5 arises from mutations of the *HNF-1β* gene on chromosome 17q21 [614]. HNF-1 beta, also known as transcription factor 2 (TCF 2) is a transcription factor, which is involved in early stages of embryonic development of several organs, including the urinary and genital tracts, the liver and bile ducts as well as the pancreas [769, 789, and 790].

MODY 5 is one of the less common forms of MODY. The glucose tolerance is normal in the first decade, and glycemic worsens with increasing age. Apart from hyperglycemia, patients with MODY show genital tract abnormalities, renal diseases such as dysplastic kidneys, renal cysts associated with diabetes in adult patients, familial glomelurocystic kidney disease, and oligomeganephronia. Most patients show increased levels of liver enzymes without any clinical symptoms [769].

MODY 6

MODY 6 arises from mutations of the gene for transcription factor referred to as neurogenic differentiation 1 (NEUROD1). The gene is on chromosome 2q32 [614]. NEUROD1 promotes transcription of the insulin gene as well as some genes involved in the formation of β-cells and parts of the nervous system [763]. This is one of the rarer forms of MODY. Only 3 kindreds with mutations causing MODY 6 have been identified so far. In both, some of the members had more typical type 2 diabetes rather than MODY and one of them fits the definition of MODY with evidence of defective insulin secretion from β-cells [791].

MODY 7

MODY 7 is due to mutations in the *KLF11* gene on chromosome 2p25 [614] for Kruppel-like factor 11. It regulates exocrine cells growth and behaves like a tumor suppressor for pancreatic malignancy [792]. It was also reported to play a role in glucose signalling in β-cells of pancreas. Its gene variants are associated with MODY 7 [792].

MODY 8

MODY 8 is due to mutation in the *CEL* gene on chromosome 9q34.3 [614] for carboxyl-ester lipase. It controls both exocrine and endocrine function of pancreas. The patients had abdominal pain and presence of a spectrum of faecal elastase deficiency [793].

MODY 9

MODY 9 is due to mutations in the *PAX4* gene on chromosome 7q32. It is a transcription factor for β-cell development. Pathological mutations in *PAX4* are considered as a subtype of MODY [768].

Neonatal Diabetes Mellitus

Neonatal diabetes mellitus (NDM) is defined as insulin-sensitive hyperglycemia occurring in the first months of life, lasting for more than 2 weeks and requiring insulin for management [794, 795]. NDM is rare, with an incidence of approximately 1 in 500 000 births [794]. It is considered distinct from autoimmune type 1 diabetes, which manifests after the first 3 to 6 months of life [796]. Antibodies to insulin or islet cells and other markers of autoimmune type 1 diabetes are absent. Neonatal diabetes mellitus forms two separate forms that vary in the length of insulin dependency in the premature stage of the disease. In about 50% of cases of neonatal diabetes mellitus, diabetes is transient and resolves at a median age of 3 months (Transit Neonatal Diabetes Mellitus, TNDM). The other 50% of cases of neonatal diabetes mellitus are permanent (Permanent Neonatal Diabetes Mellitus, PNDM) [792].

The etiology of neonatal diabetes mellitus is genetically heterogeneous, producing abnormal development or absence of pancreas or islets, decreased β-cell mass secondary to increased β-cell apoptosis or destruction, and β-cell dysfunction that limits insulin secretion [798]. On the other hand, variable patterns for NDM (i.e. for TNDM and for PNDM) suggest differing underlying mechanisms.

Transient Neonatal Diabetes Mellitus is a form of neonatal diabetes that appears in the first six weeks of life and usually ends by 18 months. Approximately one third of patients with neonatal diabetes mellitus have transient disease that resolves after several months, with no further recurrence even after many years of follow-up; approximately one fourth of patients with NDM have transient NDM followed by occurrence from 7 to 20 years [794].

Transient neonatal diabetes mellitus has been associated with the overexpression of the genes in the 6q24 locus [799 – 802]. There are also mutations in the *KCNJ11* and *ABCC8* genes [798]. There are 3 known mechanisms that may cause TNDM 90% of the cases: a) paternal uniparental disomy of chromosome 6 – there are two chromosome 6 homologues where each homologues acquires a copy of genes in the 6q24 locus. This is inherited from paternal side [800 – 802]; b) duplication of 6q24 on the paternal allele [800, 803]; 3) 6q24 methylamine defect in the maternal copy of the promoter that may be implicated in the pathogenic mechanism of diabetes.

There are multiple imprinted genes in region 6q24 including *ZAC* (zinc finger protein which regulates apoptosis and cell cycle arrest – also called *LOT1*, for loss of transformation [805] and *HIMAI* (hydatiform mole-associated and imprinted – also called *PLAGL1*, for pleromorphic adenoma of the salivary gland gene like 1). *HIMAI* is an untranslated RNA of undetermined function. *ZAC* is a zinc-finger transcription factor [806] with multiple functions such as: a coactivator with p53 of Apaf1 (apoptotic protease activation factor 1), transcription [807, 808], regulation the histone acetyl transferase activity of p300 [809], coactivator or corepressor of several nuclear hormone receptors [810]. Little is known about the specific role (s) of *ZAC* or *HYMAI* during pancreatic islet development. Overexpression of *ZAC* in cell lines resulted in a decreased rate of cell replication, increased apoptosis, and G1 arrest [805, 811]. Overexpression of *ZAC* could be anticipated to reduce growth rate and subsequently β-cell mass [798]. *ZAC* regulates the expression of receptor 1 of the pituitary adenylate cyclase activating polypeptide, a potential insulin secretagogue and an important mediator of autocrine control of insulin secretion [804].

Transient neonatal diabetes mellitus is characterized by intrauterine growth retardation, dehydration, small gestational age at birth, and failure to thrive [813 – 816]. In patients with transient neonatal diabetes mellitus, the β-cell is preserved and able to secrete insulin through the stimulatory G protein pathway while exhibiting a specific defect of insulin secretion after glucose stimulation. By Valerio and colleagues [816] lack of treatment leads to long-lasting hyperglycemia without the risk of ketoacidosis but associated with microangiopathy in adult life.

Permanent Neonatal Diabetes Mellitus can occur alone (isolated) or as part of a larger genetic syndrome. In PNDM, diabetes develops within days to months after birth and persists throughout life. The hallmark of PNDM is hyperglycemia early in life, but without the period of remission that defines TNDM. Permanent neonatal diabetes mellitus is known to have many different genetic causes, several of which have been identified. To date, 13 genes involved in pancreatic development, β-cell apoptosis, or dysfunction have been identified as being able to give rise to PNDM [798].

In islet development the genes involved are: *TCF2/HNF1β*. *PTF1A*, *PDX1/IPF1*(< 1% of cases), *GLIS3*, *ZAC*; in reduced β-cell mass are involved genes: *EIF2AK3*, *INS* (about 20% of cases), *FOXP3*; and in β-cell dysfunction – *GCK* (about 4% of cases), *ABCC8* (about 19% of cases), *SLC2A2*, *SLC19A2*, *KCNJ11* (about 30% of cases) [798, 817]. Isolated PNDM has been associated with mutations in at least five genes. These genes are: *KCNJ11, ABCC8, INS, GCK,* and *PDX1*. Syndromic cases are caused by mutations in different genes. Two of these involved genes are known to be responsible in the heterozygous state for two distinct MODY syndromes. Mutations in *PDX1/IPF-1* and *GCK*, that cause MODY 4 and MODY 2, respectively, in the heterozygous condition produce PNDM in the homozygous state. Of note, TNDM has been seen in children with two MODY 5 (*HNFβ/TCF2*) mutations [798].

The K$_{ATP}$ channels are encoded by the genes *KCNJ11* and *ABCC8* [818]. These channels regulate insulin secretion. The mutations in these genes mostly reduce the response of the channel to ATP, which prevents channel closure and consequently insulin secretion. Familial cases in the case of *KCNJ11* gene show autosomal dominant inheritance. Patients with PNDM as a result of *ABCC8* mutations show autosomal recessive inheritance [819]. Heterozygous mutations in the insulin gene (*INS*) have been identified [820 – 823]. Most mutations are located within the A or B chains of insulin and are predicted to interfere with the formation of disulfide bridges between cysteine residues, either by replacing a cysteine residue or introducing an additional cysteine residue into the insulin molecule [817].

This type of monogenic neonatal diabetes mellitus involves the progressive death of β-cells. These mutations show autosomal dominant inheritance. The enzyme glucokinase is considered the glucose sensor of the β-cells. Heterozygous *GCK* gene mutations produce familial, mild, non-progressive hyperglycemia, and homozygous or compound heterozygous *GCK* gene mutations preventing the β-cells from secreting insulin in response to hyperglycemia [824, 825].

The remaining known genetic causes of neonatal diabetes mellitus are uncommon. Complete deficiency of transcription factor IPF1 due to mutations in the *IPF1* gene, has been described in two patients with pancreatic agenesis to date [826, 827]. Homozygous mutations in *PTF1A* have been identified in several patients with pancreatic and cerebellar hypoplasia/agenesis from two consanguineous families [828. 829]. All of them died during infancy due to central respiratory failure [798]. GLIS3 is a transcriptional regulator that has recently been shown to be involved inthe production of a complex syndrome including neonatal diabetes mellitus, congenital hypothyroidism and dysmorphic features [830, 831]. To date, homozygous mutations in the *GLIS3* gene have been identified in four probands from three unrelated consanguineous families [798]. IPEX (Immune dysregulation, Polyendocrinopathy, Enteropathy, X-linked) syndrome is a multisystemic disorder that presents in hemizygous males with a mutation in the *FOXP3* gene [832]. Heterozygous carrier females remain asymptomatic.

Intrauterine growth retardation, hyperglycemia, sever dehydration, osmotic polyuria, and failure to thrive are all associated with PNDM.

Type A Insulin Resistance

The term type A syndrome was originally applied to lean adolescent female patients with severe insulin resistance, acanthosis nigricans, severe ovarian hyperandrogenism, and decreased insulin binding to circulating leukocytes [833]. Type A syndrome (type A insulin resistance) is currently used for both female and male patients with severe inherited insulin resistance and acanthosis nigricans in the absence of autoantibodies to the insulin receptor [834, 835].

The mechanism of type A insulin resistance syndrome is either a defect in insulin receptor itself or postreceptor abnormality [836]. Several investigations have been reported various mutations of insulin receptor gene in this disorder [837 – 839], which cause decreased receptor number, decreased binding affinity, or abnormality in signal transduction due to a kinase defect. Biallelic mutations in both alleles of the insulin receptor gene give rise to various very rare syndromes characterized by severe insulin resistance, with a strong genotype-phenotype correlation existing among patients [840, 841]. The first insulin receptor mutations were identified in 1988, and since then over 50 disease-causing insulin receptor mutations have described [842, 843]. The vast majority of these mutations are found in association with extreme insulin resistance syndromes [844]. It is possible to classify mutations in the insulin receptor gene into at least five classes, based upon the molecular mechanism whereby the mutation impairs the function of receptor [845, 846].

Class 1

Decreased receptor biosynthesis. Several mutations have been identified that impair receptor biosynthesis, such as: nonsense mutations [847 – 849], deletion mutations that result in premature chain termination [839, 850], and few of the nonsense mutations have been demonstrated to cause an 80% – 90% decrease in the level of insulin receptor mRNA [848, 849].

Class 2

Impaired transport of receptors to the cell surface. Expression studies demonstrated that substitution of Arg for His^{209}, substitution of Lys for Asn^{15}, and a mutation substitution valine for phenylalanine at position 382 in the α-subunit of the insulin receptor, impair transport of receptors through the endoplasmic reticulum and Golgi apparatus to the cell surface [849, 851, and 852].

Class 3

Decreased affinity of insulin binding. Many different types of mutations are known to decrease the affinity of insulin binding. For example, the Ser^{735} mutation inhibits the cleavage of the precursor into two separate subunits and decreases affinity with which the receptor binds insulin [853 – 855].

Class 4

Defects in receptor tyrosine kinase activity. At least five missense mutations have been identified in the intracellular domain of β-subunit of the insulin receptor [856 – 860].

Class 5

Accelerated degradation of the insulin receptor. With normal insulin receptors, decreasing the pH from 7,8 to 6,0 causes a tenfold acceleration in the rate at which insulin dissociates from its receptor. Missense mutations such as Lys^{460}, Asn^{462}, cause insulin resistance by accelerating the rate of receptor degradation [849, 861]. The cause of insulin resistance is a decrease in the number of insulin receptors on the surface of target cells that results from an accelerated rate of receptor degradation [846].

Family studies indicate an autosomal dominant or autosomal recessive pattern of inheritance of the type A insulin resistance syndrome, with variable penetrance [833, 835]. It appears that most patients with type A insulin resistance syndrome do not possess insulin receptor mutations, implying the presence of other critical primary defects in insulin signaling [844, 862]. In addition to mutations of the insulin receptor gene, a transmembrane protein named PC-1 and lamin A have been proposed as the cause of the type A insulin resistance syndrome [843, 863, and 864].

Patients with type A insulin resistance usually developing in adolescence are almost exclusively female, also suffering from acanthosis nigricans, hyperandrogenism and polycystic ovary syndrome. It does not typically occur in diabetes, although impaired glucose tolerance or diabetes may develop at a later stage. Paradoxically, many of the patients with type A insulin resistance present with hypoglycemia [865]. Postpubertal females have evidence of mild to severe androgen excess of ovarian origin, ranging from hirsutism, acne, oligoamenorrhoea and infertility to frank virilism with markedly elevated testosterone levels. Additional, but not invariable, features of the type A insulin resistance include short stature, acral hypertrophy, accelerated linear growth, muscle cramps, and retinitis pigmentosa [833 – 835, and 866]. Type A insulin resistance variants involve insulin resistance and clinical features similar to acromegaly (pseudoacromegaly), but without the increase in growth hormone or IGF-1 [866, 867].

Mutations have been identified in the insulin receptor gene in patients with several distinct syndromes: leprechaunism, the Rabson-Mendenhall syndrome, and the type A insulin resistance. Because the clinical syndromes do not correlate with the type of mutation, it seems most likely that it is the severity of insulin resistance that determines the clinical manifestation. The mechanism by which insulin elicits its multiple biologic responses in target cells is extremely complex [846].

Type B Insulin Resistance

Type B insulin resistance is caused by autoantibodies (immunoglobulin G, IgG) to the insulin receptor. Such antibodies affect insulin action through a direct inhibition of access to the insulin binding site, a desensitization of one or more steps subsequent to insulin binding, an acceleration of receptor degradation, or a combination thereof [868]. Insulin receptor antibodies have a regulatory effect on plasma membrane $(Ca^{2+}+Mg^{2+})ATPase$, which antagonizes that of insulin. By Nagy and colleagues [871] this effect of the antibodies might explain in part their diabetogenic effects. At maximal insulin resistance, the insulin receptor concentration is thought to be normal, but probably with reduced affinity. The blocking antibodies are believed to be polyclonal [874]. It is a rare disease that responds in an unpredictable manner to immunosuppressive therapies; therefore, there are no treatment guidelines for the use of immunosuppressive agents for patients with the disease [869, 870]. In contrast to the typical early onset of the type A insulin resistance, patients afflicted with the type B insulin resistance are commonly middle-aged at presentation. The mean age of onset is about 40 years, but it has been seen as early as at age 12 and as late as at 78 [870]. As seen in other autoimmune disorders, the disease is more common in females (a female predominance, 80%). The disease has been noted in many ethnic groups but is most common in African American [869, 870]. Fluctuating hyper- and hypoglycemia is observed. Some patients have hypoglycemia as the primary metabolic feature. Anti-insulin-receptor antibodies can cause spontaneous hypoglycemia as a result of an insulinomimetic effect [872, 873]. Some patients present initially with hyperglycemia and subsequently develop spontaneous hypoglycemia. Also patients with concurrent fasting hypoglycemia and postprandial hyperglycemia have been described [875]. Many patients show manifestations of autoimmune diseases such as arthritis, nephritis, vitiligo, alopecia areata, systemic lupus erytematosus, primary biliary cirrhosis, Hodgkin's disease, and ataxia-telangiectasia [833 – 835]. Postpubertal females often demonstrate severe insulin resistance, i.e. abnormal glucose homeostasis, acanthosis nigricans, and ovarian hyperandrogenism. Spontaneous remission of insulin resistance with disappearance of insulin receptor antibodies has been documented in a few patients [876].

Type C Insulin Resistance

Type C insulin resistance is caused by mutations at the insulin receptor gene [877] or post-binding defects in insulin action [865]. It is not commonly caused by mutations in the tyrosine kinase domain of the insulin receptor gene [877]. Type C insulin resistance is defined by the triad of hyperandrogenism, insulin resistance, acanthosis nigricans (HAIR-AN syndrome) like type A insulin resistance and unlike type A insulin resistance, often in association with obesity [835], in absence of autoimmune disease. This type of insulin resistance is found in 5% of patients with polycystic ovary syndrome [878]. The etiology of type C insulin resistance is not known. By Globerman and Karnieli [877], type C insulin resistance may be a mild form of "classic" type A insulin resistance. On the other hand, by Vidal-Puig and Moller [835] it has not yet been fully clarified whether HAIR-AN syndrome represents a distinct entity from other syndromes of severe insulin resistance, such as the type A and type B insulin resistance, or polycystic ovary syndrome.

Leprechaunism

Leprechaunism, known as Donohue's syndrome, was originally described by Donohue in 1948 who reported a female infant looking like an elf with multiple endocrine abnormalities [879]. This was presented as a case of "dysendocrinism". In 1954 a similar child was born to the same family and Donohue and Uchida proposed the term "leprechaunism" for this condition [880].

Leprechaunism is a rare autosomal recessive disorder associated with extreme insulin resistance with paradoxical hypoglycemia [881]. The most severe form of insulin resistance occurs in leprechaunism, where there are homozygous or compound heterozygous mutations in the regulatory or coding domains of the insulin receptor, resulting in what is effectively a functionally null receptor [12]. A number of different mutations in the insulin receptor gene have been reported.

Leprechaunism is characterized by severe intrauterine and postnatal growth retardation and failure to thrive, lipoatrophy, dysmorphic features (globular eyes, large ears, micrognathia) and acanthosis nigricans. These infants have hyperinsulinemia, often associated with glucose intolerance or frank diabetes mellitus, in addition to fasting hypoglycemia. Affected female infants commonly have hirsutism and clitoromegaly, whereas affected males have penile enlargement, dysmorphic lungs, renal disease, breast hyperplasia, thick skin with lack of subcutaneous fat and distended abdomen. The majority of babies with leprechaunism may die within the first 2 years of life although a few may survive until adolescence [880].

Rabson-Mendenhall Syndrome

Rabson-Mendenhall syndrome is very rare syndrome associated with severe insulin resistance, initially described by Mendenhall [882]. Rabson-Mendenhall syndrome is also the result of mutations of the insulin receptor, and is inherited as autosomal recessive trait.

Patients with Rabson-Mendenhall syndrome present in childhood with severe insulin resistance and diabetes mellitus, acanthosis nigricans, abnormal nails and dentition, accelerated linear growth, precocious pseudopuberty and pineal hyperplasia [882]. Prognosis is generally poor, mainly due to the development of severe microvascular complications of diabetes. Patients with Rabson-Mendenhall syndrome survive beyond 1 year of age and, with time, develop constant hyperglycemia followed by diabetic ketacidosis and death. It is caused by progressive decline in insulin levels, which become insufficient to prevent glucose synthesis in the liver and prevent release of fatty acid by adipocytes [883].

Polycystic Ovary Syndrome

Polycystic ovary syndrome (PCOS) is an endocrine-metabolic syndrome. It is a steroid-related disorder of unknown etiology that affects approximately 5% to 10% of all women of reproductive age [897 – 899]. Its clinical manifestations include oligoamenorrhoea, hirsutism, acne, infertility, hyperandrogenism, high levels of luteinizing hormone with normal levels of follicle stimulating hormone, altered gonadotropin dynamics, chronic anovulation, and polycystic ovaries [900, 901]. The syndrome is associated with increased risk of endometrial carcinoma [902]. The syndrome has a significant metabolic impact. It is now well established that PCOS represents a complex trait similar to type 2 diabetes mellitus and obesity. Polycystic ovary syndrome is also associated with hyperinsulinemia, glucose intolerance, abnormal blood lipid levels, and obesity, which constitute the metabolic syndrome [903]. In addition, β-cell insulin secretory defects are present in women with PCOS [917, 918]. PCOS is also associated with profound peripheral insulin resistance, conferring an increased risk for the development of type 2 diabetes mellitus at an early age [897, 904, and 905]. One-third to one-half of the women who have polycystic ovary syndrome also have metabolic syndrome, and insulin resistance may be the pathogenic link between the 2 syndromes [906, 907]. Women with PCOS are at substantially higher risk for impaired glucose tolerance and type 2 diabetes, with combined prevalence rates of 35% – 40% for glucose intolerance [905, 908]. Insulin resistance and subsequent hyperinsulinemia are found in 50% – 70% of PCOS women [904]. Hyperinsulinemic insulin resistance is a nearly universal feature of PCOS and occurs in both obese and lean women with the disorder. The prevalence of metabolic syndrome in women with PCOS is high among all age groups. This increased prevalence appears to be independent of body weight [910]. About 10% of women with PCOS have been found to have type 2 diabetes mellitus [908]. Studies from Scandinavian population have found a five fold higher prevalence of diabetes among women with PCOS compared with controls [909]. Insulin resistance and hyperinsulinemia play important roles in the pathogenesis of polycystic ovary syndrome.

Insulin resistance in polycystic ovary syndrome appears to be selective, affecting metabolic but not mitogenic actions of insulin in cultured skin fibroblasts [911]. Insulin resistance in PCOS may only disturb the metabolic effects of insulin signaling, and either not affect or enhance the mitogenic effects of insulin signaling [911, 914].

Not all tissues in PCOS women are insulin resistant; the insulin resistance seems to be tissue selective [912]. Insulin resistance has been reported in muscle, adipose tissue, and in the liver [904, 913]; however, it has not been reported in the ovary itself [912]. Hence the "paradox" in polycystic ovary syndrome: whereas some tissues are insulin resistant, other tissues are insulin sensitive [915]. The abnormalities observed in PCOS differ from those reported in other insulin resistant states consistent with the hypothesis that PCOS is a genetically unique disorder states consistent with the hypothesis that PCOS is a genetically unique disorder conferring an increased risk for type 2 diabetes [916].

The molecular mechanisms underlying insulin resistance in peripheral tissues in polycystic ovary syndrome remain under intensive investigation. The molecular mechanisms of insulin resistance in PCOS differ from those in other common conditions such as obesity and type 2 diabetes [914]. There is a postbinding defect in insulin signaling in adipocytes [913, 919] and skeletal muscle [920]. Insulin resistance in polycystic ovary syndrome is associated with a unique postbinding defect in insulin receptor signaling due to a complex interaction between intrinsic (genetically determined) and environmental factors [916]. In addition, extrinsic factors including inflammatory mediators, adipokines, androgens, free fatty acids, amino acids, and increased glucose levels, have been all implicated in the pathogenesis of insulin resistance in polycystic ovary syndrome [922].

Recent studies of skeletal muscle in PCOS have provide evidence for the interaction of intrinsic defects in insulin signaling with factors in the *in vivo* environment in the pathogenesis of insulin resistance in this tissue [921]. *In vivo* studies of PCOS patients revealed significant reduction in insulin-mediated glucose uptake [920]. Impaired insulin-stimulated glucose uptake in skeletal muscle of women with PCOS is associated with decreased IRS-1-associated PI3-kinase activation [920]. The expression of insulin receptors, IRS-1, and p85 regulatory subunit of PI3-kinase was normal but that of IRS-2 was significantly increased in skeletal muscle *in vivo*. Basal IRS-1 associated PI3-kinase activity was normal but insulin-mediated IRS-1-associated PI3-kinase activity was significantly decreased [920]. *In vitro* studies revealed that expression of insulin receptor β-subunit, IRS-2, and p85 regulatory subunit of PI3-kinase were similar to that of controls [916]. GLUT 4 expression was normal in skeletal muscle of PCOS patients, whereas basal and insulin-stimulated glucose transport and GLUT 1 abundance were significantly increased in cultured myotubes from women with PCOS [916]. Phosphorylation of IRS-1 on Ser^{312}, a key regulatory site, was significantly increased in PCOS. Insulin signaling via IRS-2 was also decreased in myotubes from women with PCOS [916]. On the other hand, impaired insulin signaling in skeletal muscle in PCOS is selective for glucose metabolic pathways: mitogenic signaling via the mitogen activated protein kinase ERK1/2 is enhanced [914]. The observations provide support for the hypothesis that enhanced serine phosphorylation of IRS-1 is an important mechanism for insulin resistance in PCOS [914].

Women with PCOS are often obese and have upper-body fat distribution for which androgens and insulin resistance seem to have synergistic effect [923]. Adipose tissue of PCOS women also exhibits a defect in glucose uptake. A decrease in glucose uptake was found in both obese and nonobese women with PCOS *in vivo* and *in vitro* [913]. Studies have revealed modest but significant decreases in maximal insulin-stimulated rates of glucose utilization *in vivo* and in isolated adipocytes [919]. The number of insulin receptors in adipocytes of women with PCOS was normal [913, 919]. Basal autophosphorylation of the insulin receptor β-subunit was also normal [924]. A decrease in IRS-1 tyrosine expression and phosphorylation in insulin resistant PCOS women were found and tyrosine phosphorylation of IRS-2 was also decreased [925]. The expression of GLUT 4 was significantly decreased in adipocytes from PCOS women, independently of obesity [926]. According to Diamanti-Kandarakis and Papavassiliou [923] the observed diminished insulin sensitivity in PCOS patients cannot be explained by defective binding at receptor level. It must be a step downstream from receptor binding in the insulin signal-transduction pathway that is defective.

Glycogen synthase activity is constitutively inhibited by phosphorylation by glycogen synthase kinase-3. When activated by the insulin-signaling cascade, protein kinase B serine phosphorylates glycogen synthase kinase-3 and following glycogen synthase activity to increase [927]. Insulin-stimulated glycogen synthesis may be impaired in PCOS [911, 928]. According to Liberman and Eldar-Finkelman [929] glycogen synthase kinase-3 may inhibit insulin signaling by inducing serine phosphorylation of IRS-1. Chang and colleagues [927] demonstrated reduced insulin-stimulated glucose uptake in PCOS adipocytes compared to control. PCOS adipocytes displayed higher tyrosine phosphorylation and lower insulin-stimulated serine phosphorylation of glycogen synthase kinase-3β, suggesting glycogen synthase kinase-3β overactivity. These data, by authors, implicate glycogen synthase kinase-3 hyperactivity in the pathogenesis of PCOS. Glycogen synthase kinase-3β is hyperactivated and resistant to downregulation by insulin in PCOS [927]. It is to note that glycogen synthase kinase-3 protein levels and activity are increased in muscle from patients with type 2 diabetes mellitus [930, 931].

Fibroblasts do not belong to the group of classic target cells of insulin. On the other hand, fibroblast cultures have been used in an attempt to exclude environmental factors influencing the insulin action in them. Therefore, the defects of insulin signal transduction that are present in fibroblasts serve as a good model to study intrinsic defects of intracellular insulin activity. The number of insulin receptors and their affinity for ligand in fibroblast cultures in women with PCOS were normal [911, 932]. Increased basal autophosphorylation of serine residues of the insulin receptor β-subunit was present in ~ 50% of the fibroblastic cultures of patients with PCOS, and insulin-stimulated tyrosine autophosphorylation of the insulin receptor β-subunit was decreased [932]. In the same study ~ 50% of women with PCOS had normal basal and insulin-stimulated autophosphorylation of insulin receptors, despite a similar degree of insulin resistance of the PCOS-Ser patients [932]. This implies that there might be a defect downstream of the insulin receptor in the cascade of insulin-signaling pathway [933]. Insulin-stimulated glycogen synthesis in cultured skin fibroblasts of PCOS women was found reduced while the mitogenic activity of insulin was normal [911]. This indicates that a selective abnormality might affect the metabolic and not the mitogenic insulin activity [911]. IRS-1 expression and IRS-1 associated PI3-kinase activity in cultured fibroblasts from PCOS women were normal [911]. These data suggest that the defect leading to reduced glycogen synthesis lies in a different pathway or at steps that are downstream of IRS-1 mediated PI3-kinase activation [911]. Activation of protein kinase B is normal in PCOS cultured fibroblasts, whereas glycogen synthase kinase-3 phosphorylation is reduced [933].

Hyperinsulinemic PCOS women exhibit a significant decrease of GLUT 4 protein levels compared with control endometria [934]. Mioni and colleagues [935] showed differences in endometrial GLUT 4 level between nonhyperinsulinemic and hyperinsulinemic women with PCOS. This difference was more drastic in obese women compared with lean women [936]. Fornes and colleagues [934] showed a defect in the insulin-signaling pathway at the level of IRS-1, AS160 (Rab-GAP), and GLUT 4 in PCOS endometria from patients with hyperinsulinemia, which can lead to impairment in glucose uptake.

Diabetes Mellitus Associated with Extrapancreatic Conditions [817]

Walcott-Rallison syndrome is rare autosomal recessive syndrome due to mutations in *EIF2AK3* (eukaryotic translation initiation factor alpha 2-kinase 3) gene encoding the protein PERK (pancreatic endoplasmic reticulum kinase) [884]. It is characterized by early-onset diabetes mellitus, hepatic and renal failure, developmental delay and induction β-cell apoptosis [885, 886].

Fanconi-Bickel syndrome is a rare autosomal recessive syndrome due to mutations in the *SLC2A2* gene encodes glucose transporter GLUT 2 in pancreatic β-cells. The syndrome is characterized by abnormal metabolism of glucose and galactose, accumulation of glycogen in the liver and kidneys [887], fasting hypoglycemia, and postprandial hyperglycemia. Neonatal diabetes mellitus has been described [888, 889].

Roger's syndrome. Thiamine-responsible megaloblastic anemia (TRMA) is an autosomal recessive disorder. The syndrome is due to the mutations in THTR1 (thiamine transporter), encoded by *SLC19A2* gene [890]. This disease is characterized by diabetes mellitus, megaloblastic anemia and sensorineural deafness. Diabetes mellitus results as a consequence of diminished insulin secretion.

Wolfram syndrome is an autosomal recessive disorder due to mutations in the *WFS1* and *WFS2* genes [891, 892]. Diabetes mellitus is insulin deficient and presents at a mean age of 6 years. Over time other features develop and patients with Wolfram syndrome die at a median age of 30 years.

Alström syndrome is an autosomal-recessively inherited disorder. The syndrome is due to mutations in *ALMS1* gene of unknown function [893], and is characterized by retinitis pigmentosa, deafness, obesity, diabetes mellitus, hyperlipidemia, insulin resistance and hypertension [894].

Bardet-Biedl syndrome is an autosomal-recessively inherited syndrome. It has been linked to at least 12 different genetic loci, referred to as *BBS1* to *BBS12* [895]. Heterozygous carriers exhibit an increased risk for obesity, hypertension, diabetes mellitus, and renal disease. Syndrome is characterized by mental retardation, pigmentary retinopathy, obesity, diabetes mellitus, polydactyly, renal dysplasiahepatic fibrosis, and hypogonadism [896].

REFERENCES

[1]   Kahn C, Rosenthal A. Immunologic reactions to insulin: Insulin allergy, insulin resistance and the autoimmune insulin syndrome. Diabetes Care 1979;2:283-295
[2]   Ship JC, Stone DB. Insulin resistance and insulin allergy. In: Fajan SS, Sussman KE (eds.). Diabetes mellitus: Diagnosis and treatment. American Diabetes Association, New York. 1971:173-179
[3]   Kahn CR, Goldstein BJ, Reddy SS. Heredity and acquired syndromes of insulin resistance. In: Pickup J, Williams G (eds.). Textbook of diabetes. Blackwell Science, London. 1991:276-285
[4]   Chisholm DJ, Campbell LV, Kraegen EW. Pathogenesis of the insulin resistance syndrome (syndrome X). Clin Exp Pharmacol Physiol 1997;24:782-784
[5]   Kashyap SR, DeFronzo RA. The insulin resistance syndrome: physiological considerations. Diabetes Vasc Dis Res 2007;4:13-19
[6]   DeFronzo RA. Lilly Lecture. The triumvirate: beta cell, muscle, liver. A collusion responsible for NIDDM. Diabetes 1988;37:667-687
[7]   DeFronzo RA, Bonadonna RC, Ferrannini E. Pathogenesis of NIDDM. A balanced overview. Diabetes Care 1992;15:318-368
[8]   Bailey CJ. Treating insulin resistance: future prospects. Diabetes Vasc Dis Res 2007;4:20-31
[9]   DeFronzo RA. Pathogenesis of type 2 diabetes: metabolic and molecular implications for identifying diabetes genes. Diabetes Rev 1997;5:117-269
[10] Saltiel AR, Kahn CR. Insulin signalling and the regulation of glucose and lipid metabolism. Nature 2001; 414:799-806
[11] Stern MP. Strategies and prospects for finding insulin resistance genes. J Clin Invest 2000;106,3:323-327

[12]   Taylor SI. Lilly Lecture: Molecular mechanisms of insulin resistance. Lessons from patients with mutations in the insulin-receptor gene. Diabetes 1992; 41:1473-1490

[13]   Zeyda M, Stulnig TM. Obesity, inflammation, and insulin resistance – a mini-review. Gerontology 2009;55:379-386

[14]   Moller DE, Flier JS. Insulin resistance – mechanism, syndromes, and implications. N Engl J Med 1991;325:938-948

[15]   Krook A, O'Rahilly S. Mutant insulin receptors in syndromes of insulin resistance. Baillier's Clin Endocrinol Metab 1996;10:97-122

[16]   Krentz AJ. Fortnightly Review: Insulin resistance. BMJ 1996;313:1385-1389

[17]   Shulman GI. Cellular mechanisms of insulin resistance. J Clin Invest 2000;106:171-176

[18]   Gerich JE, Dailey G. Advances in diabetes for the millennium: understanding insulin resistance. MedGenMed 2004;6,Suppl.1:11-21

[19]   Michael MD, Kulkarni RN, Postic C, *et al.* Loss of insulin signaling in hepatocytes leads to serve insulin resistance and progressive hepatic dysfunction. Mol Cell 2000;6:87-94

[20]   Miyake K, Ogawa W, Matsumoto M, Nakamura T, Sakaue H, Kasuga M. Hyperinsulinemia, glucose intolerance, and dyslipidemia induced by acute inhibition of phosphoinositide 3-kinase signaling in the liver. J Clin Invest 2002;110:1483-1491

[21]   Kasuga M. Insulin resistance and pancreatic β cell failure. J Clin Invest 2006;116,7:1756-1760

[22]   Trayhurn P, Bing C, Woods IS. Adipose tissue and adipokines – energy regulation from the human perspective. J Nutr 2006;136:1935S-1939S

[23]   Reaven GM. Banting Lecture 1988: role of insulin resistance in human disease. Diabetes 1988;37:1595-1607

[24]   Rader DJ. Effect of insulin resistance, dyslipidemia, and intra-abdominal adiposity on the development of cardiovascular disease and diabetes mellitus. Am J Med 2007;120,3A:S12-S18

[25]   Tataranni PA. Pathophysiology of obesity-induced insulin resistance and type 2 diabetes mellitus. Eur Rev Med Pharmacol Sc 2002;6:27-32

[26]   Haffner SM. Abdominal obesity, insulin resistance, and cardiovascular risk in pre-diabetes and type 2 diabetes. Eur Heart J Suppl 2006;8,Suppl.8:B20-B25

[27]   Lelliott C, Vidal-Puig AJ. Lipotoxicity, an imbalance between lipogenesis de novo and fatty acid oxidation. Int J Obes Relat Metab Disord 2004;28,Suppl.4:S22-S28

[28]   Schrauwen P, Hesseling MK. Oxidative capacity, lipotoxicity, and mitochondrial damage in type 2 diabetes. Diabetes 2004;53:1412-1417

[29]   Fonseca-Alaniz MH, Takada J, Alonso-Vale MIC, Lima FB. Adipose tissue as an endocrine organ: from theory to practice. J Pediatr (Rio J) 2007;83,Suppl.5:S192-S203

[30]   Lafontan M, Langin D. Lipolysis and lipid mobilization in human adipose tissue. Prog Lipid Res 2009, doi:10.1016/j.plipres.2009.05.001

[31]   Trayhurn P, Beattie JH. Physiological role of adipose tissue: white adipose tissue as an endocrine and secretory organ. Proc Nutr Soc 2001;60:329-339

[32]   Kerskow EE, Flier JS. Adipose tissue as an endocrine organ. J Clin Endocrinol Metab 2004;89:2548-2556

[33]   Lafontan M, Berlan M. Do regional differences in adipocyte biology provide new pathophysiological insights? Trends Pharmacol Sci 2003;24:276-283

[34]   Trayhurn P, Wood IS. Adipokines: inflammation and the pleiotropic role of white adipose tissue. Br J Nutr 2004;92:347-355

[35]   Bastard JP, Maachi M, Lagathu E, *et al.* Recent advances in the relationship between obesity, inflammation and insulin resistance. Eur Cytokine Netw 2006;17:4-12

[36]   Antuna-Puente B, Feve B, Fellahi S, Bastard J.-P. Adipokines: The missing link between insulin resistance and obesity. Diabetes Metabol 2008;34:2-11

[37]   Miyazaki Y, DeFronzo RA. Visceral fat dominant distribution in male type 2 diabetic patients is closely related to hepatic insulin resistance, irrespective of body type. Cardiovasc Diabetology 2009;8:44, doi:10.1186/1475-2840-8-44

[38]   Wagenknecht LE, Langefeld CD, Scherzinger AI, *et al.* Insulin sensitivity, insulin secretion, and abdominal fat: the Insulin Resistance Atherosclerosis Study (IRAS) family study. Diabetes 2003;52:2490-2496

[39]   Gastaldelli A, Miyazaki Y, Pettiti M, *et al.* Metabolic effects of visceral fat accumulation in type 2 diabetes. J Clin Endocrinol Metab 2002;87:5098-5103

[40]   Roden M, Price TB, Perseghin G, *et al.* Mechanism of free fatty acid-induced insulin resistance in humans. J Clin Invest 1996;97:2859-2865

[41]   Abate N, Garg A, Peshock RM, Stray-Gundersen J, Adams-Huet B, Grundy SM. Relationship of generalized and regional adiposity to insulin sensitivity in men with NIDDM. Diabetes 1996;45:1684-1693

[42] Bays H, Mandarino L, DeFronzo RA. Role of the adipocyte, free fatty acids, and ectopic fat in pathogenesis of type 2 diabetes mellitus: peroxisomal proliferator-activated receptor agonists provide a rational therapeutic approach. J Clin Endocrinol Metab 2004;89:463-478

[43] Bjorbaek C, Kahn BB. Leptin signaling in the central nervous system and periphery. Recent Prog Horm Res 2004;59:305-331

[44] Friedman JM, Halaas JL. Leptin and the regulation of body weight in mammals. Nature 1998;395:763-770

[45] Elmquist JK, Elias CE, Saper CB. From lesions to leptin: hypothalamic control of food intake and body weight. Neuron 1999;22:221-232

[46] Fruhbeck G, Gómez-Ambrosi J, Muruzabal J, Burrel MA. The adipocyte: a model for integration of endocrine and metabolic signalling in energy metabolism regulation. Am J Physiol Endocrinol Metabol 2001;280:E827-847

[47] Correia ML, Rahmouni K. Role of leptin in the cardiovascular and endocrine complications of metabolic syndrome. Diabetes Obesity Metabol 2006;8:603-610

[48] Lembo G, Vecchione C, Fratta L, Argenziano L, Trimarco B, Lembo G. Leptin induces direct vasodilation through distinct endothelial mechanisms. Diabetes 2000;49:293-297

[49] Rabe K, Lehrke M, Parhofer KG, Broedl UC. Adipokines and insulin resistance. Mol Med 2008;14,11-12:741-751

[50] Tartaglia L, Dembski M, Weng X, *et al.* Identification and expression cloning of a leptin receptor, ob-R. Cell 1996;83:1263-1271

[51] Howard JK, Flier JS. Attenuation of leptin and insulin signaling by SOCS proteins. Trend Endocrinol Metab 2006;17:365-371

[52] Niswender KD, Morrison CD, Clegg DJ. Insulin activation of phosphatidylinositol 3-kinase in the hypothalamic arcuate nucleus: a key mediator of insulin-induced anorexia. Diabetes 2003;52:227-231

[53] Caro JF, Kolaczynski JW, Nyce MR, *et al.* Decreased cerebrospinal-fluid/serum leptin ratio in obesity: a possible mechanism for leptin resistance. Lancet 1996;348:159-161

[54] Guerre-Millo M. Adipose tissue and adipokines: for better or worse. Diabetes Metab 2004;30:13-19

[55] Heymsfield SB, Greenberg AS, Fujioka K, *et al.* Recombinant leptin for weight loss in obese and lean adults: a randomized, controlled, dose-escalation trial. JAMA 1999;282:1568-1575

[56] Morioka T, Asilmaz E, Hu J, *et al.* Disruption of leptin receptor expression in the pancreas directly affects beta cell growth and function in mice. J Clin Invest 2007;117:2860-2868

[57] Kieffer TJ, Habener JF. The adipoinsular axis: effects of leptin on pancreatic beta-cells. Am J Physiol Endocrinol Metab 2000;278:E1-E14

[58] Munzberg H, Myers MG Jr. Molecular and anatomical determinants of central leptin resistance. Nat Neurosci 2005;8:566-570

[59] Oral EA, Simha V, Ruiz E, *et al.* leptin-replacement therapy for lipodystrophy. N Engl J Med 2002;346:570-578

[60] Simha V, Szczepaniak LS, Wagner AJ, DePaoli AM, Garg A. Effect of leptin replacement on intrahepatic and intramyocellular lipid content in patients with generalized lipodystrophy. Diabetes Care 2003;26:30-35

[61] Unger RH. Minireview: weapons of lean body mass destruction: the role of ectopic lipids in the metabolic syndrome. Endocrinol 2003; 144:5159-5165

[62] Hotamisligil GS, Shargill NS, Spiegelman BM. Adipose expression of tumor necrosis factor-alpha – direct role in obesity-linked insulin resistance. Science 1993;259:87-91

[63] Hotamisligil GS. Molecular mechanisms of insulin resistance and the role of the adipocyte. Int J Obes Relat Metab Disord 2000;24:S23-S27

[64] Moller DE. Potential role of TNF-alpha in the pathogenesis of insulin resistance and type 2 diabetes. Trends Endocrinol Metab 2000;11:212-217

[65] Ahima RS, Flier JS. Adipose tissue as an endocrine organ. Trends Endocrinol Metab 2000;11:327-332

[66] Sethi JK, Hotamisligil GS. The role of TNF alpha in adipocyte metabolism. Semin Cell Dev Biol 1999;10:19-29

[67] Langin D. Adipose tissue lipolysis as a metabolic pathway to define pharmacological strategies against obesity and the metabolic syndrome. Pharmacol Res 2006;53:482-491

[68] Jaworski K, Sarkadi-Nagy E, Duncan RE, Ahmadian M, Sul HS. Regulation of triglyceride metabolism. IV. Hormonal regulation of lipolysis in adipose tissue. Am J Physiol Gastrointest Liver Physiol 2007;293:G1-G4

[69] Prins JB, Niesler CU, Winterford CM. Tumor necrosis factor-alpha induces apoptosis of human adipose cells. Diabetes 1997;46:1939-1944

[70] Jellema A, Plat J, Mensink RP. Weight reduction, but not a moderate intake of fish oil, lowers concentrations of inflammatory markers and PAI-3 antigen in obese men during the fasting and postprandial state. Eur J Clin Invest 2004;34:766-773

[71] Hotamisligil GS, Arner P, Caro JF, Atkinson RL, Spiegelman BM. Increased adipose tissue expression of tumor necrosis factor-α in human obesity and insulin resistance. J Clin Invest 1995;95:2409-2415

[72] Hotamisligil GS, Peraldi P, Budavari A, Ellis R, White MF, Spiegelman BM. IRS-1-mediated inhibition of insulin receptor tyrosine kinase activity in TNF-α- and obesity-induced insulin resistance. Science 1996;271:665-668

[73] Bernstein LE, Berry J, Kim S, Canavan B, Grinspoon SK. Effects of etanercept in patients with the metabolic syndrome. Arch Intern Med 2006;166:902-908

[74] Dominguez H, Storgaard H, Rask-Madsen E, et al. Metabolic and vascular effects of tumor necrosis factor-alpha blockade with etanercept in obese patients with type 2 diabetes. J Vasc Res 2005;42:517-525

[75] Arner P. The adipocyte in insulin resistance: Key molecules and the impact of the thiazolidinediones. Trends Endocrinol Metab 2003;14:137-145

[76] Lorenzo M, Fernández-Veledo S, Vila-Bedmar R, Garcia-Guerra L, De Alvaro C, Nieto-Vazquez I. Insulin resistance induced by tumor necrosis factor-α in myocytes and brown adipocytes. J Anim Sci 2008;86,E Suppl.:E94-E104

[77] White MF. Insulin signaling in health and disease. Science 2003;302:1710-1711

[78] Pirola L, Johnston AM, Van Obberghen E. Modulation of insulin action. Diabetologia 2004;47:170-184

[79] Arner P. Differences in lipolysis between human subcutaneous and omental adipose tissues. Ann Med 1995;27:435-438

[80] Kadowaki T, Yamauchi T. Adiponectin and adiponectin receptors. Endocr Rev 2005;26:439-451

[81] Pajvani UB, Du X, Combs TP. Structure-function studies of the adipocyte-secreted hormone Acrp30/adiponectin. Implications for metabolic regulation and bioactivity. J Biol Chem 2003;278:9073-9085

[82] Yamauchi T, Kamon J, Ito Y, et al. Cloning of adiponectin receptors that mediate antidiabetic metabolic effects. Nature 2003;423:762-769

[83] Tsuchida A, Yamauchi T, Ito Y, et al. Insulin/Foxo1 pathway regulates expression levels of adiponectin receptors and adiponectin sensitivity. J Biol Chem 2004;279:30817-30822

[84] Yamauchi T, Nio Y, Maki T, et al. Target disruption of AdipoR1 and AdipoR2 cause abrogation of adiponectin binding and metabolic actions. Nat Med 2007;13:332-339

[85] Lihn AS, Bruun JM, He G, Pedersen SB, Jensen PF, Richelsen B. Lower expression of adiponectin mRNA in visceral adipose tissue in lean and obese subjects. Mol Cell Endocrinol 2004;219:9-15

[86] Yamauchi T, Kamon J, Minokoshi Y, et al. Adiponectin stimulates glucose utilization and fatty-acid oxidation by activating AMP-activated protein kinase. Nat Med 2002;8:1288-1295

[87] Ouchi N, Kihara S, Arita Y, et al. Adiponectin, an adipocyte-derived plasma protein, inhibits endothelial NF-kappaB signalling through a cAMP-dependent pathway. Circulation 2000;102:1296-1301

[88] Hotta K, Funahashi T, Bodkin NL, et al. Circulating concentrations of the adipocyte protein adiponectin are decreased in parallel with reduced insulin sensitivity during the progression to type 2 diabetes in rhesus monkeys. Diabetes 2001;50:1126-1133

[89] Lindsay RS, Funahashi T, Hanson RL, et al. Adiponectin and development of type 2 diabetes in the Pima Indian population. Lancet 2002;360:57-58

[90] Spranger J, Krok A, Mohlig M, et al. Adiponectin and protection against type 2 diabetes mellitus. Lancet 2003;361:226-228

[91] Mohamed-Ali V, Pinkney JH, Coppack SW. Adipose tissue as an endocrine and paracrine organ. Int J Obes Relat Metab Disord 1998;22:1145-1158

[92] Fried SK, Bunkin DA, Greenberg AS. Omental and subcutaneous adipose tissues of obese subjects release interleukin-6: depot difference and regulation by glucocorticoid. J Clin Endocrinol Metab 1998;83:847-850

[93] Fain JW, Madan AK, Hiler ML, Cheema P, Bahouth SW. Comparison of the release of adipokines by adipose tissue, adipose tissue matrix, and adipocytes from visceral and subcutaneous abdominal adipose tissues of obese humans. Endocrinol 2004;14:52273-52282

[94] Maachi M, Pieroni L, Bruckert E, et al. Systemic low grade inflammation is related to both circulating and adipose tissue TNF-α, leptin and IL-6 levels in obese women. Int J Obes 2004;28:993-997

[95] Ridker PM. Clinical application of C-reactive protein for cardiovascular disease detection and prevention. Circulation 2003;107:363-369

[96] Yudkin JS, Kumari M, Humphries SE, Mohamed-Ali V. Inflammation, obesity, stress and coronary hart disease: is interleukin-6 the link? Atherosclerosis 2000;148:209-214

[97] Pedersen BK, Febbraio MA. Point: interleukin-6 does have a beneficial role in insulin sensitivity and glucose homeostasis. J Appl Physiol 2007;102:814-816

[98] Mooney RA. Counterpoint: interleukin-6 does have a beneficial role in insulin sensitivity and glucose homeostasis. J Appl Physiol 2007;102:816-818

[99] Bastard JP, Jardel C, Bruckert E, *et al.* Elevated levels of interleukin 6 are reduced in serum and subcutaneous adipose tissue of obese women after weight loss. J Clin Endocrinol Metab 2000;85:3338-3342

[100] Bastard JP, Maachi M, Van Nhieu JT, *et al.* Adipose tissue IL-6 content correlates with resistance to insulin activation of glucose uptake both *in vivo* and in vitro. J Clin Endocrinol Metab 2002;87:2084-2089

[101] Pickup JC, Mattock MB, Chusney GD, Burt D. NIDDM as a disease of the innate immune system: association of acute-phase reactants and interleukin-6 with metabolic syndrome X. Diabetologia 1997;40:1286-1292

[102] Kern PA, Ranganathan S, Li C, Wood L, Ranganathan G Adipose tissue tumor necrosis factor and interleukin-6 expression in human obesity and insulin resistance. Am J Physiol Endocrinol Metab 2001;280:E745-E751

[103] Filg H, Hotamisligil GS. Nonalcoholic fatty liver disease: Cytokine-adipokine interplay and regulation of insulin resistance. Gastroenterol 2006;131:934-945

[104] Senn JJ, Klover PJ, Nowak IA, *et al.* Suppressor of cytokine signaling-3 (SOCS-3), a potential mediator of interleukin-6-dependent insulin resistance in hepatocytes. J Biol Chem 2003;278:13740-13746

[105] Kroder G, Bossenmaier B, Kellerer M, *et al.* Tumor necrosis factor-alpha- and hyperglycemia-induced insulin resistance: Evidence for different mechanisms and different effects on insulin signalling. J Clin Invest 1996;97:1471-1477

[106] Mooney RA, Senn J, Cameron S, *et al.* Suppressors of cytokine signaling-1 and -6 associate with and inhibit the insulin receptor. A potential mechanism for cytokine-mediated insulin resistance. J Biol Chem 2001;276:25889-25893

[107] Lagathu C, Bastard JP, Auclair M, Maachi M, Capeau J, Caron M. Chronic Interleukin-6 (IL-6) treatment increased IL-6 secretion and induced insulin resistance in adipocyte: Prevention by Rosiglitazone. Biochem Biophys Res Commun 2003;311:372-379

[108] Rieusset J, Bouzakri K, Chevillotte E, *et al.* SOCS (Suppressor Of Cytokine Signaling)-3 expression and insulin resistance in skeletal muscle of obese and Type 2 diabetic patients. Diabetes 2004;53:2232-2241

[109] Klover PJ, Zimmers TA, Koniaris LG, Mooney RA. Chronic exposure to interleukin-6 causes hepatic insulin resistance in mice. Diabetes 2003;52:2784-2789

[110] Senn JJ, Klover PJ, Nowak IA, Mooney RA. Interleukin-6 induces cellular insulin resistance in hepatocytes. Diabetes 2002;51:3391-3399

[111] Rotter V, Nagaev I, Smith U. Interleukin-6 (IL-6) induces insulin resistance in 3T3-L1 adipocytes and is, like IL-8 and tumor necrosis factor-alpha, overexpressed in human fat cells from insulin-resistant subjects. J Biol Chem 2003;278:45777-45784

[112] Carey AL, Steinberg GR, Macaulay SL, *et al.* Interleukin-6 increases insulin-stimulated glucose disposal in humans and glucose uptake and fatty acid oxidation *in vitro* via AMP-activated protein kinase. Diabetes 2006;55:2688-2697

[113] Al Khalili L, Bouzakri K, Glund S, Lönnquist F, Koistinen HA, Krook A. Signaling specificity of interleukin-6 action on glucose and lipid metabolism in skeletal muscle. Mol Endocrinol 2006;20:3364-3375

[114] Kim HJ, Higashimori T, Park SY, *et al.* Differential effects of interleukin-6 and -10 on skeletal muscle and liver insulin action in vivo. Diabetes 2004;53:1060-1067

[115] Inoue H, Ogawa W, Asakawa A, *et al.* Role of hepatic STAT3 in brain-insulin action on hepatic glucose production. Cell Metab 2006;3:267-275

[116] Wallenius V, Wallenius K, Ahren B, *et al.* Interleukin-6-deficient mice develop mature-onset obesity. Nat Med 2002;8:75-79

[117] Wallenius K, Wallenius V, Sunter D, Dickson SL, Jansson JO. Intracerebroventricular interleukin-6 treatment decreases body fat in rats. Biochem Biophys Res Commun 2002;293:560-565

[118] Steppan CM, Bailey ST, Bhat S, *et al.* The hormone resistin links obesity to diabetes. Nature 2001;409:307-312

[119] Kim KH, Lee K, Moon YS, Sul HS. A cysteine-rich adipose tissue-specific secretory factor inhibits adipocyte differentiation. J Biol Chem 2001;276:11252-11256

[120] Jackson MB, Osei SY, Ahima SR. The endocrine role of adipose tissue: focus on adiponectin and resistin. Curr Opin Endocrinol Diab 2005;12:163-170

[121] Rajala MW, Obici S, Scherer PE, Rossetti L. Adipose-derived resistin and gut-derived resistin-like molecule-beta selectively impair insulin action on glucose production. J Clin Invest 2003;111:225-230

[122] Rajala MW, Qi Y, Patel HR, *et al.* Regulation of resistin expression and circulating levels in obesity, diabetes and fasting. Diabetes 2004;53:1671-1679

[123] Kaser S, Kaser A, Sandhofer A, Ebenbichler CF, Tilg H, Patsch JR. Resistin messenger-RNA expression is increased by proinflammatory cytokines in vitro. Biochem Biophys Res Commun 2003;309:286-290

[124] Konrad A, Lehrke M, Schachinger V, *et al.* Resistin is an inflammatory marker of inflammatory bowel disease in humans. Eur J Gastrol Hepatol 2007;19:1070-1074

[125] Reilly MP, Lehrke M, Wolfe ML, Rohatgi A, Lazar MA, Rader DJ. Resistin is an inflammatory marker of atherosclerosis in humans. Circulation 2005;111:932-939

[126] Yang Q, Graham TE, Mody N, *et al*. Serum retinol binding protein 4 contributes to insulin resistance in obesity and type 2 diabetes. Nature 2005;436:356-362

[127] Graham TE, Yang Q, Bluher M, *et al*. Retinol binding protein 4 and insulin resistance in lean, obese, and diabetic subjects. N Engl J Med 2006;354:2552-2563

[128] Klöting N, Graham TE, Berndt J, *et al*. Serum retinol-binding protein is more highly expressed in visceral than in subcutaneous adipose tissue and is a marker of intra-abdominal fat mass. Cell Metab 2007;6:79-87

[129] Gavi S, Stuart LM, Kelly P, *et al*. Retinol-binding protein 4 is associated with insulin resistance and body fat distribution in nonobese subjects without type 2 diabetes. J Clin Endocrinol Metab 2007;92:1886-1890

[130] Takebayashi K, Suetsugu M, Wakabayashi S, Aso Y, Inukai T. Retinol binding protein-4 levels and clinical feature of type 2 diabetes patients. J Clin Endocrinol Metab 2007;92:2712-2719

[131] Cho YM, Youn BS, Lee H, *et al*. Plasma retinol-binding protein-4 concentrations are elevated in human subjects with impaired glucose tolerance and type 2 diabetes. Diabetes Care 2006;29:2457-2461

[132] Qi Q, Yu Z, Ye X, *et al*. Elevated retinol-binding protein 4 levels are associated with metabolic syndrome in Chinese people. J Clin Endocrinol Metab 2007;92:4827-4834

[133] Munkhtulga L, Naqkayama K, Utsumi N, *et al*. Identification of a regulatory SNP in the retinol binding protein 4 gene associated with type 2 diabetes in Mongolia. Hum Genet 2007;120:879-888

[134] Craig RL, Chu WS, Elbein SC. Retinol binding protein 4 as a candidate gene for type 2 diabetes and prediabetic intermediate trails. Mol Genet Metab 2007;90:338-344

[135] Broch M, Vendrell J, Ricart W, Richart C, Fernández-Real JM. Circulating retinol-binding protein-4, insulin sensitivity, insulin secretion, and insulin disposition index in obese and nonobese subjects. Diabetes Care 2007;30:1802-1806

[136] von Eynatten M, Lepper PM, Liu D, *et al*. Retinol-binding protein 4 is associated with components of the metabolic syndrome, but not with insulin resistance, in men with type 2 diabetes or coronary artery disease. Diabetologia 2007;50:1930-1937

[137] Silha JV, Nyomba BL, Leslie WD, Murphy LJ. Ethnicity, insulin resistance, and inflammatory adipokines at high and low risk for vascular disease. Diabetes Care 2007;30:286-291

[138] Hida K, Wada J, Eguchi J, *et al*. Visceral adipose tissue-derived serine protease inhibitor: a unique insulin-sensitizing adipocytokine in obesity. Proc Natl Acad Sci USA 2005;102:10610-10615

[139] Klöting N, Berndt J, Kralisch S, *et al*. Vaspin gene expression in human adipose tissue: association with obesity and type 2 diabetes. Biochem Biophys Res Commun 2006;339:430-436

[140] Youn BS, Klöting N, Kratzsch J, *et al*. Serum vaspin concentrations in humans obesity and type 2 diabetes. Diabetes 2008;57:372-377

[141] Curat CA, Wegner V, Sengens C, *et al*. Macrophages in human visceral adipose tissue: increased accumulation in obesity and source of resistin and visfatin. Diabetologia 2006;49:744-747

[142] Fukuhara A, Matsuda M, Nishizawa M, *et al*. Visfatin: A protein secreted by visceral fat that mimics the effects of insulin. Science 2005;307:426-430

[143] Chen MP, Chung FM, Chang DM, *et al*. Elevated plasma level of visfatin/pre-B cell colony-enhancing factor in patients with type 2 diabetes mellitus. J Clin Endocrinol Metab 2006;91:295-299

[144] Haider DG, Schindler K, Schaller G, Prager G, Wotzt M, Ludvik B. Increased plasma visfatin concentrations in morbidly obese subjects and reduced after gastric banding. J Clin Endocrinol Metab 2006;91:1578-1581

[145] Fillippatos TD, Derdemezisc S, Gazi IF, *et al*. Increased plasma visfatin levels in subjects with the metabolic syndrome. Eur J Clin Invest 2008;38:71-72

[146] Berndt J, Klöting N, Kralish S, *et al*. Plasma visfatin concentrations and fat depot-specific mRNA expression in humans. Diabetes 2005;54:2911-2916

[147] Oki K, Yamane K, Kamei N, Hojima H, Kahno N. Circulating visfatin level is correlated with inflammation, but not with insulin resistance. Clin Endocrinol (Oxf) 2007;67:796-800

[148] Samal B, Sun Y, Stearns G, Xie C, Suggs S, McNiece I. Cloning and characterization of the cDNA encoding a novel pre-B cell colony-enhancing factor. Mol Cell Biol 1994;14:1431-1437

[149] Lopez-Bermejo A, Chico-Julia B, Fernandez-Balsells M, *et al*. Serum visfatin increases with progressive beta-cell deterioration. Diabetes 2006;55:2871-2875

[150] Yang R, Lee MJ, Hu H, *et al*. Identification of omentin as a novel depot-specific adipokine in human adipose tissue: possible role in modulating insulin action. Am J Physiol Endocrinol Metab 2006;290:E1253-E1261

[151] de Souza Batista CM, Yang RZ, Lee MJ, *et al*. Omentin plasma levels and gene expression are decreased in obesity. Diabetes 2007;56:1655-1661

[152] Wittamer V, Franssen JD, Vulcano M, *et al*. Specific recruitment of antigen-presenting cells by chemerin, a novel processed ligand from human inflammatory fluids. J Exp Med 2003;198:977-985

[153] Bozaoglu K, Bolton K, McMillan J, *et al.* Chemerin is a novel adipokine associated with obesity and metabolic syndrome. Endocrinol 2007;148:4687-4694

[154] Goralski KB, McCarthy TC, Hanniman EA, *et al.* Chemerin: A novel adipokine that regulates adipogenesis and adipocyte metabolism. J Biol Chem 2007;282:28175-28188

[155] Takahashi M, Takahashi Y, Takahashi K, *et al.* Chemerin enhances insulin signaling and potentates insulin-stimulated glucose uptake in 3T3-L1 adipocytes. FEBS Lett 2008;582:573-578

[156] Leinonen E, Hurt-Camejo E, Wiklund O, Hulten LM, Hiukka A, Taskinen MR. Insulin resistance and adiposity correlate with acute-phase reaction and soluble cells adhesion molecules in type 2 diabetes. Atherosclerosis 2003;166:387-394

[157] Lin Y, Rajala MW, Berger JP, Moller DE, Barzilai N, Scherer PE. Hyperglycemia-induced production of acute phase reactants in adipose tissue. J Biol Chem 2001;276:42077-42083

[158] Poitou C, Viguerie N, Cancello R, *et al.* Serum amyloid A: production by human white adipocytes and regulation by obesity and nutrition. Diabetologia 2005;48:519-528

[159] Johnson BD, Kip KE, Marroquin OC, *et al.* Serum amyloid A as a predictor of coronary artery disease and cardiovascular outcome in women: the National heart, Lung, and Blood Institute-Sponsored Women's ischemia Syndrome Evaluation (WISE). Circulation 2004;109:726-732

[160] Lau DCW, Dhillon B, Yan H, Szmitko PE, Verma S. Adipokines: molecular links between obesity and atherosclerosis. Am J Physiol Heart Circ Physiol 2005;288:H2031-H2041

[161] Scheja L, Heese B, Zitzer H, *et al.* Acute-phase serum amyloid A as a marker of insulin resistance in mice. Exp Diabetes Res 2008;230937, doi:10.1155/2008/230837

[162] Uhlar CM, Whitehead AS. Serum amyloid A, the major vertebrate acute-phase reactant. Eur J Biochem 1999;265,2:501-523

[163] Larson MA, Wei SH, Weber A, Weber AT, McDonald TL. Induction of human mammary-associated serum amyloid A3 expression by prolactin or lipopolysaccharide. Biochem Biophys Res Commun 2003;301,4:1030-1037

[164] Sjöholm K, Palming J, Olofsson LE, *et al.* A microarray search for genes predominantly expressed in human omental adipocytes: adipose tissue as a major production site of serum amyloid A. J Clin Endocrinol Metab 2005;90:2233-2239

[165] Jernäs M, Palming J, Sjöholm K, *et al.* Separation of human adipocytes by size: hypertrophic fat cells display distinct gene expression. FASEB J 2006;20:1540-1542

[166] Sjöholm K, Lundgren M, Olsson M, Eriksson JW. Association of serum amyloid A levels with adipocyte size and serum levels of adipokines: Differences between men and women. Cytokine 2009;48:260-266

[167] Walder K, Kantham L, McMillan JS, *et al.* Tanis: a link between type 2 diabetes and inflammation. Diabetes 2002;51:1859-1866

[168] Cheng N, He R, Tian J, Ye PP, Ye RD. Cutting edge: TLR2 is a functional receptor for acute-phase serum amyloid A. J Immunol 2008;181:22-26

[169] Vettor R, Milan G, Rossato M, Federspil G. Review article: adipocytokines and insulin resistance. Aliment Pharmacol Ther 2005;22,Suppl.2:3-10

[170] Cianflone K, Xia Z, Chen LY. Critical review of Acylation-stimulating protein physiology in humans and rodents. Biochim Biophys Acta 2003;1609:127-143

[171] Van Harmelen V, Reynisdottir S, Cianflone K, *et al.* Mechanisms involved in the regulation of free fatty acid release from isolated human fat cells by Acylation-stimulating protein and insulin. J Biol Chem 1999;274:18243-18251

[172] Cianflone K, Maslowska M, Sniderman AD. Acylation stimulating protein (ASP), an adipocyte autocrine: new directions. Semin Cell Dev Biol 1999;10:31-41

[173] Ahrén B, Havel PJ, Pacini G, Cianflone K. Acylation stimulating protein stimulates insulin secretion. Int J Obes 2003;27:1037-1043

[174] Cianflone K, Kalant D, Marliss EB, Gougeon R, Sniderman AD. Response of plasma ASP to a prolonged fasting. Int J Obes Relat Metab Disord 1995;19:604-609

[175] Faraj M, Jones P, Sniderman AD, Cianflone K. Enhanced dietary fat clearance in postobese women. J Lipid Res 2001;42:571-580

[176] Murray I, Sniderman AD, Havel PJ, Cianflone K. Acylation stimulating protein (ASP) deficiency alters postprandial and adipose tissue metabolism in male mice. J Biol Chem 1999;274:36219-36225

[177] Fain JN, Madan AK, Hiler ML, Cheema P, Bahouth W. Comparison of the release of adipokines by adipose tissue, adipose tissue matrix, and adipocytes from visceral and subcutaneous abdominal adipose tissues of obese humans. Endocrinol 2004;145:2273-2282

[178] Bastelica D, Morange P, Berthet B, *et al.* Stromal cells are the main plasminogen activator inhibitor-1-producing cells in human fat: evidence of differences between visceral and subcutaneous deposits. Arterioscler Thromb Vasc Biol 2002;22:173-178

[179] Dimova EY, Kietzmann T. Metabolic, hormonal and environmental regulation of plasminogen activator inhibitor-1 (PAI-1) expression: lessons from the liver. Thromb Haemost 2008;100,6:992-1006

[180] Mavri A, Stegnar M, Krebs M, Sentocnik JT, Geiger M, Binder BR. Impact of adipose tissue on plasma plasminogen activator inhibitor-1 in dieting obese women. Arterioscler Thromb Vasc Biol 1999;19:1582-1587

[181] Mavri A, Alessi MC, Bastelica D, *et al.* Subcutaneous abdominal, but not femoral fat expression of plasminogen activator inhibitor-1 (PAI-1) is related to plasma PAI-1 levels and insulin resistance and decreases after weight loss. Diabetologia 2001;44:2025-2031

[182] Juan-Vague I, Alessi MC, Vague P. Increased plasma plasminogen activator inhibitor 1 levels. A possible link between insulin resistance and atherothrombosis. Diabetologia 1991;34:457-462

[183] Bastard JP, Pieroni L, Hainque B. Relationship between plasma plasminogen activator inhibitor 1 and insulin resistance. Diabetes Metab Res Rev 2000;16:192-201

[184] Lyon CJ, Law RE, Hsueh W. Minireview: adiposity, inflammation, and atherogenesis. Endocrinol 2003;144:2195-2200

[185] Wajchenberg BL. Subcutaneous and visceral adipose tissue: their relation to the metabolic syndrome. Endocr Rev 2000;21:697-738

[186] Suzuki M, Akimoto K, Hattori Y. Glucose upregulates plasminogen activator inhibitor-1 gene expression in vascular smooth muscle cells. Life Sciences 2002;72:59-66

[187] Kopelman PG. Obesity as a medical problem. Nature 2000;404:635-643

[188] Lau DC, Schillaber G, Li ZH, Wong KL, Varzanch G, Tough SC. Paracrine interactions in adipose tissue development and growth. Int J Obes Relat Metab Disord 1996;20,Suppl.3:S16-S25

[189] Tham DM, Martin-McNulty B, Wang YX, *et al.* Angiotensis II is associated with activation of NF-κB-associated genes and downregulation of PPARs. Physiol Genomics 2002;11:21-30

[190] Celerier J, Cruz A, Lamande N, Gasc JM, Corvol P. Angiotensinogen and its cleaved derivatives inhibit angiogenesis. Hypertension 2002;39:224-228

[191] Emanueli C, Madeddu P. Renin-angiotensin and kallikrein-kinin systems coordinately modulate angiogenesis. Hypertension 2002;39:e29

[192] Ebsein W. Therapie des Diabetes mellitus, insbesondere über die Anwendung des salicylsauren Natron bei demselben. Berlin Klein Wochenschrift 1876;13:337-340

[193] Weigert C, Hennige AM, Lehman R, *et al.* Direct cross-talk of interleukin-6 and insulin signal transduction via insulin receptor substrate-1 in skeletal muscle cells. J Biol Chem 2006;281:7060-7067

[194] Ozcan U, Cao Q, Yilmaz E, *et al.* Endoplasmic reticulum stress links obesity, insulin action and type 2 diabetes. Science 2004;306:425-426

[195] Miller RS, Diaczok D, Cooke DW. Repression of GLUT4 expression by the endoplasmic reticulum stress response in 3T3-L1 adipocytes. Biochem Biophys Res Commun 2007;362:188-192

[196] Dedoussis GVZ, Kaliora AC, Panagiotakos DB. Genes, diet and type 2 diabetes mellitus: a review. Rev Diabet Stud 2007;4,1:13-24

[197] Feskens E, Bowles CH, Kromhout D. Inverse association between fish intake and risk of glucose intolerance in normoglycemic elderly men and women. Diabetes Care 1991;14:935-941

[198] Hill JO, Lin D, Yakubu F, Peters JC. Development of dietary obesity in rats: influence of amount and composition of dietary fat. Int J Obes Relat Metab Disord 1992;16:321-333

[199] Liu S, Manson JE. Dietary carbohydrates, obesity, and the "metabolic syndrome" as predictors of coronary heart disease. Curr Opin Lipidol 2001;12:395-404

[200] Romieu I, Willett CW, Stampfer MJ, *et al.* Energy intake and other determinants of relative weight. Am J Clin Nutr 1988;47:406-412

[201] Westman EC, Feineman RD, Mavropoulos JC, *et al.* Low-carbohydrate nutrition and metabolism. Am J Clin Nutr 2007;86:276-284

[202] Eaton SB, Konner M. Paleolithic nutrition: a consideration of its nature and current implications. N Engl J Med 1985;312:283-289

[203] Eaton SB. The ancestral human diet: what was it and should it be a paradigm for contemporary nutrition. Proc Nutr Soc 2006;65:1-6

[204] McAuley K, Mann J. Nutritional determinants of insulin resistance. J Lipid Res 2006;47:1668-1676

[205] Putnam J. Food consumption, prices, and expenditures, 1970-91. In Economic Research Service Washington: US Department of Agriculture, 1999

[206] Elliott SS, Keim NL, Stern JS, Teft K, Havel PJ. Fructose, weight gain, and the insulin resistance syndrome. Am J Clin Nutr 2002;76,5:911-922

[207] Bray GA, Nielsen SJ, Popkin BM. Consumption of high-fructose corn syrup in beverages may play a role in the epidemic of obesity. Am J Clin Nutr 2004;79:537-543

[208] Pagliassoti MJ, Horton TJ. Sucrose, insulin action and biologic complexity. Recent Res Devel Physiol 2004;2:337-353

[209] Schwarz JM, Neese RA, Schakleton C, Hellerstein MK. De novo lipogenesis during fasting and oral fructose ingestion in lean and obese hyperinsulinemic subjects. Diabetes 1993;42,Suppl.:A39

[210] Faeh D, Minehira K, Schwarz J, Periasami R, Seongus P, Tappy L. Effect of fructose overfeeding and fish oil administration on hepatic de novo lipogenesis and insulin sensitivity in healthy males. Diabetes 2005;54:1907-1913

[211] Lê KA, Faeh D, Stettler R, *et al.* A four-week high-fructose diet alters lipid metabolism without affecting insulin sensitivity or ectopic lipids in healthy humans. Am J Clin Nutr 2006;84:1374-1379

[212] Grant AM, Christie MR, Ashcroft SJ. Insulin release from human pancreatic islets in vitro. Diabetologia 1980;19:114-117

[213] Curry DL. Effects of mannose and fructose on the synthesis and secretion of insulin. Pancreas 1989;4:2-9

[214] Sato Y, Ito T, Udaka N, *et al.* Immunohistochemical localization of facilitated-diffusion glucose transporters in rat pancreatic islets. Tissue Cell 1996;28:637-643

[215] Lê KA, Ith M, Kreis R, *et al.* Fructose overconsumption causes dyslipidemia and ectopic lipid deposition in healthy subjects with and without a family history of type 2 diabetes. Am J Clin Nutr 2009;89:1760-1765

[216] Lê KA, Faeh D, Stettler R, *et al.* A four-week high-fructose diet on gene expression in skeletal muscle of healthy men. Diabetes and Metabol 2008;34,1:82-85

[217] Dai S, McNeill JH. Fructose-induced hypertension in rats is concentration- and duration-dependent. J Pharmacol Toxicol Methods 1995;33:101-107

[218] Erlich Y, Rosenthal T. Effect of angiotensin-converting enzyme inhibitors on fructose induced hypertension and hyperinsulinemia in rats. Clin Exp Pharmacol Physiol 1995;22,Suppl.:S347-S349

[219] Reiser S. Effects of dietary sugars in metabolic risk factors associated with heart disease. Nutr Health 1985;3:203-216

[220] Daly ME, Vale C, Walker M, Alberti KG, Mathers JC. Dietary carbohydrates and insulin sensitivity: a review of the evidence and clinical implications. Am J Clin Nutr 1997;66:1072-1085

[221] Vasdev S, Ford CA, Longerich L, Gadag V, Wadhawan S. Role of aldehydes in fructose induced hypertension. Mol Cell Biochem 1998;181:1-9

[222] Messier C, Whately K, Liang J, Du L, Puissont D. The effects of a high-fat, high-fructose, and combination diet on learning, weight, and glucose regulation in C57BL/6 mice. Beh Brain Res 2007;178:139-145

[223] Basciano H, Federico L, Adeli K. Fructose, insulin resistance, and metabolic dyslipidemia. Nutr Metab 2005;2:5, doi:10.1186/1743-7075-2-2

[224] Shafrir E, Raz I. Diabetes: mellitus or lipids? Diabetologia2003;46:433-440

[225] Romieu I, Willett WC, Stampfer MJ, *et al.* Energy intake and other determinants of relative weight. Am J Clin Nutr 1988;47:406-412

[226] Hill JO, Lin D, Yakuba F, Peters JC. Development of dietary obesity in rats: influence of amount and composition of dietary fat. Int J Obes Relat Metab Disord 1992;16:321-333

[227] Storlien LH, James DE, Burleigh KM, Chisholm DJ, Kraegen EW. Fat feeding causes widespread insulin resistance, decreased energy expenditure and obesity in rats. Am J Physiol 1986;251:E576-E583

[228] Golay A, Bobbioni E. The role of dietary fat in obesity. Int J Obes Relat Metab Disord 1997;21,Suppl.3:2-11

[229] Astrup AGK, Grunwald GK, Melanson EL, Saris WH, Hill JO. The role of low-fat diets in body weight control: a meta-analysis of ad libitum dietary intervention studies. Int J Obes Relat Metab Disord 2000;24:1545-1552

[230] Petro AE, Cotter J, Cooper DA, Peters JC, Surwit SJ, Surwit RS. Fat, carbohydrates, and calories in the development of diabetes and obesity in the C57BL/6J mouse. Metabolism 2004;53:454-457

[231] Cahová M, Vavřinková H, Kazdová L. Glucose-fatty acid interaction in skeletal muscle and adipose tissue in insulin resistance. Physiol Res 2007;56:1-15

[232] Alsaif MA, Duwaihy MMS. Influence of dietary fat quantity and composition on glucose tolerance and insulin sensitivity in rats. Nutr Res 2004;24:417-425

[233] Walz HA, Härndahl L, Wierup N, *et al.* Early and rapid development of insulin resistance, islet dysfunction and glucose intolerance after high-fat feeding in mice overexpressing phosphodiesterase 3 B. J Endocrinol 2006;189:629-641

[234] Randle PJ, Garland P, Hales C, Newsholme E. The glucose-fatty acid cycle: its role in insulin sensitivity and the metabolic disturbances of diabetes mellitus. Lancet 1963;13:786-789

[235] Shulman GI. Cellular mechanisms of insulin resistance. J Clin Invest 2000;106:171-176

[236] Petersen KF, Hendler R, Price T, *et al.* $^{13}C/^{31}P$ NMR studies on the mechanism of insulin resistance in obesity. Diabetes 1998;47:381-386

[237] Rathman DL, Shulman RG, Shulman GI. ^{31}P nuclear magnetic resonance measurements of muscle glucose-6-phosphate: evidence for reduced insulin-dependent muscle glucose transport or phosphorylation activity in non-insulin dependent diabetes mellitus. J Clin Invest 1992;89:1069-1075

[238] Rothman DL, Magnusson I, Cline G, *et al.* Decreased muscle glucose transport/phosphorylation is an early defect in the pathogenesis of non-insulin dependent diabetes mellitus. Proc Natl Acad Sci USA 1995;92:983-987

[239] Okada T, Kawano Y, Sakakibara T, Hazeki O, Uli M. Essential role of phosphatidylinositol-3-kinase in insulin induced transport and antilipolysis in rat adipocytes. Studies with a selective inhibitor wortmannin. J Biol Chem 1994;269:3568-3573

[240] Heine RJ, Mulder C, Popp-Snijders C, van der Meer J, van der Venn EA. Linoleic-acid-enriched diet: long-term effects on serum lipoprotein and apolipoprotein concentrations and insulin sensitivity in noninsulin-dependent diabetes patients. Am J Clin Nutr 1989;49:448-456

[241] Schwab US, Niskanen LK, Maliranta HM, Savalainen MJ, Kesaniemi YA, Clusitupa MI. Lauric and palmitic acid-enriched diets have minimal impact on serum lipid and lipoprotein concentrations and glucose metabolism in healthy young women. J Nutr 1995;125:466-473

[242] Summers LK, Fielding BA, Bradshaw HA, *et al.* Substituting dietary saturated fat with polyunsaturated fat changes abdominal fat distribution and improves insulin sensitivity. Diabetologia 2002;45:369-377

[243] Lovejoy JC, Smith SR, Champagne CM, *et al.* Effects of diets enriched in saturated (oleic), or trans (elaidic) fatty acids on insulin sensitivity and substrate oxidation in healthy adults. Diabetes Care 2002;25:1283-1288

[244] Marshall JA, Bessesen DH, Hamman RF. High saturated fat and low starch and fibre are associated with hyperinsulinemia in a non-diabetic population: the San Luis Valley Diabetes Study. Diabetologia 1997;40:430-438

[245] Parker DR, Weiss ST, Troisi R, Cassano PA, Vokonas PS, Landsberg L. Relationship of dietary saturated fatty acids and body habitus to serum insulin concentrations: the Normative Aging Study. Am J Clin Nutr 1993;58:129-136

[246] Feskens EJ, Loeber JG, Kromhout D. Diet and physical activity as determinants of hyperinsulinemia: the Zutphen Elderly Study. Am J Epidemiol 1994;140:350-360

[247] Vessby B, Fengblad S, Lithell H. Insulin sensitivity is related to the fatty acid composition of serum lipids and skeletal muscle phospholipids in 70-year-old man. Diabetologia 1994;37:1044-1050

[248] Storlien LH, Jenkins AB, Chisholm DJ, Pascoe WS, Khouri S, Kraegen EW. Influence of dietary fat composition on development of insulin resistance in rats. Relationship to muscle triglyceride and w-3 fatty acids in muscle phospholipids. Diabetes 1991;40:280-289

[249] Borkman M, Storlien LH, Pan DA, Jenkins AB, Chisholm DJ, Campbell LV. The relationship between insulin sensitivity and the fatty acid composition of phospholipids of skeletal muscle. N Engl J Med 1993;328:328-344

[250] Storlien LH, Kraegen EW, Chisholm DJ, Ford GL, Bruce DG, Pascoe WS. Fish oil prevents insulin resistance induced by high-fat feeding in rats. Science 1987;237:885-888

[251] Vessby B, Unsitupa M, Hermansen K, *et al.* Substituting dietary saturated for monounsaturated fat impairs insulin sensitivity in healthy men and women: the KANWU Study. Diabetologia 2001;44:312-319

[252] Pan DA, Lillioja S, Milner MR, *et al.* Skeletal muscle membrane lipid composition is related to adiposity and insulin action. J Clin Invest 1995;96:2802-2808

[253] Nugent C, Prins JB, Whitehead JP, Wentworth JB, Chatterjee VK, O'Rahilly S. Arachidonic acid stimulates glucose uptake in 3T3-L1 adipocytes by increasing GLUT1 and GLUT4 levels at the plasma membrane. J Biol Chem 2001;276:9146-9157

[254] Barroso I, Gurnell M, Crowley VE, *et al.* Dominant negative mutations in human PPARgamma associated with severe insulin resistance, diabetes mellitus and hypertension. Nature 1999;402:880-883

[255] Kliewer SA, Sundseth SS, Jones SA, *et al.* Fatty acids and eicosanoids regulate gene expression through direct interactions with peroxisome proliferator-activated receptors alpha and gamma. Proc Natl Acad Sci USA 1997;94:4318-4323

[256] Wu Z, Xie Y, Morrison RF, Bucher NL, Farmer SR. PPARgamma induces insulin-dependent glucose transporter GLUT4 in the absence of C/EBPalpha during the conversion of 3T3 fibroblasts into adipocytes. J Clin Invest 1998;101:22-32

[257] Schwartz MS, Chadha A. Type 2 diabetes mellitus in childhood: obesity and insulin resistance. J Am Osteopath Assoc 2008;108:518-524

[258] Astrup A, Dyerberg J, Selleck M, Stender S. Nutrition transition and its relationship to the development of obesit5y and related chronic diseases [review]. Obes Rev 2008;9,Suppl.1:48-52

[259] Rodriguez-Morán M, Guerrero-Romero F, Brito-Zurita O, *et al.* Cardiovascular risk factors and acculturation in Yaquis and Tepehuanos Indians from Mexico. Arch Med Res 2008;39:352-357

[260] O'Dea K. Westernization, insulin resistance and diabetes in Australian aborigines [review]. Med J Aust 1991;155:258-264

[261] Manson JE, Nathan DM, Krolewski AS, Stampfer MJ, Willett WC, Hennekens CH. A prospective study of exercise and incidence of diabetes among US male physicians. JAMA 1992;268:63-67

[262] Blair SN, Kohl HW III, Paffenbarger RS Jr, Clark DG, Cooper KH, Gibbons LW. Physical fitness and all-cause mortality. A prospective study of healthy men and women. JAMA 1989;262:2395-2401

[263] Helmrich SP, Ragland DR, Leung RW, Paffenbarger RS Jr. Physical activity and reduced occurrence of non-insulin-dependent diabetes mellitus. N Engl J Med 1991;325:147-152

[264] Wareham NJ, Wong MY, Day NE. Glucose intolerance and physical inactivity: the relative importance of low habitual energy expenditure and cardiorespiratory fitness. Am J Epidemiol 2000;152:132-139

[265] Knowler WC, Barrett-Connor E, Fowler SE, *et al.* Reduction in the incidence of type 2 diabetes with lifestyle intervention or metformin. N Engl J Med 2002;346:393-403

[266] Hwu CM, Hsio CF, Kuo SW, *et al.* Physical inactivity is an important lifestyle determinant of insulin resistance in hypertensive patients. Blood Press 2004;13,6:355-361

[267] Blanc S, Normand S, Pachiaudi C, Portrat C-O, Laville M, Gharib C. Fuel homeostasis during physical inactivity induced by bed rest. J Clin Endocrinol Metab 2000;85,6:2223-2233

[268] Carlsson S, Midthjell K, Tesfamarian MY, Grill V. Age, overweight and physical inactivity increase the risk of latent autoimmune diabetes in adults: results from the Nord-Trøndelag health study. Diabetologia 2007;50:55-58

[269] Amati F, Dubé JJ, Coen PM, Stefanovic-Racic M, Toledo FGS, Goodpaster BH. Physical inactivity and obesity underlie the insulin resistance of aging. Diabetes Care 2009;32,8:1547-1549

[270] Rogers MA, King DS, Hagberg JM, Ehsani AA, Halloszy JO. Effect of 10 days of physical inactivity on glucose tolerance in master athletes. J Appl Physiol 1990;68,5:1833-1837

[271] Stuart CA, Shangraw RE, Prince MJ, Peters EJ, Wolfe RR. Bed-rest-induced insulin resistance occurs primarily in muscle. Metabolism 1988;37:802-806

[272] Arciero PJ, Smith DL, Calles-Escandon J. Effects of short-term inactivity on glucose tolerance, energy expenditure, and blood flow in trained subjects. J Appl Physiol 1998;84:1365-1373

[273] Smorawinski J, Kaciuba-Uscilko H, Nazar K, *et al.* Effects of three-day bed rest on metabolic, hormonal and circulatory responses to an oral glucose load in endurance or strength trained athletes and untrained subjects. J Physiol Pharmacol 2000;51:279-289

[274] Hamburg NM, McMackin CJ, Huan AL, *et al.* Physical inactivity rapidly induces insulin resistance and microvascular dysfunction in healthy volunteers. Arterioscler Thromb Vasc Biol 2007;27:2650-2656

[275] Stettler K, Ith M, Acheson KJ, *et al.* Interaction between dietary lipids and physical inactivity on insulin sensitivity and on intramyocellular lipids in healthy men. Diabetes Care 2005;28:1404-1409

[276] Qi D, Rodrigues B. Glucocorticoids produce whole body insulin resistance with changes in cardiac metabolism. Am. J Physiol Endocrinol Metab 2007;292:E654-E667

[277] Schacke H, Docke WD, Asadullah K. Mechanisms involved in the side effects of glucocorticoids. Pharmacol Ther 2002;96:23-43

[278] Selatitskaya VG, Kuz'minova OI, Odintsov SV. Development of insulin resistance in experimental animals during long-term glucocorticoid treatment. Bull Exp Biol Med 2002;133:339-341

[279] Delbende C, Delarue C, Lefebvre H, *et al.* Glucocorticoids, transmitters and stress. Br J Psychiatry Suppl 1992;15:24-35

[280] Macfarlane DP, Forbes S, Walker BR. Glucocorticoids and fatty acid metabolism in humans: fuelling fat distribution in the metabolic syndrome. J Endocrinol 2008;197:189-204

[281] Chikanza IC, Kozaci D, Chernajovsky Y. The molecular and cellular basis of corticosteroid resistance. J Endocrinol 2003;179:301-310

[282] Andrews RC, Walker BR. Glucocorticoids and insulin resistance: old hormones, new targets. Clinical Science 1999;96:513-523

[283] Rooney DP, Neely RD, Cullen C, Ennis CN, Sheridan B, Atkinson AB. The effect of cortisol on glucose/glucose-6-phosphate cycle activity and insulin action. J Clin Endocrinol Metab 1994;77:1180-1183

[284] Rizza RA, Mandarino LJ, Gerich J. Cortisol-induced insulin resistance in man: impaired suppression of glucose production and stimulation of glucose utilization due to a postreceptor defect of insulin action. J Clin Endocrinol Metab 1982;54:`131-138

[285] Chavez M, Seeley RJ, Green PK, Wilkinson CW, Schwartz MW, Woods SC. Adrenalectomy increases sensitivity to central insulin. Physiol Behav 1997;62:631-634

[286] Ling ZC, Khan A, Delaunay F, *et al.* Increased glucocorticoid sensitivity in islet beta-cells: effects on glucose 6-phosphatase, glucose cycling and insulin release. Diabetologia 1998;41:634-639

[287] Delaunay F, Khan A, Cintra A, *et al.* Pancreatic beta cells are important targets for the diabetogenic effects of glucocorticoids. J Clin Invest 1997;100:2094-2098

[288] Lambillotte C, Gilon P, Henquin JC. Direct glucocorticoid inhibition of insulin secretion: an *in vitro* study of dexamethasone effects in mouse islets. J Clin Invest 1997;99:414-423

[289] Stubbs M, York DA. Central glucocorticoid regulation of parasympathetic drive to pancreatic β-cells in the obese fa/fa rat. Int J Obes 1991;15:547-553

[290] Coderre L, Valega GA, Pilch PF, Chipkin SR. *In vivo* effects of dexamethasone and sucrose on glucose transport (GLUT-4) protein tissue distribution. Am J Physiol Endocrinol Metab 1996;271:E643-E648

[291] Haber RS, Weinstein SP. Role of glucose transporters in glucocorticoid-induced insulin resistance. GLUT4 isoform in rat skeletal muscle is not decreased by dexamethasone. Diabetes 1992;41:728-735

[292] Oda N, Nakai A, Mokanu T, *et al.* Dexamethasone-induced changes in glucose transporter 4 in rat heart muscle, skeletal muscle and adipocytes. Eur J Endocrinol 1995;133:121-126

[293] Owen OE, Cahill GF Jr. Metabolic effects of exogenous glucocorticoids in fasted man. J Clin Invest 1973;52:2596-2605

[294] Weinstein SP, Paquin T, Pritsker A, Haber RS. Glucocorticoid-induced insulin resistance: dexamethasone inhibits the activation of glucose transport in rat skeletal muscle by both insulin- and non-insulin-related stimuli. Diabetes 1995;44:441-445

[295] Sakoda H, Ogihara T, Anai M, *et al.* Dexamethasone-induced insulin resistance in 3T3-L1 adipocytes is due to inhibition of glucose transport rather than insulin signal transduction. Diabetes 2000;49:1700-1708

[296] Turnbow MA, Keller SR, Rice KM, Garner CW. Dexamethasone down-regulation of insulin substrate-1 in 3T3-L1 adipocytes. J Biol Chem 1994;269:2516-2520

[297] Guillaume-Gentil C, Assimacopoulos-Jeannet F, Jeaurenaud B. Involvement of non-esterified fatty acid oxidation in glucocorticoid-induced peripheral insulin resistance *in vivo* in rats. Diabetologia 1993;36:899-906

[298] Corporeau C, Foll CL, Taouis M, Gouygou JP, Berge JP, Delarue J. Adipose tissue compensates for defect of phosphatidylinositol 3'-kinase induced in liver and muscle by dietary fish oil in fed rats. Am J Physiol Endocrinol Metab 2006;290:E78-E86

[299] Clemmons DR, Moses AC, McKay MJ, Sommer A, Rosen DM, Ruckle J. The combination of insulin-like growth factor-1 and insulin-like growth factor binding protein-3 reduces insulin requirements in type 1 diabetes: evidence for *in vivo* biologic activity. J Clin Endocrinol 2000;85:1518-1524

[300] Garcia-Estevez DA, Araujo-Vilar D, Cabezas-Cerrato J. Non-insulin-mdicated glucose uptake in several insulin-resistant states in the postabsorptive period. Diabetes Res Clin Pract 1998;39:107-113

[301] Nabarro JDN. Acromegaly. Clin Endocrinol 1993;26:481-512

[302] Ezzat S, Fornster MJ, Berchtold P, Redelmeier DA, Boerlin V, Harris AG. Acromegaly: clinical and biochemical features in 500 patients. Medicine 1994;73:233-240

[303] Ho KK, Jenkins AB, Furler SM, Borkman M, Chisholm DJ. Impact of octeroide, a long-acting somatostatin analogue, on glucose tolerance and insulin sensitivity in acromegaly. Clin Endocrinol 1992;36:271-279

[304] Kasayam S, Otsuki M, Takagi M, *et al.* Impaired β-cell function in the presence of reduced insulin sensitivity determines glucose tolerance status in acromegalic patients. Clin Endocrinol 2000;52:549-555

[305] Bramnert M, Segerlantz M, Laurila E, Daugaad JR, Manhem P, Groop L. Growth hormone replacement therapy induces insulin resistance by activating the glucose-fatty acid cycle. J Clin Endocrinol Metab 2003;88:1455-1463

[306] Rose DR, Clemmons DR. Growth hormone receptor antagonist improves insulin resistance in acromegaly. Growth Horm IGF Res 2002;12:418-424

[307] Krag MB, Gormsen LC, Guo ZK, *et al.* Growth hormone-induced insulin resistance is associated with increased intramyocellular triglyceride content but unaltered VLDL-triglyceride kinetics. Am J Physiol Endocrinol Metab 2007;292:E920-E927

[308] Bak JF, Møller N, Schmitz O. Effects of growth hormone on fuel utilization and muscle glycogen synthase activity in normal humans. Am J Physiol Endocrinol Metab 1991;260:E736-E742

[309] Christopher M, Hew FL, Oakley M, Rantzau C, Alford F. Defects of insulin action and skeletal muscle glucose metabolism in growth hormone-deficient adult persist after 24 months of recombinant human growth hormone therapy. J Clin Endocrinol Metab 1998;83:1668-1681

[310] Fowelin J, Attwall S, Lager I, Bengtsson BA. Effects of treatment with recombinant human growth hormone on insulin sensitivity and glucose metabolism in adults with growth hormone deficiency. Metabolism 1993;42:1443-1447

[311] Hwu CM, Kwok CF, Lai TY, *et al.* Growth hormone (GH) replacement reduces total body fat and normalizes insulin sensitivity in GH-deficient adults: a report of one year clinical experience. J Clin Endocrinol Metab 1997;82:3285-3292

[312] Weaver JU, Monson JP, Noonan K, *et al.* The effect of low dose recombinant growth hormone replacement on regional fat distribution, insulin sensitivity, and cardiovascular risk factors in hypopituitary adults. J Clin Endocrinol Metab 1995;80:153-159

[313] Dresner A, Laurent D, Marcucci M, *et al.* Effects of free fatty acids on glucose transport and IRS-1-associated phosphatidylinositol 3-kinase activity. J Clin Invest 1999;103:253-259

[314] Dominici FP, Cifone D, Bartke A, Turyn D. Loss of sensitivity to insulin at easily events of the insulin signaling pathway in the liver of growth hormone-transgenic mice. J Endocrinol 1999;161:383-392

[315] Kumar KVSH, Reddy CVK, Raghunath M, Modi KD. Association between thyroid hormones, insulin resistance and metabolic syndrome. Endocrine Abstracts 2009;19:P339

[316] Kumar HK, Yadov RK, Prajapati J, Reddy CVK, Raghunath M, Modi K. Association between thyroid hormones, insulin resistance and metabolic syndrome. Saudi Med J 2009;30,7:907-911

[317] Mueller A, Schöfl C, Dittrich R, *et al.* Thyroid-stimulating hormone is associated with insulin resistance independently of body mass index, and age in women with polycystic ovary syndrome. Hum Reprod 2009;24,11:2924-2930

[318] Kopp HP, Krzyzanowska K, Schernthaner GH, Kriwanek S, Schernthaner G. Relationship of androgens to insulin resistance in morbidly obese premenopausal women: studies before and after vertical banded gastroplasty. Obesity Surgery 2006;16:1214-1220

[319] Kapoor D, Malkin CJ, Channer KS, Jones TH. Androgens, insulin resistance and vascular disease in men. Clin Endocrinol 2005;63:239-250

[320] Borrisova AM, Tankova T, Kamenova P, *et al.* Effect of hormone replacement therapy on insulin secretion and insulin sensitivity in postmenopausal diabetic women. Gynecol Endocrinol 2002;16:67-74

[321] Amiel SA, Sherwin RS, Simpsons DC, Lauritano AA, Tamborlane WV. Impaired insulin action in puberty: a contributing factor to poor glycemic control in adolescents with diabetes. N Engl J Med 1986;315:215-219

[322] Holmang A, Laesson BM, Brzezinska Z, Bjorntorp P. The effects of short term testosterone exposure on insulin sensitivity in female rats. Am J Physiol 1992;262:E851-E855

[323] Tang WH, Young JB. Cardiomyopathy and heart failure in diabetes. Endocrinol Metab Clin North Am 2001;30:1031-1046

[324] Suskin N, McKelvie RS, Burns RJ, *et al.* Glucose and insulin abnormalities relate to functional capacity in patients with congestive heart failure. Eur Heart 2000;21:1368-1375

[325] Opie LH. The metabolic vicious cycle in heart failure. Lancet 2004;364:1733-1734

[326] Kannel WB, McGee DL. Diabetes and cardiovascular disease. The Framingham study. JAMA 1979;241:2035-2038

[327] Tang WHW. A critical review of anti-adrenergic therapy in patients with heart failure and diabetes mellitus. Vasc Health Risk Manag 2007;3,5:639-645

[328] Parsonage W, Hetmanski D, Cowley A. Differentiation of the metabolic and vascular effects on insulin in insulin resistance patients with chronic heart failure. Am J Cardiol 2002;89:696-703

[329] Bakris GL, Fonseca V, Katholi R, *et al.* Metabolic effects of carvedilol vs metoprolol in patients with type 2 diabetes mellitus and hypertension: a randomized controlled trial. JAMA 2004;292:2227-2236

[330] Poitout V, Robertson RP. Glucolipotoxicity: fuel excess and β-cell dysfunction. Endocrine Rev 2008;29:351-366

[331] Tataranni PA. Pathophysiology of obesity-induced insulin resistance and type 2 diabetes mellitus. Eur Rev Med Pharmacol Sci 2002;6:27-32

[332] Unger RH, Grundy S. Hyperglycemia as an inducer as well as a consequence of impaired islet cell function and insulin resistance: implications for the managements of diabetes. Diabetologia 1985;28:119-121

[333] Stumvoll M, Tataranni PA, Stefan N, Vozarova B, Bogardus C. Increased glycemia physiologically accompanies insulin resistance due to incomplete beta cell compensation. Diabetologia 2002;45:A185

[334] Yki-Jarvinen H. Glucose toxicity. Endocrine Rev 1992;13:415-431

[335] Robertson RP, Olson LK, Zhang HJ. Differentiating glucose toxicity from glucose desensitization: a new message for the insulin gene. Diabetes 1994;43:1085-1089

[336] Weir GC, Laybutt DR, Kaneto H, Bonner-Weir S, Sharma A. Beta-cell adaptation and decompensation during the progression of diabetes. Diabetes 2001;50:S154-S159

[337] Robertson RP, Harmon J, Tran POT, Poitout V. β-cell glucose toxicity, lipotoxicity, and chronic oxidative stress in type 2 diabetes. Diabetes 2004;53,Suppl.1:S119-S124

[338] Rossetti L, Giaccari A, DeFronzo RA. Glucose toxicity. Diabetes Care 1990;13:610-630

[339] Robertson RP. Chronic oxidative stress as a central mechanism for glucose toxicity in pancreatic islet beta cells in diabetes. J Biol Chem 2004;279,41:42351-42354

[340] Poitout V, Hagman D, Stein R, Artner I, Robertson RP, Harmon JS. Regulation of the insulin gene by glucose and fatty acids. J Nutr 2006;136:873-876

[341] Robertson RP, Zhang HJ, Pyzdrowski KL, Walseth TF. Preservation of insulin mRNA levels and insulin secretion in HIT cells by avoidance of chronic exposure to high glucose concentrations. J Clin Invest 1992;90:320-325

[342] Robertson RP, Hamon JS, Tanako Y, *et al.* Glucose toxicity in the β-cell: cellular and molecular mechanisms. In: Diabetes mellitus. A fundamental and clinical text. 2nd ed. Le Roith D, Taylor SI, Olefsky JM, eds. Philadelphia: Lippincott Williams and Wilkins. 2000:125-132

[343] Olson LK, Redmon JB, Towle HC, Robertson RP. Chronic exposure of HIT cells to high glucose concentrations paradoxically decreases insulin gene transcription and alters binding of insulin gene regulatory protein. J Clin Invest 1993;92:514-519

[344] Olson LK, Sharma A, Peshavaria M, *et al.* Reduction of insulin gene transcription in HIT-T15 cells chronically expressed to a supraphysiologic glucose concentration is associated with loss of STF-1 transcription factor expression. Proc Natl Acad Sci USA 1995;92:9127-9131

[345] Sharma A, Olson LK, Robertson RP, Stein R. The reduction of insulin gene transcription in HIT-T15 β-cells chronically exposed to high glucose concentration is associated with the loss of RIPE3b1 and STF-1 transcription factor expression. Mol Endocrinol 1995;9:1127-1134

[346] Morral N, Edenberg HJ, Witting SR, Altomonte J, Chu T, Brown M. Effects of glucose metabolism on the regulation of genes of fatty acid synthesis and triglyceride secretion in the liver. J Lipid Res 2007;48:1499-1510

[347] Ghiselli A, Laurenti O, De Mattia G, Maiani G, Ferro-Luzzi A. Salicylate hydroxylation as an early marker of *in vivo* oxidative stress in diabetic patients. Free Radic Biol Med 1992;13:621-626

[348] Nourooz-Zadeh J, Tajaddini-Sarmadi J, McCarthy S, Betteridge DJ, Wolff SP. Elevated levels of authentic plasma hydroperoxides in NIDDM. Diabetes 1995;44:1054-1058

[349] Rehman A, Nourooz-Zadeh J, Moller W, Tritschler H, Pereira P, Halliwell B. Increased oxidative damage to all DNA bases in patients with type II diabetes mellitus. FEBS Lett 1999;448:120-122

[350] Sakuaba H, Mizukami H, Yagihashi N, Wada R, Hanyu C, Yagihashi S. Reduced β-cell mass and expression of oxidative stress related DNA damage in the islet of Japanese type II diabetic patients. Diabetologia 2002;4:85-96

[351] Kawahito S, Kitahata H, Oshita S. Problems associated with glucose toxicity: Role of hyperglycemia-induced oxidative stress. World J Gastroenterol 2009;15,33:4137-4142

[352] Robertson RP. Oxidative stress and impaired insulin secretion in type 2 diabetes. Curr Opin Pharmacol 2006;6:615-619

[353] Grankvist K, Marklund SL, Taljedal IB. CuZn-superoxide dismutase, Mn-superoxide dismutase, catalase and glutathione peroxidase in pancreatic islets and other tissues in the mouse. Biochem J 1981;199:393-398

[354] Tiedge M, Lortz S, Drinkgern J, Lenzen S. Relation between antioxidant enzyme gene expression and antioxidative defense status in insulin-producing cells. Diabetes 1997;46:1733-1742

[355] Welsh N, Margulis B, Borg LA, *et al.* Differences in the expression of heat-shock proteins and antioxidant enzymes between human and rodent pancreatic islets: implications for the pathogenesis of insulin-dependent diabetes mellitus. Mol Med 1995;1:806-820

[356] Wolff SP, Dean RT. Glucose autoxidation and protein modification: the potential role of "autoxidative glycosylation" in diabetes. Biochem J 1987;245:243-250

[357] Hunt JV, Dean RT, Wolff SP. Hydroxyl radical production and autoxidative glycosylation: glucose autoxidation as the cause of protein damage in the experimental glycation model of diabetes mellitus and ageing. Biochem J 1988;256:205-212

[358] Kaneto H, Hu G, Fujii N, Kim S, Bonner-Weir S, Weir GC. Involvement of c-Jun N-terminal kinase in oxidative stress-mediated suppression of insulin gene expression. J Biol Chem 2002;277:30010-30018

[359] Baynes JW. Role of oxidative stress in development of complications in diabetes. Diabetes 1991;40:405-412

[360] Tiedge M, Lortz S, Munday R, Lenzen S. Complementary action of antioxidant enzymes in the protection of bioengineered insulin-producing RINm5F cells against the toxicity of reactive oxygen species. Diabetes 1998;47:1578-1585

[361] Vincent AM, Russell JW, Low P, Fledman EL. Oxidative stress in the pathogenesis of diabetic neuropathy. Endocr Rev 2004;25:612-628

[362] Baynes JW, Thorpe SR. Role of oxidative stress in diabetic complications: a new perspective on an old paradigm. Diabetes 1999;48:1-9

[363] Brunner Y, Schvartz D, Priego-Capote F, Couté Y, Sanchez JC. Glucotoxicity and pancreatic proteomics. J Proteomics 2009;71:576-591

[364] Sakai K, Matsumoto K, Nishikawa T, *et al.* Mitochondrial reactive oxygen species reduce insulin secretion by pancreatic beta-cells. Biochem Biophys Res Commun 2003;300:216-222

[365] Kaneto H, Xu G, Song KH, *et al.* Activation of the hexosamine pathway leads to deterioration of pancreatic beta-cell function through the induction of oxidative stress. J Biol Chem 2001;276:31099-31104

[366] Eriksson JW. Metabolic stress in insulin's target cells leads to ROS accumulation – a hypothetical common pathway causing insulin resistance. FEBS Lett 2007;581:3734-3742

[367] Lu B, Ennis D, Lai R, *et al.* Enhanced sensitivity of insulin-resistant adipocytes to vanadate is associated with oxidative stress and decreased reduction of vanadat (+5) to vanadyl (+4). J Biol Chem 2001;276:35589-35598

[368] Rudich A, Tirosh A, Potashnik R, Hemi R, Kanety H, Bashan N. Prolonged oxidative stress impairs insulin-induced GLUT4 translocation in 3T3-L1 adipocytes. Diabetes 1998;47:1562-1569

[369] Dokken BB, Saengsirisuwan V, Kim JS, Teachey MK, Henriksen EJ. Oxidative stress-induced insulin resistance in rat skeletal muscle: role of glycogen synthase kinase-3. Am J Physiol Endocrinol Metab 2008;294:E615-E621

[370] Kowluru RA, Chan PS. Oxidative stress and diabetic retinopathy. Exp Diabetes Res 2007;2007:43603

[371] Du Y, Miller CM, Kern TS. Hyperglycemia increases mitochondrial superoxide in retina and retinal cells. Free Radic Biol Med 2003;35:1491-1499

[372] Yamagishi S, Imaizumi T. Diabetic vascular complications: pathophysiology, biochemical basis and potential therapeutic strategy. Curr Pharm Des 2005,11:2279-2299

[373] van Dam PS. Oxidative stress and diabetic neuropathy: pathophysiological mechanisms and treatment perspectives. Diabetes Metab Res Rev 2002;18:176-184

[374] Deedwania PC. Diabetes is a vascular disease: the role of endothelial dysfunction in pathophysiology of cardiovascular disease in diabetes. Cardiol Clin 2004;22:505-509

[375] Winer N, Sowers JR. Diabetes and arterial stiffening. Adv Cardiol 2007;44:245-251

[376] Grobbe DE. How to ADVANCE prevention of cardiovascular complications in type 2 diabetes. Metabolism 2003;52:24-28

[377] Thompson CS. Animal models of diabetes mellitus: relevance to vascular complications. Curr Pharm Des 2008;14:309-324

[378] Schalh DS, Kipnis DM. Abnormalities in carbohydrate tolerance associated with elevated plasma nonesterified fatty acids. J Clin Invest 1965;44,12:2010-2020

[379] Schaffer JE. Lipotoxicity: when tissues overeat. Curr Opin Lipidol 2003;14:281-287

[380] McGarry JD. What if Minkowski had been ageusic? An alternative angle on diabetes. Science 1992;258,5083:766-770

[381] Unger RH. Lipotoxicity in the pathogenesis of obesity-dependent NIDDM. Genetic and clinical implications. Diabetes 1995;44:863-870

[382] Briaud I, Harman JS, Kelpe CL, Segu VB, Poitou V. Lipotoxicity of the pancreatic β-cell is associated with glucose-dependent esterification of fatty acids into neutral lipids. Diabetes 201;50:315-321

[383] Hagman DK, Hays LB, Parazzoli SD, Poitout V. Palmitate inhibits insulin gene expression by altering PDX-1 nuclear localization and reducing MafA expression in isolated rat islets of Langerhans. J Biol Chem 2005;280:32413-32418

[384] Kelpe CL, Moore PC, Parazzoli SD, Wicksteed B, Rhodes CI, Poitout V. Palmitate inhibition of insulin gene expression is mediated at the transcriptional level via ceramide synthesis. J Biol Chem 2003;278:30015-30021

[385] Gremlich S, Bonny C, Waeber G, Thorens B. Fatty acids decrease IDX-1 expression in rat pancreatic islets and reduce GLUT2, glucokinase, insulin and somatostatin levels. J Biol Chem 1997;272:30261-30269

[386] Rutz-Laser B, Meda P, Constant I, *et al.* Glucose-induced preproinsulin gene expression is inhibited by the free-fatty acid palmitate. Endocrinol 1999;140:4005-4014

[387] Shimabukuro M, Ohneda M, Lee Y, Unger RH. Role of nitric oxide in obesity-induced beta cell disease. J Clin Invest 1997;100:290-295

[388] Shimabukuro M, Koyama K, Lee Y, Unger RH. Leptin- or troglitazone-induced lipopenia protects islets from interleukin 1 beta cytotoxicity. J Clin Invest 1997;100:1750-1754

[389] Shimabukuro M, ZhouYT, Levi M, Unger RH. Fatty acid-induced beta cell apoptosis: a link between obesity and diabetes. Proc Natl Acad Sci USA 1998;95:2498-2502

[390] Moore PC, Ugas MA, Hagman DK, Parazzoli SD, Poitout V. Evidence against the involvement of oxidative stress in fatty acid inhibition of insulin secretion. Diabetes 2004;53:2610-2616

[391] Sako Y, Grill VE. A 48-hour lipid infusion in the rat time-dependently inhibits glucose-induced insulin secretion and β-cell oxidation through a process likely coupled to fatty acid oxidation. Endocrinol 1990;127:1580-1589

[392] Elks ML. Chronic perfusion of rat islets with palmitate suppresses glucose-stimulated insulin release. Endocrinol 1993;133:208-214

[393] Zhou YP, Grill VE. Long-term exposure of rat pancreatic islets to fatty acids inhibits glucose-induced insulin secretion and biosynthesis through a glucose-fatty acid cycle. J Clin Invest 1994;93:870-876

[394] Zhou Y-P, Grill V. Long-term exposure to fatty acids and ketones inhibits β-cell functions I human pancreatic islets of Langerhans. J Clin Endocrinol Metab 1995;80:1584-1590

[395] Mason TM, Goh T, Tchipashvili V, *et al.* Prolonged elevation of plasma free fatty acids desensitizes the insulin secretory response to glucose *in vivo* in rats. Diabetes 1999;48:524-530

[396] Paolisso G, Gambardella A, Amuto L, *et al.* Opposite effects of short- and long-term fatty acid infusion on insulin secretion in healthy subjects. Diabetologia 1995;38:1295-1299

[397] Hosokowa H, Corkey BE, Leahy JL. β-Cell hypersensitivity to glucose following 24-h exposure of rat islets to fatty acids. Diabetologia 1997;40:392-397

[398] Liu YQ, Tornheim K, Leahy JL. Fatty-acid induced β-cell hypersensitivity to glucose. Increased phosphofructokinase activity and lowered glucose-6-phosphate content. J Clin Invest 1998;101:1870-1875

[399] Liu YQ, Tornheim K, Leahy JL. Shared biochemical properties of glucotoxicity and lipotoxicity decrease citrate synthase activity and increase phosphofructokinase activity. Diabetes 1998;47:1889-1893

[400] Mahgnan C, Collins S, Berthault MF, *et al.* Lipid infusion lowers sympathetic nervous activity and leads to increased β-cell responsiveness to glucose. J Clin Invest 1999;103:413-419

[401] Zhang C-Y, Baffy G, Perret P, *et al.* Uncoupling protein-2 negatively regulates insulin secretion and is a major link between obesity, β-cell dysfunction, and type 2 diabetes. Cell 2001;105:745-755

[402] Chan CB, MacDonald PE, Saleh MC, Johns DC, Marban E, Wheeler MB. Overexpression of uncoupling protein 2 inhibits glucose-stimulated insulin secretion from rat islets. Diabetes 1999;48:1482-1486

[403] Chan CB, De Leo D, Joseph JW, *et al.* Increased uncoupling protein-2 levels in β-cells are associated with impaired glucose-stimulated insulin secretion: mechanism of action. Diabetes 2001;50:1302-1310

[404] Joseph JW, Koshkin V, Zhang CY, *et al.* Uncoupling protein 2 knockout mice have enhanced insulin secretory capacity after a high-fat diet. Diabetes 2002;51:3211-3219

[405] Briaud I, Kelpe CL, Johnson LM, Tran POT, Poitout V. Differential effects of hyperglycemia on insulin secretion in islets of Langerhans from hyperglycemic vs. normoglycemic rats. Diabetes 2002;51:662-668

[406] El-Assaad W, Buteau J, Peyot ML, *et al.* Saturated fatty acids synergize with elevated glucose to cause pancreatic β-cell death. Endocrinol 2003;144:4154-4163

[407] Maedler K, Spinas GA, Dyntar D, Moritz W, Kaiser N, Donath MY. Distinct effects of saturated and monounsaturated fatty acids on β-cell turnover and function. Diabetes 2001;50:69-76

[408] Maedler K, Oberholzer J, Bucher S, Spinas GA, Donath MY. Monounsaturated fatty acids prevent the deleterious effects of palmitate and high glucose on human pancreatic β-cell turnover and function. Diabetes 2003;52:726-733

[409] Shimabukuro M, Zhou Y-T, Levi M, Unger RH. Fatty-acid-induced β-cell apoptosis: a link between obesity and diabetes. Proc Natl Acad Sci USA 1998;95:2498-2502

[410] Lupi R, Dotta F, Marselli L, *et al.* Prolonged exposure to free fatty acids has cytostatic and pro-apoptotic effects on human pancreatic islets: evidence that β-cell death is caspase mediated, partially dependent on ceramide pathway and Bcl-2 regulated. Diabetes 2002;51:1437-1442

[411] Shimabukuro M, Higa M, Zhou YT, Wang MY, Newgard CB, Unger RH. Lipoapoptosis in β-cells of obese prediabetic *fa/fa* rats. Role of serine palmitoyltransferase overexpression. J Biol Chem 1998;273:32487-32490

[412] Roduit R, Morin J, Masse F, *et al.* Glucose down-regulates the expression of peroxisome proliferator-activated receptor-α gene in the pancreatic β-cell. J Biol Chem 2000;275:35799-35806

[413] Ruderman N, Prentki M. AMP kinase and malonyl-CoA: targets for therapy of the metabolic syndrome. Nat Rev Drug Discov 2004;3:340-351

[414] Piro S, Anello M, Di Pietro C, *et al.* Chronic exposure to free fatty acids or high glucose induces apoptosis in rat pancreatic islets: possible role of oxidative stress. Metabolism 2002;51:1340-1347

[415] Maestre I, Jordan J, Calvo S, *et al.* Mitochondrial dysfunction is involved in apoptosis induced by serum withdrawal and fatty acids in the β-cell line INS-1. Endocrinol 2003;144:335-345

[416] Wang X, Li H, De Leo D, *et al.* Gene and protein kinase expression profiling of reactive oxygen species-associated lipotoxicity in the pancreatic β-cell line MIN 6. Diabetes 2004;53:129-140

[417] Morgan D, Oliveira-Emilio HR, Keane D, *et al.* Glucose, palmitate and pro-inflammatory cytokines modulate production and activity of a phagocyte-like NADPH oxidase in rat pancreatic islets and a clonal β cell line. Diabetologia 2007;50:359-369

[418] Kelly DP, Hale DE, Rutledge SL, *et al.* Molecular basis of inherited medium-chain acyl-CoA dehydrogenase deficiency causing sudden child death. J Inherited Dis 1992;15:171-180

[419] Zhou Y-T, Grayburn P, Karim A, *et al.* Lipotoxic heart disease in obese rats: implications for human obesity. Proc Natl Acad Sci USA 2000;97:1784-1789

[420] Hiu H, Kovacs A, Ford D, *et al.* A novel mouse model of lipotoxic cardiomyopathy. J Clin Invest 2001;107:813-822

[421] Colberg SR, Simoneau JA, Thaete FL, Kelley DE. Skeletal muscle utilization of free fatty acids in women with visceral obesity. J Clin Invest 1995;95:1846-1853

[422] Pan DA, Hulbert AJ, Storlien LH. Dietary fats, membrane phospholipids and obesity. J Nutr 1994;124:1555-1565

[423] Rossetti L, Hawkins M, Chen W, Gindi J, Barzilai N. *In vivo* glucosamine infusion induces insulin resistance in normoglycemic but not in hyperglycemic conscious rats. J Clin Invest 1995;96:132-140

[424] Glick BS, Rothman JE. Possible role for fatty acyl-coenzyme A in intracellular protein transport. Nature 1987;326:309-312

[425] Griffin ME, Marcucci MJ, Cline GW, *et al.* Free fatty acid-induced insulin resistance is associated with activity of protein kinase C theta and alterations in the insulin signaling pathway. Diabetes 1999;48:1270-1274

[426] Schrauwen P. High-fat diet, muscular lipotoxicity and insulin resistance. Proc Nutr Soc 2007;66:33-41

[427] Hesselink MKC, Mensink M, Schrauwen P. Lipotoxicity and mitochondrial dysfunction in type 2 diabetes. Immun Endoc Metab Agents in Med Chem 2007;7:3-17

[428] Ibdah JA, Hyacinth P, Zhao Y, *et al.* Lack of mitochondrial trifunctional protein in mice causes neonatal hypoglycemia and sudden death. J Clin Invest 2001;107:1403-1409

[429] Garg A, Misra A. Hepatic steatosis, insulin resistance, and adipose tissue disorders. J Clin Endocinol Metab 2002;87:3019-3022

[430] Wititsuwannakul D, Kim KH. Mechanism of palmityl coenzyme A inhibition of liver glycogen synthase. J Biol Chem 1977;252:7812-7817

[431] Brindley DN. Intracellular translocation of phosphatidate phosphorylase and its possible role in the control of glycerolipid synthesis. Prog Lipid Res 1984;23:115-133

[432] Thomas ME, Harris KPG, Walls J, *et al.* Fatty acids exacerbate tubulointerstitial injury in protein-overload proteinuria. Am J Physiol Renal Physiol 2002;283:F640-F647

[433] Sarafidis PA, Nilsson PM. The metabolic syndrome: a glance at its history. J Hypertens 2006;24:621-626

[434] Kylin E. Studien ueber das hypertonie-hyperglykämie-hyperurikämie syndrom. Zentralblatt Fuer Innere Med 1923;44:105-127

[435] DeFronzo R, Ferrannini E. Insulin resistance: A multifaceted syndrome responsible for NIDDM, obesity, hypertension, dyslipidemia and atherosclerotic cardiovascular disease. Diabetes Care 1991;14:173-194

[436] Modan M, Halkin H, Almog S, *et al.* Hyperinsulinemia: a link between hypertension, obesity and glucose intolerance. J Clin Invest 1985;75:807-817

[437] Haffner S, Valdez R, Hazuda H, Mitchell B, Morales P, Stern M. Prospective analysis of the insulin-resistance syndrome (Syndrome X). Diabetes 1992;41:715-722

[438] Meigs J, D'Agostino RS, Wilson P, Cupples L, Nathan D, Singer D. Risk variable clustering in the insulin resistance syndrome. The Framingham offspring study. Diabetes 1997;46:1594-1560

[439] Groop L, Orho-Melander M. The dysmetabolic syndrome. J Internal Med 2001;250:105-120

[440] Johnson LW, Weinstock RS. The metabolic syndrome: concepts and controversy. Mayo Clin Proc 2006;81,2:1615-1620

[441] Alberti KGMM, Zimmet PZ. Definition, diagnosis and classification of diabetes mellitus and its complications, part 1: diagnosis and classification of diabetes mellitus: provisional report of a WHO consultation. Diab Med 1998;15:539-553

[442] Isomaa B, Almgren P, Tuomi T, *et al.* Cardiovascular morbidity and mortality associated with the metabolic syndrome. Diabetes Care 2001;24:683-689

[443] Zimmet PZ. Kelly West Lecture 1991: challenges in diabetes epidemiology – from West to the rest. Diabetes Care 1992;15:232-252

[444] Gogia A, Agarwal PK. Metabolic syndrome. Indian J Med Sci 2006;60,2:72-81

[445] Balkau B, Charles MA. European Group for the Study of Insulin Resistance (EGIR). Comment on the provisional report of the WHO consultation [letter]. Diab Med 1999;16:442-443

[446] Executive Summary of The Third Report of The National Cholesterol Education Program (NCEP) Expert Panel on Detection, Evaluation, and Treatment of High Blood Cholesterol in Adults (Adult Treatment Panel III). JAMA 2001;285:2486-2497

[447] Bloomgarden ZT. American Association of Clinical Endocrinologists (AACE) consensus conference on the insulin resistance syndrome: 25-26 August 2002, Washington, DC. Diabetes Care 2003;26:1297-1303

[448] Alberti KG, Zimmet P, Shaw J. Metabolic syndrome – a new world-wide definition. A Consensus Statement from the International Diabetes Federation. Diab Med 2006;23:469-480

[449] Taslim S, Tai ES. The relevance of the metabolic syndrome. Ann Acad Med Singapore 2009;38:29-33

[450] Cornier MA, Dabelea D, Hernandez TL, *et al.* The metabolic syndrome. Endocrine Rev 2008;29:777-822

[451] Ferrennini E, Haffner SM, Mitchell BD, Stern MP. Hyperinsulinemia: the key feature of a cardiovascular and metabolic syndrome. Diabetologica 1991;34:416-427

[452] Ford ES, Giles WH, Dietz WH. Prevalence of the metabolic syndrome among US adults. Findings from the Third National Health and Nutrition Examination Survey. JAMA 2002;287:356-359

[453] Ceska R. Clinical implications of the metabolic syndrome. Diabetes Vasc Dis Res 2007;4,Suppl.3:S2-S4

[454] McFarlane SI, Banerji M, Sowers JR. Insulin resistance and cardiovascular disease. J Clin Endocrinol Metab 2001;86:713-718

[455] Ford ES, Giles WH, Mokdad AH. Increasing prevalence of the metabolic syndrome among U.S. adults. Diabetes Care 2004;27:2444-2449

[456] Bjorntorp P. Metabolic implications of body fat distribution. Diabetes Care 1991;14:1132-1143

[457] Lamarche B. Abdominal obesity and its metabolic complications: implications for the risk of ischemic heart disease. Coron Artery Dis 1998;9:473-481

[458] Freedland ES. Role of a critical visceral adipose tissue threshold (CVATT) in metabolic syndrome: implications for controlling dietary carbohydrates: a review. Nutr Metabol 2004;1,12, doi:10. 1186/1743-7075-1-12

[459] Lorenzo C, Williams K, Hunt KJ, Haffner SM. The National Cholesterol Education Program – Adult Treatment Panel III, International Diabetes Federation, and World Health Organization definitions of the metabolic syndrome as predictors of incident cardiovascular disease and diabetes. Diabetes Care 2007;30:8-13

[460] Paoletti R, Bolego C, Poli A, Cignarella A. Metabolic syndrome, inflammation and atherosclerosis. Vasc Health Risk Manag 2006;2,2:145-152

[461] Gill H, Mugo M, Whaley-Connell A, Stump C, Sowers JR. The key role of insulin resistance in the cardiometabolic syndrome. Am J Med Sci 2005;330,6:290-294

[462] Ryysy L, Hakkinen AM, Goto T, *et al.* Hepatic fat content and insulin action on free fatty acids and glucose metabolism rather than insulin absorption are associated with insulin requirements during insulin therapy in type 2 diabetic patients. Diabetes 2000;49:749-758

[463] Seppala-Lindroos A, Vehkavaara S, Hakkinen AM, *et al.* Fat accumulation in the liver is associated with defects in insulin suppression of glucose production and serum free fatty acids independent of obesity in normal men. J Clin Endocrinol Metab 2002;87:3023-3028

[464] Adiels M, Taskinen MR, Packard C, *et al.* Overproduction of large VLDL particles is driven by increased liver fat content in men. Diabetologia 2006;49:755-765

[465] Malmstrom R, Packard CJ, Caslake M, *et al.* Defective regulation of triglyceride metabolism by insulin in the liver in NIDDM. Diabetologia 1997;40:454-462

[466] Kotronen A, Yki-Järvinen H. Fatty liver. A novel component of the metabolic syndrome. Arterioscler Thromb Vasc Biol 2008;28:27-38

[467] Petersen KF, Dufour S, Savage DB, *et al.* The role of skeletal muscle insulin resistance in the pathogenesis of the metabolic syndrome. PNAS 2007;104,31:12587-12594

[468] Sniderman AD, Lamarche B, Tilley J, *et al.* Hypertriglyceridemic hyperapoB in type 2 diabetes. Diabetes Care 2002;25:579-582

[469] Turner RC, Millns H, Neil HAW, *et al.* Risk factors for coronary artery disease in non-insulin dependent diabetes mellitus: United Kingdom Prospective Diabetes Study (UKPDS 23). BMJ 1998;316:823-828

[470] Lamarche B, Tchernof A, Mooriania S, *et al.* Small, dense low-density lipoprotein particles as a predictor of the risk of ischemic heart disease in men. Prospective results from the Quebec Cardiovascular Study. Circulation 1997;95:69-75

[471] Austin MA, Edwards KL. Small, dense low density lipoproteins, the insulin resistance syndrome and noninsulin-dependent diabetes. Curr Opin Lipidol 196;7:167-171

[472] Eckel RH, Grundy SM, Zimet PZ. The metabolic syndrome. Lancet 2005;365:1415-1428

[473] McGarry JD. Banting lecture 2001: dysregulation of fatty acid metabolism in the etiology of type 2 diabetes. Diabetes 2002;51:7-18

[474] Kahn BB, Flier JS. Obesity and insulin resistance. J Clin Invest 2000;106:473-481

[475] Jocken JW, Langin D, Smit E, *et al.* Adipose triglyceride lipase and hormone-sensitive lipase protein expression is decreased in the obese insulin-resistant state. J Clin Endocrinol Metab 2007;92:2292-2299

[476] Bergman RN, Kim SP, Hsu IR, *et al.* Abdominal obesity: role in the pathophysiology of metabolic disease and cardiovascular risk. Am J Med 2007;120:S3-S8

[[477] Lewis GF, Steiner G. Acute effects of insulin in the control of VLDL production in humans. Implications for the insulin-resistant state. Diabetes Care 1996;19:390-393

[478] Ginsberg HN, Zhang YL, Hernandez-Ono A. Regulation of plasma triglycerides in insulin resistance and diabetes. Arch Med Res 2005;36:232-240

[479] Jiang J, Torok N. Nonalcoholic steatohepatitis and the metabolic syndrome. Metab Syndr Relat Disord 2008;6:1-7

[480] Ferrannini E, Buzzigoli G, Bonadonna R, *et al.* Insulin resistance in essential hypertension. N Engl J Med 1987;317:350-357

[481] Bonora E, Capaldo B, Perin PC, *et al.* Hyperinsulinemia and insulin resistance are independently associated with plasma lipids, uric acid and blood pressure in non-diabetic subjects. The GISIR database. Nutr Metab Cardiovasc Dis 2007;18:624-631

[482] Laakso M, Sarlund H, Mykkanen L. Essential hypertension and insulin resistance in non-insulin-dependent diabetes. Eur J Clin Invest 1989;19:518-526

[483] Tooke JE, Hannemann MM. Adverse endothelial function and the insulin resistance syndrome. J Intern Med 2000;247:425-431

[484] Kuroda S, Uzu T, Fujii T, *et al.* Role of insulin resistance in the genesis of sodium sensitivity in essential hypertension. J Hum Hypertens 1999;13:257-262

[485] Hanley AJ, Karter AJ, Festa A, *et al.* Factor analysis of metabolic syndrome using directly measured insulin sensitivity: the Insulin Resistance Atherosclerosis Study. Diabetes 2002;51:2642-2647

[486] Sowers JR. Insulin resistance and hypertension. Am J Physiol Circ Physiol 2004;286:H1597-H1602

[487] Sowers JR, Haffner S. Treatment of cardiovascular and renal risk factors in the diabetic hypertensive. Hypertension 2002;40:781-788

[488] Dzau VJ. Theodore Cooper Lecture: Tissue angiotensis and pathobiology of vascular disease: a unifying hypothesis. Hypertension 2001;37:1047-1052

[489] Jager J, Gremeaux T, Cormont M, Le Marchand-Brustel Y, Tanti JF. Interleukin-1β-induced insulin resistance in adipocytes through down-regulation of insulin receptor substrate-1 expression. Endocrinol 2007;148:241-251

[490] Norata GD, Ongari M, Garlaschelli K, Raselli S, Grigore L, Catapano AL. Plasma resistin levels correlate with determinants of the metabolic syndrome. Eur J Endocrinol 2007;156:279-284

[491] Bahia L, Aguiar LG, Villela N, *et al.* Relationship between adipokines, inflammation, and vascular reactivity in lean controls and obese subjects with metabolic syndrome. Clinics 2006;61:433-440

[492] Xydakis AM, Case CC, Jones PH, *et al.* Adiponectin, inflammation, and the expression of the metabolic syndrome in obese individuals: the impact of rapid weight loss through caloric restriction. J Clin Endocrinol Metab 2004;89:2697-2703

[493] Van Guilder GP, Hoetzer GL, Greiner JJ, Stauffer BL, Desouza CA. Influence of metabolic syndrome on biomarkers of oxidative stress and inflammation in obese adults. Obesity (Silver Spring) 2006;14:2127-2131

[494] Choi KM, Ryu OH, Lee KW, *et al.* Serum adiponectin, interleukin-10 levels and the inflammatory markers in the metabolic syndrome. Diabetes Res Clin Pract 2007;75:235-240

[495] Gonzalez AS, Guerrero DB, Soto MB, Diaz SP, Martinez-Olmos M, Vidal O. Metabolic syndrome, insulin resistance and the inflammation markers C-reactive protein and ferritin. Eur J Clin Nutr 2006;60:802-809

[496] Ridker PM, Buring JE, Cook NR, Rifai N. C-reactive protein, the metabolic syndrome, and the risk of incident cardiovascular events: an 8-year follow-up of 14,719 initially healthy American women. Circulation 2003;107:391-397

[497] Hung J, McQuillan BM, Chapman CM, Thompson PL, Beilby JP. Elevated interleukin-18 levels are associated with the metabolic syndrome independent of obesity and insulin resistance. Arterioscler Thromb Vasc Biol 2005;25:1268-1273

[498] Mertens I, Verrjken A, Michiels JJ, Van der Planken M, Ruige JB, Van Gaal LF. Among inflammation and coagulation markers, PAI-1 is a true component of the metabolic syndrome. Int J Obes (Lond) 2006;30:1308-1314

[499] Deepa R, Velmurugan K, Arvind K, *et al.* Serum levels of interleukin 6, C-reactive protein, vascular cell adhesion molecule 1, and monocyte chemotactic protein 1 in relation to insulin resistance and glucose intolerance – the Chennai Urban Rural Epidemiology Study (CURES). Metabolism 2006;55:1232-1238

[500] Duncan BB, Schmidt MI, Pankow JS. Low-grade systemic inflammation and the development of type 2 diabetes mellitus: the atherosclerosis risk in communities study. Diabetes 2003;52:1799-1805

[501] Bahia L, Aguiar LG, Villela N, *et al.* Relationship between adipokines, inflammation, and vascular reactivity in lean controls and obese subjects with metabolic syndrome. Clinics 2006;61:433-440

[502] Choi KM, Ryu OH, Lee KW, *et al.* Serum adiponectin, interleukin-10 levels and inflammatory markers in the metabolic syndrome. Diabetes Res Clin Pract. 2007;75:235-240

[503] Yokota, Oritani K, Takahashi I, *et al.* Adiponectin, a new member of the family of soluble defense collagens, negatively regulates the growth of myelomonocytic progenitors and the functions of macrophages. Blood 2000;96:1723-1732

[504] Verma S, Li SH, Wang CH, *et al.* Resistin promotes endothelial cells activation: further evidence of adipokine-endothelial interaction. Circulation 2003;108:736-740

[505] Juahan-Vague I, Alessi MC. PAI-1, obesity, insulin resistance and risk of cardiovascular events. Thromb. Haemost 1997;78:656-660

[506] Thompson SG, Kienast J, Pyke SD, Haverkate F, Van de Loo JC. Haemostatic factors and the risk of Myocardial infarction or sudden death in patients with angina pectoris. N Engl J Med 1995;332:635-641

[507] Kannel WB, Anderson K, Wilson PW. White blood cell count and cardiovascular disease: insights from the Framingham Study. JAMA 1992;257:1253-1256

[508] Munro JM, Cotran RS. Biology of disease: atherogenesis and inflammation. Lab Invest 1988;58:249-261

[509] Yarnell JW, Baker IA, Sweetnam PM, *et al.* Fibrinogen, viscosity and white blood cell count are major risk factors for ischemic heart disease: the Caerphilly Speedwell Collaborative Heart Disease studies. Circulation 1991;83:836-844

[510] Hansson GK. Inflammation, atherosclerosis, and coronary artery disease. N Engl J Med 2005;352:1685-1695

[511] Randle PJ, Garland PB, Hales CN, Newsholme EA. The glucose fatty-acid cycle. Its role in insulin sensitivity and the metabolic disturbances of diabetes mellitus. Lancet 1963;1:785-789

[512] Schalach DS, Kipnis DM. Abnormalities in carbohydrate tolerance associated with elevated plasma nonesterified fatty acids. J Clin Invest 1965;44:2010-2020

[513] Laakso M. Gene variants, insulin resistance and dyslipidemia. Curr Opin Lipidol 2004;15:115-120

[514] Draper N, Echwald SM, Lavery GG, *et al.* Association studies between microsatellite markers within the gene encoding human 11β-hydroxysteroid dehydrogenase type 1 and body mass index, waist to hip ration, and glucocorticoid metabolism. J Clin Endocrinol Metab 2002;87:4984-4990

[515] Heid IM, Wagner SA, Gohlke H, *et al.* Genetic architecture of the APM1 gene and its influence on adiponectin plasma levels and parameters of the metabolic syndrome in 1,727 healthy Caucasians. Diabetes 2006;55:375-384

[516] Kawamura T, Egusa G, Okubo M, Imazu M, Yamakido M. Association of β3-adrenergic receptor gene polymorphism with insulin resistance in Japanese-American men. Metabolism 1999;48:1367-1370

[517] Frittitta L, Barrata R, Spampinato D. The Q121K PC-1 variant and obesity have additive and independent effects in causing insulin resistance. J Clin Endocrinol Metab 2001;86:5888-5891

[518] Baroni MG, Arca M, Sentinelli F. The G972R variant of the insulin receptor substrate-1 (IRS-1) gene, body fat distribution and insulin resistance. Diabetologia 2001;44:367-372

[519] Gonzales-Sanchez JL, Martinez-Larrad MT, Saez ME, Zabena C, Martinez-Calatrava MJ, Serrano-Rios M. Endothelial nitric oxide synthase haplotypes are associated with features of metabolic syndrome. Clin Chem 2007;53:91-97

[520] Foulis AK, McGill M, Farquharson MA. Insulitis in type 1 (insulin-dependent) diabetes mellitus in man – macrophages, lymphocytes, and interferon-gamma containing cells. J Pathol 1991;165:97-103

[521] Todd JA. From genome to aetiology in a Multifactorial disease type-1 diabetes. BioAssays 1999;21:164-173

[522] Gilespie KM. Type 1 diabetes: pathogenesis and prevention (Review). CMAJ 2006;175:165-170

[523] Onkamo P, Vaananen S, Karvonen M, *et al.* Worldwide increase in incidence of Type 1 diabetes – the analysis of the data on published incidence trends. Diabetologia 1999;42:1395-1403

[524] Gottlieb PA, Eisenbarth GS. Human autoimmune diabetes. In: Molecular pathology of autoimmune diseases. Theofilopoulos AN, Bona CA, ed. 2nd ed. Taylor and Francis, New York, London. 2002: 588-613

[525] Al-Mutairi HF, Mohsen AM, Al-Mazidi ZM. Genetics of type 1 diabetes mellitus. Kuwait Med J 2007;39,2:107-115

[526] Khardori R, Pauza ME. Type 1 diabetes mellitus: pathogenesis and advances in therapy. Int J Diab Dev Countries 2003;23:106-119

[527] Shaltout AA, Moussa MA, Qabazard M, *et al.* Further evidence for the rising incidence of childhood Type 1 diabetes in Kuwait. Diab Med 2002;19:522-525

[528] Gardner SG, Bingley PJ, Sawtell PA, *et al.* Rising incidence of insulin dependent diabetes in children aged under 5 years in the Oxford region. BMJ 1973;315:713-717

[529] EURODIAB ACE Study Group. Variation and trend in incidence of childhood diabetes in Europe. Lancet 2000;355:873-876

[530] Atkinson MA, Eisenbarth GS. Type 1 diabetes: new perspectives on disease pathogenesis and treatment. Lancet 2001;358:221-229

[531] Rabinovitch A. Autoimmune diabetes. Science Med 2000;7,3:18-27

[532] Munoz-Torres M, Jodar E, Escobar-Jimenez F, *et al.* Bone mineral density measured by dual X-ray absorptiometry in Spanish patients with insulin-dependent diabetes mellitus. Calcif Tissue Int 1996;58:316-319

[533] Miazgowski T, Czekalski S. A 2-year follow-up study on bone mineral density and markers of bone turnover in patients with long-standing insulin-dependent diabetes mellitus. Osteoporos Int 1998; 8:399-403

[534] Jehle PM, Jehle DR, Mohans S, *et al.* Serum levels of insulin-like growth factor system components and relationship to bone metabolism in type 1 and type 2 diabetes mellitus patients. J Endocrinol 1998;159:297-306

[535] Tuominen JT, Impivaara O, Puukka P, *et al.* Bone mineral density in patients with type 1 and type 2 diabetes. Diabetes Care 1999;22:1196-1200

[536] Janghorbani M, Van Dam RM, Willett WC, Hu FB. Systemic review of type 1 and type 2 diabetes mellitus and risk of fracture. Am J Epidemiol 2007, doi: 10.1093/aje/kwm106

[537] Haller MJ, Atkinson MA. Diabetes Mellitus: Etiology, presentation and management. Pediatr Clin N Am 2005;52:1553-1578

[538] Warram JH, Krolewski AS, Kahn CR. Determinants of IDDM and perinatal mortality in children of diabetic mothers. Diabetes 1988;37:1328-1334

[539] Risch N. Assessing the role of HLA-linked and unlinked determinants of disease. Am J Hum Genet 1987;40:1-14

[540] Hyttinen V, Kaprio J, Kinnunen L, Koskenvuo M, Tuomilehto J. Genetic liability of type 1 diabetes and the onset age among 22,650 young Finnish twin pairs: a nationwide follow-up study. Diabetes 2003,52:1052-1055

[541] Klein S, Sato A. The HLA System – first of two parts. N Engl J Med 2000;343:702-709

[542] Pociot F, McDermott MF. Genetics of type 1 diabetes mellitus. Genes Immun 2002;5:235-249

[543] Notkins AL. Immunologic and genetic factors in type 1 diabetes. J Biol Chem 2002;277,46:43545-43548

[544] Cudworth AG, Woodrow JC. HLA system and diabetes mellitus. Diabetes 1975;24:345-349

[545] Nerup J, Platz P, Andersen OO, *et al.* HLA antigens and diabetes mellitus. Lancet 1974;2:864-866

[546] Naredran P, Estella E, Fourlanos S. Immunology of type 1 diabetes. Q J Med 2005;98:547-556

[547] Risch N. Assessing the role of HLA-linked and unlinked determinants of disease. Am J Hum Genet 1987;40:1-14

[[548] Todd JA. Genetic analysis of type 1 diabetes using whole genome approaches. Proc Natl Acad Sci USA 1995;92:8560-8566

[549] Todd JA, Wicker LS. Genetic protection from the inflammatory disease type 1 diabetes in humans and animal models. Immunity 2001;15:387-395

[550] She JX. Susceptibility to type 1 diabetes: HLA-DQ and DR revisited. Immunol Today 1996;17:323-329

[551] Peakman M. Advance in understanding the immunopathology of type 1 diabetes mellitus. CPD Bull Immunol Allerg 2001;2:23-26

[552] Bell GI, Horita S, Karam JH. A polymorphic locus near the insulin gene is associated with insulin-dependent diabetes mellitus. Diabetes 1984:33:176-183

[553] Mein CA, Esposito L, Dunn MG, *et al.* A search for type 1 diabetes susceptibility genes in families from the United Kingdom. Nat Genet 1998;19:297-300

[554] Concannon P, Gogolin-Ewans KJ, Hinds DA, *et al.* A second-generation screen of the human genome for susceptibility to insulin-dependent diabetes mellitus. Nat Genet 1998;19:292-296

[555] Cox NJ, Wapelhorst B, Morrison VA, *et al.* Seven regions of the genome show evidence of linkage to type 1 diabetes in a consensus analysis of 767 multiplex families. Am J Hum Genet 2001:69:820-830

[556] Dorman JS, Bunker CH. HLA-DQ locus of the human leucocyte antigen complex and type 1 diabetes mellitus: a HUGE review. Epidemiol Rev 2000;22:218-227

[557] Nistico L, Buzzetti R, Pritchard LE, *et al.* The CTLA-4 gene region of chromosome 2q33 is linked to, and associated with, type 1 diabetes. Belgian Diabetes Registry. Hum Mol Genet 1996;5:1075-1080

[558] Ueda H, Howson JM, Esposit L, *et al.* Association of the T-cell regulatory gene CTLA4 with susceptibility to autoimmune disease. Nature 2003;423:506-511

[559] Bottini N, Musumeci L, Alonso A, *et al.* A functional variant of lymphoid tyrosine phosphatase is associated with type 1 diabetes. Nat Genet 2004;36:337-338

[560] Vella A, Cooper JD, Lowe CE, *et al.* Localization of a type 1 diabetes locus in the IL2RA/CD25 region by use of tag single-nucleotide polymorphism. Am J Hum Genet 2005;76:773-779

[561] Smyth DJ, Cooper JD, Bailey R, *et al.* A genome-wide association study of nonsynonymous SNPs identifies a type 1 diabetes locus in the interferon-induced helicase (IFIH1) region. Nat Genet 2006;38:617-619

[562] Najentsev S, Cooper JD, Godfrey L, *et al.* Analysis of the vitamin D receptor gene sequence variants in type 1 diabetes. Diabetes 2004;53:2709-2712

[563] Hakonarson H, Grant SF, Bradfield JP, *et al.* A genome-wide association study identifies KIAAO350 as a type 1 diabetes gene. Nature 2007;448:591-594

[564] Temple IK. Imprinting in human disease with special reference to transient neonatal diabetes and Beckwith-Wiedemann syndrome. Endocr Rev 2007;12:113-123

[565] Mehers KL, Gillespie KM. The genetic basis for type 1 diabetes. British Med Bull 2008;88:115-129

[566] Foulis AK, Farquharson MA, Hardman R. Aberrant expression of Class II major histocompatibility complex molecules by B cells and hyperexpression of Class I major histocompatibility complex molecules by insulin containing islets in Type 1 (insulin-dependent) diabetes mellitus. Diabetologia 1987;30:333-343

[567] Santamaria P, Nakhleh RE, Sutherland DE, Barbosa JJ. Characterization of T lymphocytes infiltrating human pancreas allograft affected by isletitis and recurrent diabetes. Diabetes 1992;41,1:53-61

[568] Bottazzo GF, Florin-Christensen A, Doniach D. Islet-cell antibodies in diabetes mellitus with autoimmune polyendocrine deficiencies. Lancet 1974;2,7892:1279-1283

[569] Baekkeskov S, Aanstoot HJ, Christgau S, *et al.* Identification of the G4K autoantigen in insulin-dependent diabetes as the GABA-synthesizing enzyme glutamic acid decarboxylase. Nature 1990;347,6289:151-156

[570] Lan MS, Wasserfall C, Maclaren NK, Notkins AL. IA-2, a transmembrane protein of the protein tyrosine phosphatase family, is a major autoantigen in insulin-dependent diabetes mellitus. Proc Natl Acad Sci USA 1996;93,13:6367-6370

[571] Saeki K, Zhu M, Kubosaki A, Xie J, Lan M, Notkins AL. Target disruption of the protein tyrosine phosphatase-like molecule IA-2 results in alterations in glucose tolerance tests and insulin secretion. Diabetes 2002;51:1842-1850

[572] Hyoty H. Enterovirus infections and type 1 diabetes. Ann Med 2002;34:138-147

[573] Honeyman MC, Coulson BS, Stone NL, *et al.* Association between rotaviruses infection and pancreatic islet autoimmunity in children at risk of developing type 1 diabetes. Diabetes 2000;49:1319-1324

[574] Yoon J-W, Jun H-S. Viruses in type 1 diabetes: brief review. ILAR Journal 2004;45,3:343-348

[575] Umpierrez GE, Latif KA, Murphy MB, *et al.* Thyroid dysfunction in patients with type 1 diabetes: a longitudinal study. Diabetes Care 2003;26:1181-1185

[576] Iughetti L, Bulgarelli S, Forese S, Lorini R, Balli F, Bernasconi SJ. Endocrine aspects of coeliac disease. Pediatr Endocrinol Metab 2003;16:805-818

[577] Zelissen PM, Bast EJ, Croughs RJ. Associated autoimmunity in Addison's disease. Autoimmun 1995;8:121-130

[578] Neufeld M, Maclaren N, Blizzard R. Autoimmune polyglandular syndrome. Pediatr Ann 1980;9:154-162

[579] Neufeld M, Maclaren NK, Blizzard RM. Two types of autoimmune Addison's disease associated with different polyglandular autoimmune (PGA) syndromes. Medicine (Baltimore) 1981:60:355-362

[580] Furlanos S, Dolta F, Greenbaum CJ, *et al.* Latent autoimmune diabetes in adults (LADA) should be loss latent. Diabetologia 2005;48:2206-2212

[581] Naik RG, Palmer JP. Latent autoimmune diabetes in adults (LADA) Rev Endocr Metab Disord 2003,4:233-241

[582] Kobayashi T, Tamemoto K, Nakanishi K, *et al.* Immunogenetic and clinical characterization of slowly progressive IDDM. Diabetes Care 1993;16:78-788

[583] Tuomi T, Groop LC, Zimmet PZ, Rowley MJ, Knowles W, Mackay IR. Antibodies to glutamic acid decarboxylase reveal latent autoimmune diabetes mellitus in adults with a non-insulin-dependent onset of disease. Diabetes 1993;42:359-362

[584] Carlsson S, Midthjell K, Tesfamarin MY, Grill V. Age, overweight and physical inactivity increase the risk of latent autoimmune diabetes in adults: results from the Nord-Trøndelag health study. Diabetologia 2007;50:55-58

[585] Leslie RDG, Williams R, Pozzilli P. Clinical review: type 1 diabetes and latent autoimmune diabetes in adults: one end of the rainbow. J Clin Endocrinol Metab 2006;91:1654-1659

[586] Genovese S, Bonifacion E, McNally JM, *et al.* Distinct cytoplasmic islet cell antibodies with different risk for type 1 (insulin-dependent) diabetes mellitus. Diabetologia 1992;35:385-388

[587] Gianani R, Pugliese A, Bonner-Weir S, *et al.* Prognostically significant heterogeneity of cytoplasmic islet cell antibodies in relatives of patients with type 1 diabetes. Diabetes 1992;41:347-353

[588] Stenström G, Gottsäter A, Bakhtadze E, Berger B, Sundkvist G. Latent autoimmune diabetes in adults. Definition, prevalence, β-cell function, and treatment. Diabetes 2005;54:S68-S72

[589] Gale EA. Latent autoimmune diabetes in adults: a guide for the perplexed. Diabetologia 2005;48:2195-2199

[590] Carlsson S, Midthjell K, Grill V, Nord-Trøndelag Study. Smoking is associated with an increased risk of type 2 diabetes but a decreased risk of autoimmune diabetes in adults: an 11-year follow-up of incidence of diabetes in the Nord-Trøndelag Study. Diabetologia 2004;47:1953-1956

[591] Bandurska-Stankiewicz E, Praszkiewicz I, Surdykowski L. Latent autoimmune diabetes in adults – LADA diabetes. Diabetologia Dośw Klin 2006;6,4:173-181

[592] Turner R, Stratton I, Horton V, *et al.* UKPDS 25: autoantibodies to islet-cell cytoplasm and glutamic acid decarboxylase for prediction of insulin requirement in type 2 diabetes. UK Prospective Diabetes Study Group. Lancet 1997;350:1288-1293

[593] Nabhan F, Emanuele MA. Latent autoimmune diabetes of adulthood. Postgraduate Med 2005;117:7-12

[594] Palmer JP, Hirsch IB. Latent autoimmune diabetes of adults, type 1.5, adult-onset, and type 1 diabetes. Diabetes Care 2003;26:536-538

[595] Naik RG, Palmer JP. Latent autoimmune diabetes in adults (LADA). Rev Endocr Metab Disord 2003;4:233-241

[596] Palmer JP, Hampe CS, Chiu H, Goel A, Brooks-Worrell BM. Is latent autoimmune diabetes in adults distinct from type 1 diabetes or just type 1 diabetes at an older age? Diabetes 2005;54,Suppl.2:S62-S67

[597] Hosszufalasi N, Vatay A, Rajczy K. Similar genetic features and different islet cell autoantibody pattern of latent autoimmune diabetes in adults (LADA) compared with adult-onset type 1 diabetes with rapid progression. Diabetes Care 2003;26:452-457

[598] Caputo M, Cerrone GE. HLA-DQB1 genotyping in latent autoimmune diabetes of adults (LADA). Medicine (B. Aires) 2005;65:235-240

[599] Petrone A, Bugawan TL, Mesturino CA, *et al.* The distribution of HLA class II susceptible/protective haplotypes could partially explain the low incidence of type 1 diabetes in continental Italy (Lazio region). Tissue Antigens 2001;58:385-394

[600] Vatay A, Rajczy K, Pozsonyi E, *et al.* Differences in the genetic background of latent autoimmune diabetes in adults (LADA) and type 1 diabetes mellitus. Immunol Lett 2002;84:109-115

[601] Cerna M, Novota P, Kolostova K, *et al.* HLA in Czech adult patients with autoimmune diabetes mellitus: comparison with Czech children with type 1 diabetes and patients with type 2 diabetes. Eur J Immunogenet 2003;30:401-407

[602] Hornum L, Markholst H. New autoimmune genes and the pathogenesis of type 1 diabetes. Curr Diabetes Rep 2004;4:135-142

[603] Bach JF. The effect of infections on susceptibility to autoimmune and allergic diseases. N Engl J Med 2002;347:911-920

[604] Leslie RD, Delli Castelli M. Age-dependent influences on the origins of autoimmune diabetes: evidence and implications. Diabetes 2004;53:3033-3040

[605] Salvetti M, Ristori G, Bamprezzi R, Pozzilli P, Leslie RDG. Twins: mirrors of the immune system. Immunology Today 2000;21:342-347

[606] Lin Y, Sun Z. Current views on type 2 diabetes. J Endocrinol 2010.204:1-11

[607] Martin BC, Warram JH, Krolewski AS, Bergman RN, Soeldner JS, Kahn RN. Role of glucose and insulin resistance in development of type 2 diabetes mellitus: results of a 25-year follow-up study. Lancet 1992;340:925-929

[608] Butler AE, Janson J, Bonner-Weir S, Ritzel R, Rizza RA, Buttler PC. β-Cell deficient and increased β-cell apoptosis in humans with type 2 diabetes. Diabetes 2003;52:102-110

[609] Hossain P. Kawar B, El Nahas M. Obesity and diabetes in the developing world – a growing challenge. N Engl J Med 2007;356:213-215

[610] Tuomilehto J, Lindström J, Eriksson JG, *et al.* Prevention of type 2 diabetes mellitus by changes in lifestyle among subjects with impaired glucose tolerance. N Engl J Med 2001;344:1343-1350

[611] Knowler WC, Barrett-Connor E, Fowler SE, *et al.* Reduction in the incidence of type 2 diabetes with lifestyle intervention or metformin. N Engl J Med 2002;346:393-403

[612] Staiger H, Machicao F, Fritsche A, Häing H-U. Pathomechanisms of type 2 diabetes genes. Endocrine Rev 2009;30,6:557-585

[613] Poulsen P, Kyvik KO, Vaag A, Beck-Nielsen H. Heritability of type II (non-insulin-dependent) diabetes mellitus and abnormal glucose tolerance – a population-based twin study. Diabetologia 1999;42:139-145

[614] Doria A, Patti M-E, Kahn CR. The emerging genetic architecture of type 2 diabetes. Cell Metabol 2008;8:186-200

[615] Majithia AR, Florez CJ. Clinical translation of genetic predictors for type 2 diabetes. Curr Opin Endocrinol Diab Obes 2009;16:100-106

[616] Ridderstrale M, Groop L. Genetic dissection of type 2 diabetes. Mol Cell Endocrinol 2009;297:10-17

[617] Keshavarz P, Inoue H, Sakamoto Y, *et al.* No evidence for association of ENPP1 (PC-1) K121Q variant with risk of type 2 diabetes in a Japanese population. J Hum Genet 2006;51:559-566

[618] Chandalia M, Grundy SM, Adams-Huet B, Abate N. Ethnic differences in the frequency of ENPP1/PC1 121Q genetic variant in the Dallas Heart Study cohort. J Diabetes Complications 2007;21:143-148

[619] Neel JV. Diabetes mellitus: a "thrifty" genotype rendered detrimental by "progress". Am J Hum Genet 1962;14:353-362

[620] Beck-Nielsen H, Groop LC. Metabolic and genetic characterization of pre-diabetic states. Sequence of events leading to non-insulin-dependent diabetes mellitus. J Clin Invest 1994;94:1714-1721

[621] Chakravarthy MV, Booth FW. Eating, exercise, and "thrifty" genotypes: connecting the dots toward on evolutionary understanding of modern chronic diseases. J Appl Physiol 2004;96:3-10

[622] Deeb SS, Fajas L, Nemoto M, Pihlajamäki J, Mykkänen L. A Pro12Ala substitution in PPARγ2 is associated with decreased receptor activity, lower body mass index and impaired insulin sensitivity (letter). Nat Genet 1998;20:284-287

[623] Horikawa Y, Oda N, Cox NJ, *et al.* Genetic variation in the gene encoding calpain-10 is associated with type 2 diabetes mellitus. Nat Genet 2000;26:163-175

[624] Walston J, Silver K, Bogardus C, *et al.* Time of onset of non-insulin-dependent diabetes mellitus and genetic variation in the β3-adrenergic-receptor gene. N Engl J Med 1995;333:343-347

[625] Arslanian SA, Kalhan SC. Correlations between fatty acid and glucose metabolism: potential explanation of insulin resistance of puberty. Diabetes 1994;43:908-914

[626] Schwartz MS, Chadka A. Type 2 diabetes mellitus in childhood: obesity and insulin resistance. J Am Oseopath Assoc 2008;108:518-524

[627] Leahy JL. Pathogenesis of type 2 diabetes mellitus. Arch Med Res 2005;36:197-209

[628] Virally M, Blicklé J-F, Girand J, Halimi S, Simon D, Guillausseau P-J. Type 2 diabetes mellitus: epidemiology, pathophysiology, unmet needs and therapeutic perspectives. Diabetes Metabol 2007;33:231-244

[629] Porksen N. The *in vivo* regulation of pulsatile insulin secretion. Diabetologia 2002;45:3-20

[630] Polonsky KS, Sturis J, Van Cauter E. Temporal profiles an clinical significance of pulsatile insulin secretion. Horm Res 1998;49:178-184

[631] Polonsky KS, Given BD, Hirsch LJ, *et al.* Abnormal patterns of insulin secretion in non-insulin-dependent diabetes mellitus. N Engl J Med 1988;318:1231-1239

[632] O'Rahilly S, Turner RC, Matthews DR. Impaired pulsatile secretion of insulin in relatives of patients with non-insulin-dependent diabetes. N Engl J Med 1988;318:1225-1230

[633] Perley MJ, Kipnis DM. Plasma insulin responses to oral and intravenous glucose: studies in normal and diabetic subjects. J Clin Invest 1967;46:1954-1962

[634] Cerasi E, Luft R. The plasma insulin response to glucose infusion in healthy subjects and in diabetes mellitus. Acta Endocrinol (Kbh) 1967;55:278-304

[635] Fujta Y, Herrow AL, Seltzer HS. Conformation of impaired early insulin response to glycemic stimulus in non-obese mild diabetes. Diabetes 1975;24:17-27

[636] Luzi L, DeFronzo RA. Effect of loss of first-phase insulin secretion on hepatic glucose production and tissue glucose disposal in humans. Am J Physiol 1989;257:241-246

[637] Rebrin K, Steil GM, Mittelman SD, Bergman RN. Causal linkage between insulin suppression of liver glucose output in dogs. J Clin Invest 1996;98:741-749

[638] Getty L, Hamilton-Wessler M, Ader M, Dea MK, Bergman RN. Biphasic insulin secretion during intravenous glucose tolerance test promotes optimal interstitial insulin profile. Diabetes 1999;47:1941-1947

[639] Butler AE, Janson J, Bonner-Weir S, Ritzel R, Rizza RA, Butler PC. Beta-cell deficit and increased beta-cell apoptosis in humans with type 2 diabetes. Diabetes 2003;52:102-110

[640] Yoon KH, Ko SH, Cho JH, *et al.* Selective beta-cell loss and alpha-cell expression in patients with type 2 diabetes mellitus in Korea. J Clin Endocrinol Metab 2003;88:2300-2308

[641] Opie EL. The relation of diabetes mellitus to lesion of the pancreas: hyaline degeneration of the islets of Langerhans. J Exp Med. 1901;5:527-540

[642] Weichselbaum A, Strangl E. Zur Kenntnis der feineren Veränderungen des Pankreas bei Diabetes mellitus. Wien Klein Wochenschr 1901;14:968-972

[643] Westermark P, Wernstedt C, Wilabder E, Sletten K. A novel peptide in the calcitonin gene related peptide family as an amyloid fibril protein in the endocrine pancreas. Biochem Biophys Res Commun 1986;140:827-831

[644] Westrermark P, Wernstedt C, Wilander E, Hayden DW, O'Brien TD, Johnson KH. Amyloid fibrils in human insulinoma and islets of Langerhans of the diabetic cat are derived from a neuropeptide-like protein is also present in normal islet cells. Biochem Biophys Res Commun 1986;140:827-831

[646] Hull RL, Westermark GT, Westermark P, Kahn SE. Islet amyloid: a critical entity in the pathogenesis of type 2 diabetes. J Clin Endocrinol Metabol 2004;89,8:3629-3643

[647] Butler AE, Janson J, Soeller WC, Butler PC. Increased beta-cell apoptosis prevents adaptative increase in beta-cell mass in mouse model of type 2 diabetes: evidence for role of islet amyloid formation rather than direct action of amyloid. Diabetes 2003;52:2304-2314

[648] Porte D Jr, Kahn SE. β-cell dysfunction and failure in type 2 diabetes. Potential mechanisms. Diabetes 2001;50,Suppl.1:S160-S163

[649] Saito K, Yaginuma N, Takahashi T. Differential volumetry of A, B, and D cells in the pancreatic islets of diabetic and nondiabetic subjects. Tohoku J Exp Med 1979;129:273-283

[650] McLean N, Ogilvie RF. Quantitative estimation of the pancreas islet tissue in diabetic subjects. Diabetes 1955;4:367-376

[651] Westermark P, Wilander E. The influence of amyloid deposits on the islet volume in maturity onset diabetes mellitus. Diabetologia 1978;15:417-421

[652] Harding HP, Ron D. Endoplasmic reticulum stress and the development of diabetes: a review. Diabetes 2002;51,Suppl.3:S455-S461

[653] Donath MY, Halban PA. Decreased beta-cell mass in diabetes: significance, mechanisms and therapeutic implications. Diabetologia 2004;47:581-589

[654] Robertson RP, Harmon J, Tran PO, Poitout V. Beta-cell glucose toxicity, lipotoxicity, and chronic oxidative stress in type 2 diabetes. Diabetes 2004;4,Suppl.1:S119-S124

[655] Schrauwen P, Hesselin MK, Oxidative capacity, lipotoxicity, and mitochondrial damage in type 2 diabetes. Diabetes 2004;53:1412-1417

[656] Wajchenberg BL. β-cell failure in diabetes and preservation by clinical treatment. Endocrine Rev 2007;28,2:187-218

[657] Bjornholm M, Zierath JR. Insulin signal transduction in human skeletal muscle: identifying the defects in type II diabetes. Bioch Soc Trans 2005;33:354-357

[658] Hahn CR. Banting Lecture. Insulin action, diabetogenes, and the cause of type II diabetes. Diabetes 199;43:1066-1084

[659] Mauvais-Jarvis F, Kahn CR. Understanding the pathogenesis and treatment of insulin resistance and type 2 diabetes mellitus: what can we learn from transgenic and knockout mice? Diabetes Metabol (Paris) 2000;26:533-448

[660] Kido Y, Nakae J, Accili D. Clinical review 125: The insulin receptor and its cellular targets. J Clin Endocrinol Metab 2001;86:972-979

[661] Stumvoll M, Goldstein BJ, van Haeften TW. Type 2 diabetes: principles of pathogenesis and therapy. Lancet 2005;365:1333-1346

[662] Zierath JR, Krook A, Wallberg-Henriksson H. Insulin action and insulin resistance in human skeletal muscle. Diabetologia 2000;43:821-835

[663] Hotamisligil GS, Shargill NS, Spiegelman BM. Adipose expression of tumor necrosis factor-alpha: direct role in obesity-linked insulin resistance. Science 1993;259:8791

[664] Frittitta L, Youngren JE, Sbraccia P, *et al.* Increased adipose tissue PC-1 protein content, but not tumor necrosis factor-alpha gene expression, is associated with a reduction of both whole body insulin sensitivity and insulin receptor tyrosine-kinase activity. Diabetologia 1997;40:282-289

[665] Moller DE. Potential role of TNF-alpha in the pathogenesis of insulin resistance and type 2 diabetes. Trends Endocrinol Metab 2000;11:212-217

[666] Bandyopadhyay G, Standaert ML, Galloway L, Moscat J, Farese RV. Evidence for involvement of protein kinase C (PKC)-zeta and noninvolvement of diacylglycerol-sensitive PKCs in insulin-stimulated glucose transport in L6 myotubes. Endocrinol 1997;138:4721-4731

[667] De Fea K, Roth RA. Protein kinase C modulation of insulin receptor substrate-1 tyrosine phosphorylation requires serine 612. Biochemistry 1997;36:12939-12947

[668] Aguirre V, Uchida T, Yenush L, Davis R, White MF. The c-Jun NH_2-terminal kinase promotes insulin resistance during association with insulin receptor substrate-1 and phosphorylation of Ser(307). J Biol Chem 2000;275:9047-9054

[669] Yu C, Chen Y, Clinc GW, *et al.* Mechanism by which fatty acids inhibit insulin activation of insulin receptor substrate-1 (IRS-1)-associated phosphatidylinositol 3-kinase activity in muscle. J Biol Chem 2002;277:50230-50236

[670] Zhande R, Mitchell JJ, Wu J, Sun XJ. Molecular mechanism of insulin-induced degradation of insulin receptor substrate 1. Mol Cell Biol 2002;22:1016-1026

[671] Worm D, Vinten J, Staehr P, Henriksen JF, Handberg A, Beck-Nielsen H. Altered basal and insulin-stimulated phosphotyrosine phosphatase (PTPase) activity n skeletal muscle from NIDDM patients compared with control subjects. Diabetologia 1996;39:1208-1214

[672] Ahmad F, Azevedo JL, Cortright R, Dohm GL, Goldstein BJ. Alterations in skeletal muscle protein-tyrosine phosphatase activity and expression in insulin-resistant human obesity and diabetes. J Clin Invest 1997;100:449-458

[673] Bandyopadhyay D, Kusari A, Kenner KA, *et al.* Protein-tyrosine phosphatase 1 B complexes with the insulin receptor *in vivo* and is tyrosine phosphorylated in the presence of insulin. J Biol Chem 1997;272:1639-1645

[674] Elchebly M, Payette P, Michaliszyn E, *et al.* Increased insulin sensitivity and obesity in mice lacking the protein tyrosine phosphatase-1B gene. Science 1999;283:1544-1548

[675] Kelley DE, Simoneau JA. Impaired free fatty acid utilization by skeletal muscle in non-insulin-dependent diabetes mellitus. J Clin Invest 1994;94:2349-2356

[676] Blaak EE, van Aggel-Leijssen DP, Wagenmakers AJ, Saris WH, van Baak MA. Impaired oxidation of plasma-derived fatty acids in type 2 diabetic subjects during moderate-intensity exercise. Diabetes 2000;49:2102-2107

[677] Blaak EE, Wagenmakers AJ, Glatz JF, *et al.* Plasma FFA utilization and fatty acid-binding protein content are diminished in type 2 diabetic muscle. Am J Physiol Endocrinol Metab 2000;279:E146-E154

[678] Boden G. Free fatty acids, insulin resistance, and type 2 diabetes mellitus. Proc Assoc Am Physic 1999;111:241-248

[679] Santomauro AT, Boden G, Silva ME, *et al.* Overnight lowering of free fatty acids with Acipimox improves insulin resistance and glucose tolerance in obese diabetic and nondiabetic subjects. Diabetes 1999;48:1836-1841

[680] Phielix E, Mensink M. Type 2 diabetes mellitus and skeletal muscle metabolic function. Physiol Behav 2008;94,2:252-258

[681] Shepherd PR, Kahn BB. Glucose transporters and insulin action – implications for insulin resistance and diabetes mellitus. N Engl J Med 1999;341:248-257

[682] Gimeno RE, Klaman LD. Adipose tissue as an active endocrine organ: recent advances. Cur Opin Pharmacol 2005;5:122-128

[683] Lazar MA. How obesity causes diabetes: not a tall tale. Science 2005;307:373-375

[684] Wellen KE, Hotamisligil GS. Inflammation, stress, and diabetes. J Clin Invest 2005;115:1111-1119

[685] Fritsche L, Weigert C, Haring HU, Lehman R. How insulin receptor substrate proteins regulate the metabolic capacity of the liver – implications for health and disease. Cur Med Chem. 2008;15:1316-1329

[686] Taniguchi CM, Ucki K, Kahn R. Complementary roles of IRS-1 and IRS-2 in the hepatic regulation of metabolism. Indian J Med Res 2005;115:718-727

[687] Dong X, Park S, Lin X, Coops K, Yi X, White MF. Irs 1 and Irs 2 signaling is essential for hepatic glucose homeostasis and systemic growth. J Clin Invest 2006;116:101-114

[688] Simmgen M, Knauf C, Lopez M, *et al.* Liver-specific deletion of insulin receptor substrate 2 does not impair hepatic glucose and lipid metabolism in mice. Diabetologia 2006;49:552-561

[689] Kraine MR, Tisch RM. The role of environmental factors in insulin dependent diabetes mellitus: an unresolved issue. Environ Health Persp 1999;107:777-781

[690] Otton R, Mendonça JR, Curi R. Diabetes causes marked changes in lymphocyte metabolism. J Endocrinol 2002;174:55-61

[691]   Pavelic K, Bernacki RJ, Vuk-Pavlovic S. Insulin-modulated interleukin-2 production by murine splenocytes and T-cell hybridoma. J Endocrinol 1987;114:89-94

[692]   Chang FY, Shaio MF. Decreased cell-mediated immunity in patients with non-insulin-dependent diabetes mellitus. Diabetes Res Clin Pract 1995;28:137-146

[693]   Pickup JC, Chusney GD, Thomas SM, Burt D. Plasma interleukin-6, tumor necrosis factor alpha and blood cytokine production in type 2 diabetes. Life Sci 2000;67:291-295

[694]   Piątkiewicz P, Szablewski L, Czech A, Tatoń J, Oleszczak B, Kasprzycka M. The investigation of glucose transport into lymphocytes in healthy subjects and in diabetic patients. Med Metab 2002;6:15-21

[695]   Piątkiewicz P, Czech A, Tatoń J, et al. Glucose transport into lymphocytes in healthy subjects and in patients with type 2 diabetes mellitus. Med Metab 2003;7:12-17

[696]   Szablewski L, Piątkiewicz P, Oleszczak B, Nowak Ł, Sobczyk A, Grytner-Zięcina B. The effect of insulin therapy in patients with type 2 diabetes mellitus on the deoxy-D-glucose uptake by lymphocytes of peripheral blood. Expt Clin Diabetol 2004;4:217-223

[697]   Szablewski L, Oleszczak B, Mrozikiewicz-Rakowska B, Karnafel W, Grytner-Zięcina B. Deoxy-D-glucose transport into lymphocytes, granulocytes and erythrocytes in patients with type 2 diabetes mellitus. Expt Clin Diabetol 2007;7:245-255

[698]   Szablewski L. Disturbances of deoxy-D-glucose transport into selected peripheral blood cells in patients with type 2 diabetes mellitus. The effect of illness and type of therapy on glucose transporters in these cells. Warsaw Med Univ Ed. 2006. (in polish)

[699]   Szablewski L, Sobczyk-Kopcioł A, Oleszczak B, Mrozikiewicz-Rakowska B, Karnafel W, Grytner-Zięcina B. Expression of glucose transporters in peripheral blood cells in patients with type 2 diabetes mellitus depending on the mode of therapy. Expt Clin Diabetol 2007;7:204-212

[700]   Szablewski L, Sobczyk-Kopcioł A, Oleszczak B, Grytner-Zięcina B. GLUT 4 is expressed in circulating lymphocytes of diabetic patients. A method of detect early prediabetic stages. Diabetol Croatica 2007;36:69-76

[701]   Sobczyk-Kopcioł A, Szablewski L, Oleszczak B et al. Expression of selected glucose transporters in peripheral blood lymphocytes in patients with type 2 diabetes mellitus managed with insulin. Expt Clin Diabetol 2008;8:159-164

[702]   Szablewski L, Raszka K, Oleszczak B. The influence of hyper- and hypoglycemia on glucose uptake into human circulating lymphocytes. An in vitro study. Expt. Clin Diabetol 2007;7:131-138

[703]   Maassen JA, Janssen GM, t'Hart LM. Molecular mechanisms of mitochondrial diabetes (MIDD). Ann Med 2005;37:213-221

[704]   Maassen JA, t'Hart LM, Janssen GMC, Reiling E, Romijn JA, Lemkes HH. Mitochondrial diabetes and its lessons for common Type 2 diabetes. Bioch Soc Trans 2006;34,5:819-823

[705]   van den Ouweland JM, Lemkes HH, Ruitenbeek W, et al. Mutation in mitochondrial tRNA(Leu)(UUR) gene in a large pedigree with maternally transmitted type II diabetes mellitus and deafness. Nat Genet 1992;1:368-371

[706]   Guillasseau PJ, Massin P, Dubois-LaForgue D, et al. Maternally inherited diabetes and deafness: a multicenter study. Ann Intern Med 2001;134,9Pt1:721-728

[707]   Saker PJ, Hattersley AT, Barrow B, et al. UKPDS 21: low prevalence of the mitochondrial transfer RNA gene (tRNA(Leu(UUR))) mutation at position 3243 bp in UK Caucasian type 2 diabetic patients. Diab Med 1997;14,1:42-45

[708]   Maassen JA, t'Hart LM, Van Essen E, et al. Mitochondrial diabetes: molecular mechanisms and clinical presentation. Diabetes 2004;53,Suppl.1:S103-S109

[709]   Hayashi T, Yrayama O, Kawai K, et al. Laughter regulates gene expression in patients with type 2 diabetes. Psychother Psychosom 2006;75:62-65

[710]   Metzger BE. 1990 overview of GDM. Accomplishment of the last decade-challenges for the future. Diabetes 1991;40,Suppl.2:1-2

[711]   Avery MD, Rossi MA. Gestational diabetes. J Nurse-Midwifery 1994;39,2,Suppl.:9S-19S

[712]   Cheung NW, Byth K. The population health significance of gestational diabetes. Diabetes Care 2003;26:2005-2009

[713]   Cheung NW. The management of gestational diabetes. Vasc Health Risk Manag 2009;5:153-164

[714]   Catalano PM, Tyzbir ED, Roman NM. Longitudinal changes in insulin release and insulin resistance in non-obese pregnant women. Am J Obstet Gynecol 1991;165:1667-1672

[715]   Catalano PM, Tyzbir ED, Wolfe RR, Roman NM, Amini SB, Sims EAH. Longitudinal changes in basal hepatic glucose production and suppression during insulin infusion in normal pregnant women. Am J Obstet Gynecol 1992;167:913-919

[716]   Catalano PM, Tyzbir ED, Wolfe, et al. Carbohydrate metabolism during pregnancy in control subjects and women with gestational diabetes. Am J Physiol 1993;264:E60-E67

[717]   Butt NF. Carbohydrate and lipid metabolism in pregnancy: normal compared with gestational diabetes mellitus. Am J Clin Nutr 2000;71,Suppl:1256S-1261S

[718] Kühl C. Aetiology of gestational diabetes. Bailliers Clin Obstet Gynaecol 1991;5:279-292

[719] Lesser KB, Carpenter MW. Metabolic changes associated with normal pregnancy and pregnancy complicated by diabetes mellitus. Semin Perinatol 1994;8:399-406

[720] Cousins L, Rigg L, Hollingsworth D. The 24-hour excursion and diurnal rhythm of glucose, insulin, and C-peptide in normal pregnancy. Am J Obstet Gynecol 1980;136:483-488

[721] Kalhan SC, D'Angelo LJ, Savin SM, Adam PAJ. Glucose production in pregnant women at term gestation. Sources of glucose for human fetus. J Clin Invest 1979;63:388-394

[722] Assel B, Rossi K, Kalhan S. Glucose metabolism during fasting through human pregnancy: comparison of tracer method with respiratory colorimetry. Am J Physiol 1993;265:E351-E356

[723] Maresh M. Screening for gestational diabetes mellitus. Sem Fetal Neonatal Med 2005;10:317-323

[724] Perkins JM, Dunn JP, Jagasia SM. Perspectives in gestational diabetes mellitus: a review of screening, diagnosis, and treatment. Clin Diabetes 2007;25,2:57-62

[725] Wagaarachchi PT, Fernand L, Premachadra P, Fernand DJS. Screening based on risk factors in an Asian population. J Obstet Gynaecol 2001;21:32-34

[726] Lain KY, Catalano PM. Metabolic changes in pregnancy. Clin Obstet Gynecol 2007;50:938-948

[727] Watanabe RM, Black MH, Xiang AH, Allayee H, Lawrence JM, Buchanan TA. Genetics of gestational diabetes mellitus and type 2 diabetes. Diabetes Care 2007;30,Suppl.2:S134-S140

[728] Dorner G, Plagemann A, Reinagel H. Familial diabetes aggregation in type I diabetes: gestational diabetes an apparent risk factor for increased diabetes susceptibility in the offspring. Exp Clin Endocrinol 1987;89:84-90

[729] McLellan JA, Barrow BA, Levy JC, *et al.* Prevalence of diabetes mellitus and impaired glucose tolerance in parents of women with gestational diabetes. Diabetologia 1995;38:693-698

[730] Martin AO, Simpson JL, Ober C, Freinkel N. Frequency of diabetes mellitus in mothers of probands with gestational diabetes: possible maternal influence on the predisposition to gestational diabetes. Am J Obstet Gynecol 1985;151:471-475

[731] Freinkel N, Metzger BE, Phelps RL, *et al.* Gestational diabetes mellitus: a syndrome with phenotypic and genotypic heterogeneity. Horm Metab Res 1986;18:427-439

[732] Ober C, Xiang KS, Thisted RA, Indovina KA, Wason CJ, Dooley S. Increased risk for gestational diabetes associated with insulin receptor and insulin-like growth factor II restriction fragment length polymorphism. Genet Epidemiol 1989;6:559-569

[733] Stoffel M, Bell KL, Blackburn CL, *et al.* Identification of glucokinase mutations in subjects with gestational diabetes mellitus. Diabetes 1993;42:937-940

[734] Chiu KC, Go RC, Aoki M, *et al.* Glucokinase gene in gestational diabetes mellitus: population association study and molecular scanning. Diabetologia 1994;37:104-110

[735] Saker PJ, Hattersley AT, Barrow B, *et al.* High prevalence of a missense mutation of the glucokinase gene in gestational diabetic patients due to a founder-effect in a local population. Diabetologia 1996;39:1325-1328

[736] Ellard S, Beards F, Allen LI, *et al.* A high prevalence of glucokinase mutations in gestational diabetic subjects selected by clinical criteria. Diabetologia 2000;43:250-253

[737] Catalano PM, Tyzbir ED, Sims EAH. Incidence and significance of islet cell antibodies in women with previous gestational diabetes mellitus. Diabetes Care 1990;13:478-482

[738] Catalano PM, Kirwan JP, Haugel-de Mouzon S, King J. Gestational diabetes and insulin resistance: role in short- and long-term implications for mother and fetus. J Nutr 2003;133:1674S-1683S

[739] Ryan EA, O'Sullivan MJ, Skyler JS. Insulin action during pregnancy. Studies with the euglycemic clamp technique. Diabetes 1985;34:380-389

[740] Catalano PM, Bernstein IM, Wolfe RR, Srikanta S, Sims EAH. Subclinical abnormalities of glucose metabolism in subjects with previous gestational diabetes. Am J Obstet Gynecol 1986;155:1255-1263

[741] Koukkou E, Watts GF, Lowy C. Serum lipid, lipoprotein and apolipoprotein changes in gestational diabetes mellitus: a cross-sectional and prospective study. J Clin Pathol 1996;49:634-637

[742] Carr DB, Utzschneider KM, Hull RL, *et al.* Gestational diabetes mellitus increases the risk of cardiovascular disease in women with a family history of type 2 diabetes. Diabetes Care 2006;29:2078-2083

[743] Scollan-Kolippoulis M, Guadagno S, Walker E. Gestational diabetes management: guidelines to a healthy pregnancy. Nurse Pract 2006;31:14-19

[744] Langer O, Mazze R. The relationship between large-for-gestational age infants and glycemic control in women with gestational diabetes. Am J Obstet Gynecol 1988;159:1478-1483

[745] Hod M, Merlob P, Friedman S, *et al.* Gestational diabetes mellitus: A survey of perinatal complications in the 1980s. Diabetes 1991;40,Suppl.2:74-78

[746] Ecker JL, Greenberg JA, Norwitz ER, *et al.* Birth weight as a predictor of branchial plexus injury. Obstet Gynecol 1997;89:643-647

[747] Jang HC, Cho HC, Min YK, *et al.* Increased macrosomia and perinatal morbidity independent of maternal obesity and advanced age in Korean women with GDM. Diabetes Care 1997;20:1582-1588

[748] Persson B, Hanson U. Neonatal morbidities in gestational diabetes mellitus. Diabetes Care 1998;21,Suppl.2:B79-B84

[749] Hapo Study Cooperative Research Group. Hyperglycaemia and adverse pregnancy outcomes. N Engl J Med 2008;358:1991-2002

[750] Garner P. Type 1 diabetes mellitus and pregnancy. Lancet 1995;346:157-161

[751] Sepe SJ, Connell FA, Geiss LS, *et al.* Gestational diabetes: Incidence, maternal characteristics and perinatal outcome. Diabetes 1985;34,Suppl.2:13-16

[752] Beischer NA, Wein P, Sheedy MT, *et al.* Identification and treatment of women with hyperglycaemia diagnosed during pregnancy can significantly reduce perinatal mortality rates. Aus NZ J Obstet Gynaecol 1996;36:239-247

[753] Schaefer U, Songaster G, Xiang A, *et al.* Congenital malformations in offspring of women with hyperglycemia first detected during pregnancy. Am J Obstet Gynecol 1997;177:1165-1171

[754] Schmidt MI, Spichler ER, Duncan BB, *et al.* Gestational diabetes mellitus diagnosed with a 2-h 75-g oral glucose tolerance test and adverse pregnancy outcomes. Diabetes Care 2001;24:1151-1155

[755] Silverman BL, Rizzo TA, Cho NH, Metzger BE. Long-term effects of the intrauterine environment. Diabetes Care 1998;21,Suppl.2:B142-B149

[756] Langer O, Conway DL. Level of glycemia and perinatal outcome in pregestational diabetes. J Matern Fetal Med 2000;9:35-41

[757] Tattersall RB. Mild familial diabetes with dominant inheritance. Q J Med 1974;43:339-357

[758] Tattersall RB, Fajans SS. A difference between the inheritance of classical juvenile-onset and maturity-onset type diabetes of young people. Diabetes 1975;24:44-53

[759] Agarwal SK, Khatri S, Prakash N, Singh NP, Snuradha S, Prakash A. Maturity onset diabetes of young. J Indian Acad Clin Med 2002;3,2:271-277

[760] Johnson JD. Pancreatic beta-cell apoptosis in maturity onset diabetes of the young. Canad J Diab 2007;31,1:67-74

[761] Frongel P, Zouali H, Vionnet N, *et al.* Familial hyperglycaemia due to mutations in glucokinase: definition of a subtype of diabetes mellitus. N Engl J Med 1993;328:697-702

[762] Mohan V, Ramachandran A, Snehlata C, *et al.* High prevalence of maturity onset diabetes of the young (MODY) among Indians. Diabetes Care 1985;8:371-374

[763] Fajans SS, Bell GI, Polonsky KS. Molecular mechanisms and clinical pathophysiology of maturity-onset diabetes of the young. N Engl J Med 2001;345:971-980

[764] Mitchell SM, Frayling TM. The role of transcription factors in maturity-onset diabetes of the young. Mol Genet Metab 2002;77:35-43

[765] Froguel P, Zouali H, Vionnet N, *et al.* Familial hyperglycemia due to mutations in glucokinase. Definition of a subtype of diabetes mellitus. N Engl J Med 1993;328:697-702

[766] Sladek FM, Zhong WM, Lai E, Darnell JE Jr. Liver-enriched transcription factor HNF-4 is a novel member of the steroid hormone receptor superfamily. Genes Dev 1990;4:2353-2365

[767] Kuo CJ, Conley PB, Chen L, Sladek FM, Darnell JE Jr, Crabtree GR. A transcriptional hierarchy involved in mammalian cell-type specification. Nature 1992;355:457-461

[768] Nyunt O, Wu JY, McGown I, *et al.* Investigating maturity onset diabetes of the young. Clin Biochem Rev 2009;30:67-74

[769] Olek K. Maturity-onset diabetes of the young: an update. Clin Lab 2006;52:593-598

[770] Yamagata K, Ruruta H, Oda N, *et al.* Mutations in the hepatocyte nuclear factor-4α gene in maturity onset diabetes of the young (MODY1). Nature 1996;384:458

[771] Rehman HU. Diabetes mellitus in the young. J R Soc Med 2001;94:65-67

[772] Bulman M, Dronsfield MJ, Frayling T, *et al.* A non sense mutation in HNF-4α gene in a UK pedigree with MODY. Diabetologia 1997;40:859-863

[773] Linder T, Gragnoli C, Faruta H, *et al.* Hepatic function in a family with a nonsense mutation (R154x) in HNF-4α/MODY 1 gene. J Clin Invest 1997;100:1400-1405

[774] Herman WH, Fajans SS, Oritz FJ, *et al.* Abnormal insulin secretion, not resistance, is the genetic or primary defect of MODY in the RW pedigree. Diabetes 1994;43:40-46

[775] Weissglass-Volkov D, Huertos-Vazquez A, Suviolahti E, *et al.* Common hepatic nuclear factor-4alpha variants are associated with high serum lipid levels and the metabolic syndrome. Diabetes 2006;55:1970-1977

[776] Kapor RR, Locke J, Coclough K, *et al.* Persistent hyperinsulinemic hypoglycemia and maturity-onset diabetes of the young due to heterozygous HNF4A mutations. Diabetes 2008;57:1659-1663

[777] Fajans SS. Heterogeneity between various families with NIDDM of MODY type. In: Kobberling J, Tattersall R (eds). The genetics of Diabetes mellitus. London: Academic Press, 1982:251-601

[778] Froguel P, Velho G. Maturity-onset diabetes of the young. Curr Opin Pediatr 1994;6:482-485

[779] Matschinsky FM. Glucokinase as glucose sensor and metabolic signal generator in pancreatic beta-cells and hepatocytes. Diabetes 1990;39:647-652

[780] Appleton M, Ellard S, Bulman M, *et al.* Clinical characteristics of the HNF-1α (MODY3) and GCK mutations. Diabetologia 1997;40:A161

[781] Hattersley AT, Turner RC, Permitt MA, *et al.* Linkage of type 2 diabetes to the glucokinase gene. Lancet 1992;339:1307-1310

[782] Page RC, Hattersley AT, Ley JC, *et al.* Clinical characteristics of subjects with a missense mutation in glucokinase. Diabetes Med 1995;12:209-217

[783] Velho G, Froguel P, Clement K, *et al.* Primary pancreatic β cell secretory defect caused by mutations in GCK gene in kindreds of MODY. Lancet 1992;340:444-448

[784] Hattersley AT. GCK mutations and type 2 diabetes. In: Lightman S ed. Horizons in Medicine. Vol.7, Bristol: Blackwell Science 1996:440-449

[785] Gloyn AL. Glucokinase (GCK) mutations in hyper- and hypoglycemia: maturity-onset diabetes of the young, permanent neonatal diabetes and hyperinsulinemia of infancy. Hum Mutat 2003;22:353-362

[786] Velho G, Vaxillaire M, Boccio V, Charpentier G, Froguel P. Diabetes complications in NIDDM kindreds linked to MODY 3 locus on chromosome 12 q. Diabetes Care 1996;19:915-919

[787] Hattersley AT. Maturity-onset diabetes of the young: clinical heterogenity explained by genetic heterogeneity. Diabetes Med. 1998;15:15-24

[788] Stoffers DA, Zinkin NT, Stanojevic V, Clarke WL, Habener JF. Pancreatic agenesis attributable to a single nucleotide deletion in the human IFF1 gene coding sequence. Nat Genet 1997;15:106-110

[789] Ryffel GU. Mutations in the human genes encoding the transcription factors of the hepatocyte nuclear factor (HNF) 1 and HNF4 families: functional and pathological consequences. J Mol Endocrinol 2001;2,1:11-29

[790] Iwasaki N, Okabe I, Momoi MY, *et al.* Splice site mutation in the hepatocyte nuclear factor-1 beta gene, IVS2nt+1G>A, associated with maturity onset diabetes of the young, renal dysplasia and bicornuate uterus. Diabetologia 2001;44,3:387-388

[791] Malecki MT, Jhala US, Antonellis A, *et al.* Mutations in NEUROD1 are associated with the development of type 2 diabetes mellitus. Nat Genet 1999;23:323-328

[792] Neve B, Fernandez-Zapico ME, Ashkenazi-Katalan V, *et al.* Role of transcription factor KLF11 and its diabetes-associated gene variants in pancreatic beta cell function. Proc Natl Acad Sci USA 2005;102:4807-4812

[793] Raeder H, Johansson S, Holm PI, *et al.* Mutations in the CEL VNTR cause a syndrome of diabetes and pancreatic exocrine dysfunction. Nat Genet 2006;38:54-62

[794] von Muhlendahl KE, Herkenhoff H. Long-term course of neonatal diabetes. N Engl J Med 1995;333:704-708

[795] Shield JP. Neonatal diabetes: new insights into aetiology and implications. Horm Res 2000;53,Suppl.1:7-11

[796] Hathout EH, Sharkey J, Racine M, *et al.* Diabetic autoimmunity in infants and pre-schoolers with type 1 diabetes. Pediatr Diabetes 2000;1:131-134

[797] Hutchinson JH, Keavy AJ, Kerr MM. Congenital temporary diabetes mellitus. MJ 1962;2:436-440

[798] Aguilar-Bryan L, Bryan J. Neonatal diabetes mellitus. Endocrine Rev 2008;29:265-291

[799] Shield JPH. Neonatal diabetes mellitus. Pediatr Diabetes 2002;2:109-112

[800] Gardner RJ, Robinson DO, Lamont L, Shield JP, Temple JK. Paternal uniparental disomy of chromosome 6 and transient neonatal diabetes mellitus. Clin Genet 1998;54:522-525

[801] Hermann R, Laine AP, Johansson C, *et al.* Transient but not permanent neonatal diabetes mellitus is associated with paternal uniparental isodisomy of chromosome 6. Pediatrics 2000;105:49-52

[802] Hermann R, Soltesz G. Paternal uniparental isodisomy of chromosome 6 in transient neonatal diabetes mellitus. Eur J Pediatr 1997;156:740

[803] Das S, Lese CM, Song M, *et al.* Partial paternal uniparental disomy of chromosome 6 in an infant with neonatal diabetes, macroglossia, and craniofacial abnormalities. Am J Hum Genet 2000;57:1586-1591

[804] Arima T, Drewell RA, Arney KL, *et al.* A conserved imprinting control region at the HYMAI/ZAC domain is implicated in transient neonatal diabetes mellitus. Hum Mol Genet 2001;10:1475-1483

[805] Varrault A, Ciani E, Apiou F, *et al.* hZAC encodes a zinc finger protein with antiproliferative properties and maps to a chromosomal region frequently lost in cancer. Proc Natl Acad Sci USA 1998;95:8835-8840

[806] Hoffmann A, Ciani E, Boeckardt J, Holsboer F, Journot L, Spengler D. Transcriptional activities of the zinc finger protein Zac are differentially controlled by DNA binding. Mol Cell Biol 2003;23:988-1003

[807] Huang SM, Schonthal AH, Stallcup MR. Enhancement of p53-dependent gene activation by the transcriptional coactivator Zac1. Oncogene 2001;20:2134-2143

[808] Rozenfeld-Granot G, Krishnamurthy J, Kannen K, *et al.* A positive feedback mechanism in the transcriptional activation of Apaf-1 by p53 and coactivator Zac-1. Oncogene 2002;21:1469-1476

[809] Hoffmann A, Barz T, Spengler D. Multitasking C2H2 zinc fingers link Zac DANN binding to coordinated regulation of p300-histone acetyltransferase activity. Mol Cell Biol 2006;26:5544-5557

[810] Huang SM, Stallcup MR. Mouse Zac1, a transcriptional coactivator and repressor for nuclear receptors. Mol Cell Biol 2000;20:1855-1867

[811] Spengler D, Villalba M, Hoffmann A, *et al.* Regulation of apoptosis and cell cycle arrest by Zac1, a novel zinc finger protein expressed in the pituitary gland and the brain. EMBO J 1997;16:2814-2825

[812] Ferguson AW, Milner RDG. Transient neonatal diabetes mellitus in sibs. Arch Dis Child 1970;45:80-83

[813] Schiff D, Colle E, Stern L. Metabolic and growth patterns in transient neonatal diabetes. N Engl J Med 1972;287:119-122

[814] Blethen SL, White NH, Santiago JV, *et al.* Plasma somatostatins, endogenous insulin secretions, and growth in transient neonatal diabetes mellitus. JCEM 1981;52:144-147

[815] Salerno MC, Gasparini N, Sandomerico ML, *et al.* Two interesting cases of transient neonatal diabetes mellitus. J Pediatr Endocrinol 1994;7:47-52

[816] Valerio G, Franzese A, Salerno M, *et al.* β-cell dysfunction in classic transient neonatal diabetes is characterized by impaired insulin response to glucose but normal response to glucagon. Diabetes Care 2004;27,10:2405-2408

[817] Rubio-Cabezas Ó, Argente J. Current insights into the genetic basis of diabetes mellitus in children and adolescent. J Pediatr Endocrinol Metab 2008;21:917-940

[818] Miki T, Seino S. Roles of K_{ATP} channels as metabolic sensor in acute metabolic changes. J Moll Cell Cardiol 2005;38:917-925

[819] Ellard S, Flanagan SE, Girard CA, *et al.* Permanent neonatal diabetes caused by dominant, recessive, or compound heterozygous SUR1 mutations with opposite functional effects. Am J Hum Genet 2007;81:375-382

[820] Edhill EL, Flanagan SE, Path AM, *et al.* Insulin mutation screening in 1044 patients with diabetes: mutations in the INS gene are a common cause of neonatal diabetes but a rare cause of diabetes diagnosed in childhood or adulthood. Diabetes 2008;57:1034-1042

[821] Støy J, Edghill EL, Flanagan SE, *et al.* Insulin gene mutations as a cause of permanent neonatal diabetes. Proc Natl Acad Sci USA 2007;104:15040-15044

[822] Polak M, Dechaume A, Cavé H, *et al.* Heterozygous missense mutations in the insulin gene are linked to permanent diabetes appearing in the neonatal period or in early-infancy: a report from the French ND (Neonatal Diabetes) Study Group. Diabetes 2008;57:1115-1119

[823] Molven A, Ringdal M, Nordbø AM. Mutations in the insulin gene can cause MODY and autoantibody-negative type 1 diabetes. Diabetes 2008;57:1131-1135

[824] Njølstad PR, Barbetti F, Undlien DE, *et al.* Neonatal diabetes mellitus due to complete glucokinase deficiency. N Engl J Med 2001;344:1588-1592

[825] Njølstad PR, Sagen JV, Bjørkhaug L, *et al.* Permanent neonatal diabetes caused by glucokinase deficiency: inborn error of the glucose-insulin signaling pathway. Diabetes 2003;52:2854-2860

[826] Stoffers DA, Zinkin NT, Stanojevic V, Clarke WL, Habener JF. Pancreatic agenesis attributable to a single nucleotide deletion in the human IPF1 gene coding sequence. Nat Genet 1997;15:106-110

[827] Schwitzgebel VM, Mamin A, Brun T, *et al.* Agenesis of human pancreas due to decreased half-life of insulin promoter factor. J Clin Endocrinol Metab 2003;88:4398-4406

[828] Hoveyda N, Shield P, Garrett C, *et al.* Neonatal diabetes mellitus and cerebellar hypoplasia/agenesis: report of a new recessive syndrome. J Med Genet 1999;36:700-704

[829] Sellick GS, Barker KT, Stolte-Dijkstra I, *et al.* Mutations in PTF1A cause pancreatic and cerebellar agenesis. Nat Genet 2004;36:1301-1305

[830] Taha D, Barbar M, Kanaan H, Williamson Balfe J. Neonatal diabetes mellitus, congenital hypothyroidism, hepatic fibrosis, polycystic kidneys, and congenital glaucoma: a new autosomal recessive syndrome? Am J Med Genet 2003;122:269-273

[831] Senée V, Chelaha C, Duchatelet S, *et al.* Mutations in GLIS3 are responsible for a rare syndrome with neonatal diabetes mellitus and congenital hypothyroidism. Nat Genet 2006;38:682-687

[832] Wildin RS, Smyk-Pearson S, Filipovich AH. Clinical and molecular features of the immunodysegulation, polyendocrinopathy, enteropathy, X linked (IPEX) syndrome. J Med Genet 2002;39:537-545

[833] Kahn CR, Flier JS, Bar RS, *et al.* The syndromes of insulin resistance and acanthosis nigricans: insulin receptor disorders in man. N Engl J Med 1976;294:739-745

[834] Mantzoros CS, Flier JS. Insulin resistance: the clinical spectrum. In: Mazzaferi E, ed. Advances in endocrinology and metabolism. St. Louis: Mosby-Year Book 1995;6:193-232

[835] Vidal-Puig A, Moller DE. Insulin resistance: Classification, prevalence, clinical manifestations, and diagnosis. In: Azziz R, Nestler JE Dewailly D, eds. Androgen excess disorders in women. Philadelphia: Lippincott Raven 1997:227-236

[836] Ishihama H, Suzuki Y, Muramatsu K, *et al.* Long term follow up in type A insulin resistant syndrome treated by insulin-like growth factor I. Arch Dis Child 1994;71:144-146

[837] Kobayashi M, Sasaoka T, Shigeta Y, *et al.* Insulin resistance by unprocessed insulin proreceptors: point mutation at the cleavage site. Biochem Biophys Res Commun 1988;153:657-663

[838] Imano E, Kadowaki H, Kadowaki T, *et al.* Two patients with insulin resistance due to decreased levels of insulin-receptor mRNA. Diabetes 1991;40,5:548-555

[839] Taira M, Hashimota N, Yoshida S, *et al.* Human diabetes associated with a deletion of the tyrosine kinase domain of the insulin receptor. Science 1989;245:63-66

[840] Longo N, Wang Y, Smith SA, Langley SD, DiMeglio LA, Giannella-Neto D. Genotype-phenotype correlation in inherited severe insulin resistance. Hum Mol Genet 2002;11:1465-1475

[841] Musso C, Cochran E, Moran SA, *et al.* Clinical course of genetic diseases of the insulin receptor (type A and Rabson-Mendenhall syndromes): a 30-year prospective. Medicine (Baltimore)2004;83:209-222

[842] Wiwanitkit V. Weak linkage in insulin receptor: Identification of mutation prone point. Diabetes Metab Syndr Clin Res Rev 2008;2,2:105-108

[843] Baynes KCR, Whitehead I, Krook A, O'Rahilly S. Molecular mechanisms of inherited insulin resistance. Q J Med 1997;90:557-562

[844] Moller DE, Cohen O, Yamagucchi Y, *et al.* Prevalence of mutations of the insulin receptor gene in subjects with features of the type A syndrome of insulin resistance. Diabetes 1994;43:247-255

[845] Taylor SI, Kadowaki T, Kadowaki H, Accili D, Cama A, McKeon C. Mutations in insulin-receptor gene in insulin-resistant patients. Diabetes Care 1990;13:257-279

[846] Accili D, Barbetti F, Cama A, *et al.* Mutations in the insulin receptor gene in patients with genetic syndromes of insulin resistance and acanthosis nigricans. J Invest Dermatol 1992;98:77S-81S

[847] Kadowaki T, Bevins CL, Cama T, *et al.* Two mutant alleles of the insulin gene in a patient with extreme insulin resistance. Science 1988;240:784-790

[848] Kadowaki T, Kadowaki H, Taylor SI. A nonsense mutation causing decreased levels of insulin receptor mRNA: detection by a simplified technique for direct sequencing of genomic DNA amplified by polymerase chain reaction. Proc Natl Acad Sci USA 1990;87:658-662

[849] Kadowaki T, Kadowaki H, Rechler MM, *et al.* Five mutant alleles of the insulin receptor gene in patients with genetic forms of insulin resistance. J Clin Invest 1990;86:254-264

[850] Shimada F, Taira M, Suzuki Y, *et al.* Insulin-resistant diabetes associated with partial deletion of insulin-receptor gene. Lancet 1990;335:1179-1181

[851] Kadowaki T, Kadowaki H, Accili D, Taylor SI. Substitution of lysine for asparagine-15 in the human insulin receptor impairs intracellular transport of the receptor to the cell surface and decreases the affinity of insulin binding. J Biol Chem 1990;265:19143-19150

[852] Accili D, Frapier C, Mostha L. A mutation in the insulin receptor gene that impairs transport of the receptor to the plasma membrane and causes insulin resistant diabetes. EMBO J 1989;8:2509-2517

[853] Yoshimasa Y, Seino S, Whittaker J, *et al.* Insulin-resistant diabetes due to a point mutation that prevents insulin proreceptor processing. Science 1988;240:784-787

[854] Kobayashi M, Sasaoka T, Takata Y, *et al.* Insulin resistance by unprocessed insulin proreceptors point mutations at the cleavage site. Biochem Biophys Res Commun 1988;153:657-663

[855] Kobayashi M, Sasaoka T, Takata Y, Hisatomi A, Shigeta Y. Insulin resistance by uncleaved insulin proreceptor. Emergence of binding site by trypsin. Diabetes 1988;37:653-656

[856] Odawara M, Kadowaki T, Yamamoto R, *et al.* Human diabetes associated with a mutation in the tyrosine kinase domain of the insulin receptor. Science 1989;245:66-68

[857] Moller DE, Flier JS. Detection of an alteration in the insulin-receptor gene in patients with insulin resistance, acanthosis nigricans, and the polycystic ovary syndrome (type A insulin resistance). N Engl J Med 1988;319:1526-1529

[858] Moller DE, Yokota A, Ginsberg-Fellner F, Flier JS. Functional properties of a naturally occurring $Trp^{1200} \rightarrow Ser^{1200}$ mutation of the insulin receptor. Mol Endocrinol 1990;4:1183-1191

[859] Moller DE, Yokota A, White MF, Pazianos AG, Flier JS. A naturally occurring mutation of insulin receptor Ala^{1132} impairs tyrosine kinase function and is associated with dominantly inherited insulin resistance. J Biol Chem 1990;265:14979-14985

[860] Cama A, Sierra M, Ottin L, *et al.* A mutation in the tyrosine kinase domain of the insulin receptor causing insulin resistance in an obese woman. J Clin Endocrinol Metab 1991;73:894-901

[861] Kadowaki H, Kadowaki T, Cama A, *et al.* Mutagenesis of lysine-460 in the human insulin receptor: effects upon receptor recycling and site-site interaction among binding sites. J Biol Chem 1990;265:21285-21296

[862] Krook A, Kumar S, Laing I, Boulton AJM, Wass JAH, O'Rahilly S. Molecular scanning of the insulin receptor gene in syndromes of insulin resistance. Diabetes 1994;43:357-368

[863] Sbraccia P, Goodman PA, Maddux BA, *et al.* Production of an inhibitor of insulin receptor tyrosine kinase in fibroblasts from a patient with insulin resistance and NIDDM. Diabetes 1991;40:295-299

[864] Young J, Morbois-Trabut L, Conzinet B, *et al.* Type A insulin resistance syndrome revealing a novel lamin A mutation. Diabetes 2005;54:1873-1878

[865] McDonald A, Williams RM, Reagan FM, Semple RK, Dunger DB. IGF-1 treatment of insulin resistance. Eur J Endocrinol 2007;157:S51-S56

[866] Tritos NA, Mantzoros CS. Syndromes of severe insulin resistance. J Clin Endocrinol Metab 1998;83,9:3025-3030

[867] Muačević-Katanec D, Profozić V, Metelko Ž. The importance of determining the presence and degree of insulin resistance in the general population and in some clinical states. Diabetol Croatica 2005;34,1:3-12

[868] Flier JS. Syndrome of insulin resistance. In Principles and Practice of Endocrinology and Metabolism. Becker KL (ed) Philadelphia, JB Lippincott 2nd Ed. 1995:1249-1259

[869] Page KA, Dejardin S, Kahn CR, Kulkarni RN, Herold KC, Inzucchi SE. A patient with type B insulin resistance syndrome, responsive to immune therapy. Natur Cln Pract Endocrinol Metab 2007;3,12:835-840

[870] Magsino CH, Spencer J Insulin receptor antibodies and insulin resistance. Southern Med J 1999;92,7:717-719

[871] Nagy K, Grunberer G, Levy J. Insulin antagonistic effects of insulin receptor antibodies on plasma membrane $(Ca^{2+}+Mg^{2+})$ATPase activity: a possible etiology of type B insulin resistance. Endocrinol 1990;126:45-52

[872] Arioglu E, Anderwelt A, Diabo C, Bele M, Taylor SI, Gorden P. Clinical course of the syndrome of autoantibodies to the insulin receptor (Type B insulin resistance): a 28-year perspective. Medicine (Baltimore) 2002;81:87-100

[873] Taylor SI, Barbetti F, Accili D, Roth J, Gorden P. Syndromes of autoimmunity and hypoglycemia. Endocrinol Metab Clin North Am 1989;18:123-143

[874] Tran HA, Reeves GE. Treatment of type B insulin resistance wit immunoglobulin: novel use of an old therapy. Med J Australia 2009;190,3:168

[875] Yamashi H, Yamaguchi Y, Fujita N, *et al.* Anti-insulin receptor autoantibodies in a patient with type B insulin resistance and fasting hypoglycemia. Acta Diabetol 2000;37:189-196

[876] Flier JS, Bar RS, Muggeo M, *et al.* The evolving clinical course of patients with insulin receptor autoantibodies: spontaneous remission or receptor proliferation with hypoglycemia. J Clin Endocrinol Metab 1978;47:985-995

[877] Globerman H, Karnieli E. Analysis of the insulin receptor gene tyrosine kinase domain in obese patients with hyperandrogenism, insulin resistance and acanthosis nigricans (type C insulin resistance). Int J Obes 1998;22:349-353

[878] Flier JS, Eastman RC, Minaker KL, Matteson D, Rowe JW. Acanthosis nigricans in obese women with hyperandrogenism characterization of an insulin-resistant state distinct from the type A and B syndromes. Diabetes 1985;34:101-107

[879] Donohue WL. Clinicopathologic conference at the Hospital for Sick Children on "Dysendocrinism". J Pediatr 1948;32:739-748

[880] Donohue WL, Uchida I. Leprechaunism: a euphemism for a rare familial disorder. J Pediatr 1954;45:505-519

[881] Al-Gazali LI, Khalil M, Devadas K. A syndrome of insulin resistance resembling leprechaunism in five sibs of consanguineous parents. J Med Genet 1993;30:470-475

[882] Mendenhall EN. Tumor of the pineal gland with high insulin resistance. J Indiana State Med Assoc 1950;43:32-36

[883] Longo N, Wang Y, Pasquali M. Progressive decline in insulin levels in Rabson-Mendenhall syndrome. J Clin Endocrinol Metab 1999;84:2623-2629

[884] Herbert TP. PERK in the life and death of the pancreatic beta-cell. Biochem Soc Trans 2007;35:1205-1207

[885] Delepine M, Nicolino M, Barrett T, Golamaully M, Lathrop GM, Julier C. EIF2AK3, encoding translation inhibition factor 2-alpha kinase3, is mutated in patients with Wolcott-Rallison syndrome. Nat Genet 2000;25:406-409

[886] SeneeV, Vatem KM, Delepine M, *et al.* Walcott-Rallison syndrome: clinical, genetic, and functional study of EIF2AK3 mutations and suggestion of genetic heterogenity. Diabetes 2004;53:1876-1883

[887] Santer R, Schneppenheim R, Dombrowski A, Gotze H, Steinmann B, Schaub J. Mutations in GLUT2, the gene for the liver-type glucose transporter, in patients with Fanconi-Bickel syndrome. Nat Genet 1997;17:324-326, erratum 1998;18:298

[888] Kentrup H, Altmuller J, Pfaffle R, Heimann G. Neonatal diabetes mellitus with hypergalactosemia. Eur J Endocrinol 1999;141:379-381

[889] Yoo HW, Shin YL, Seo EJ, Kim GH. Identification of a novel mutation in the GLUT2 gene in a patient with Fanconi-Bickel syndrome presenting with neonatal diabetes mellitus and galactosemia. Eur J Pediatr 2002;161:351-353

[890] Labay V, Raz T, Baron D, *et al.* Mutations in SLC19A2 cause thiamine-responsive megablastic anaemia associated with diabetes mellitus and deafness. Nat Genet 1999;22:300-304

[891] Khanim F, Kirk J, Latif F, Barrett TG. WFS1/wolframin mutations, Wolfram syndrome, and associated diseases. Hum Genet 2001;17:357-367

[892] Amr S, Heisey C, Zhang M, *et al.* A homozygous mutation in a novel zinc-finger protein, ERIS, is responsible for Wolfram syndrome 2. Am J Hum Genet 2007;81:673-683

[893] Hearn T, Renforth GL, Spalluto C, *et al.* Mutation of ALMS1, a large gene with a tandem repeat encoding 47 amino acids, causes Alström syndrome. Nat Genet 2002;31:79-83

[894] Alstrom CH, Hallgren B, Nilsson LB, Asander H. Retinal degeneration combined with obesity, diabetes mellitus and neurogenous deafness: a specific syndrome (not hitherto described) distinct from the Laurence-Moon-Bardet-Biedl syndrome: a clinical endocrinological and genetic examination based on a large pedigree. Acta Psychiatr Neurol Scand Suppl 1959;129:1-35

[895] Stoetzel C, Muller J, Laurier V, *et al.* Identification of a novel BBS gene (BBS12) highlights the major role of a vertebrate-specific branch of chaperonin-related proteins, in Bardet-Biedl syndrome. Am J Hum Genet 2007;80:1-11

[896] Beales PL, Elcioglu N, Woolf AS, Parker D, Flinter FA. New criteria for improved diagnosis of Bardet-Biedl syndrome: results of a population survey. J Med Genet 1999;36:437-446

[897] Dunaif A. Insulin resistance and the polycystic ovary syndrome: mechanism and implications for pathogenesis. Endocr Rev 1997;18:774-800

[898] Diamanti-Kandarakis E, Kouli CR, Bergiele AT, *et al.* A survey of the polycystic ovary syndrome in the Grek island of Lesbos: hormonal and metabolic profile. J Clin Endocrinol Metab 1999;11:4006-4011

[899] Azziz R, Woods KS, Reyna R, Key TJ, Knochenhauer ES, Yildiz BO. The prevalence and features of the polycystic ovary syndrome in an unselected population.

[900] El-Mazny A, Abou-Salem N, El-Sherbiny W, El-Mazny A. Insulin resistance, dyslipidemia, and metabolic syndrome in women with polycystic ovary syndrome. Int J Gynecol Obstet 2010;109:239-241

[901] Unluturk U, Harmanci A, Kocaefe C, Yildiz BO. The genetic basis of the polycystic ovary syndrome: a literature review including discussion of PPAR-γ. PPAR Res 2007;ID 49109, doi: 101155/2007/49109

[902] Hardiman P, Pillay OS, Atiomo W. Polycystic ovary syndrome and endometrial carcinoma. Lancet 2003;361:1810-1812

[903] Dokras A, Bochner M, Hallinrake E, Markham S, Vanvoorhis B, Jagasia DH. Screening women with polycystic ovarian syndrome for metabolic syndrome. Obstet Gynecol 2005;106,1:131-137

[904] Dunaif A, Segal KR, Futterweit W, Dobrjansky A. Profound peripheral insulin resistance, independent of obesity, in polycystic ovary syndrome. Diabetes 1989;38:1165-1174

[905] Legro RS, Kunselman AR, Dodson WC, Dunaif A. Prevalence and predictors of risk for type 2 diabetes mellitus and impaired glucose tolerance in polycystic ovary syndrome: a prospective study in 254 affected women. J Clin Endocrinol Metab 1999;84:165-169

[906] Azziz R. How prevalent is metabolic syndrome in women with polycystic ovary syndrome? Nat Clin Pract Endocrinol Metab 2006;2,3:132-133

[907] Essah PA, Nestler JE. The metabolic syndrome in polycystic ovary syndrome. J Endocrinol Invest 2006;29,3:270-280

[908] Ehrmann DA, Barnes RB, Rosenfield RL, Cavaghan MK, Imperial J. Prevalence of impaired glucose tolerance and diabetes in women with polycystic ovary syndrome. Diabetes Care 1999;22:141-146

[909] Daqhlgren E, Johansson S, Lindstedt G, *et al.* Women with polycystic ovary syndrome wedge resected in 1956 to 1965: a long-term follow-up focusing on natural history and circulating hormones. Fertil Steril 1992;57:505-513

[910] Essah PA, Nestler JE. Metabolic syndrome in women with polycystic ovary syndrome. Fertil Steril 2006;86,Suppl.1:S18-S19

[911] Book CB, Dunaif A. Selective insulin resistance in the polycystic ovary syndrome. J Clin Endocrinol Metab 1999;84:3110-3116

[912] Bremer AA, Miller WL. The serine phosphorylation hypothesis: a unifying mechanism for hyperandrogenemia and insulin resistance. Fertil Steril 2008;89,5:1039-1048

[913] Dunaif A, Segal KR, Shelley DR, Green G, Dobrjansky A, Licholai T. Evidence for distinctive and intrinsic defects in insulin action in polycystic ovary syndrome. Diabetes 1992;41:1257-1266

[914] Corbould A, Zhao H, Mirzoeva S, Aird F, Dunaif A. Enhanced mitogenic signaling in skeletal muscle of women with polycystic ovary syndrome. Diabetes 2006;55:751-759

[915] Poretsky L. On the paradox of insulin-resistant states. Endocr Rev 1991;12:3-13

[916] Corbould A, Kim Y-B, Youngren JF, *et al.* Insulin resistance in the skeletal muscle of women with PCOS involves intrinsic and acquired defects in insulin signaling. Am J Physiol Endocrinol Metab 2005;228:E1047-E1054

[917] Ehrmann DA, Sturis J, Byrne MM, Karrison T, Rosenfield RL, Polonsky KS. Insulin secretory defects in polycystic ovary syndrome. Relationship to insulin sensitivity and family history of non-insulin-dependent diabetes mellitus. J Clin Invest 1995;96:520-527

[918] Dunaif A, Finegood DT. β-Cell dysfunction independent of obesity and glucose intolerance in the polycystic ovary syndrome. J Clin Endocrinol Metab 1996;81:92-947

[919] Ciaraldi TP, el-Roeiy A, Madar Z, Reichart D, Olefsky JM, Yen SS. Cellular mechanism of insulin resistance n polycystic ovarian syndrome. J Clin Endocrinol Metab 1992;75:577-583

[920] Dunaif A, Wu X, Lee A, Diamanti-Kandarakis E. Defects in insulin receptor signaling *in vivo* in the polycystic ovary syndrome (PCOS). Am J Physiol Endocrinol Metab 2001;281:E392-E399

[921] Corbould A, Dunaif A. The adipose cell lineage is not intrinsically insulin resistant in polycystic ovary syndrome. Metabol 2007;56,5:716-722

[922] Peppa M, Koliaki C, Nikolopoulos P, Raptis SA. Skeletal muscle insulin resistance in endocrine disease. J Biomed Biotech 2010, ID 527850, doi:10.1155/2010/527850

[923] Diamanti-Kandarakis E, Papavassiliou AG. Molecular mechanisms of insulin resistance in polycystic ovary syndrome. Trends Mol Med 2006;12,7:324-332

[924] Futterweit W. Polycystic ovary syndrome: clinical perspectives and management. Obstet Gynecol Surv 1999;54:403-413

[925] Diamanti-Kandarakis E, Argyrakopoulou G, Economou F, Kandarakis E, Koutsiliens M. Defects in insulin signaling pathways in ovarian steroidogenesis and other tissues in polycystic ovary syndrome (PCOS). J Steroid Biochem Mol Biol 2008;109:242-246

[926] Rosenbaum D, Haber RS, Dunaif A. Insulin resistance in polycystic ovary syndrome: decreased GLUT4 glucose transporters in adipocytes. Am J Physiol 1993;264,2Pt1:E197-E202

[927] Chang W, Goodarzi MO, Williams H, Magoffin DA, Pall M, Azziz R. Adipocytes from women with polycystic ovary syndrome demonstrate altered phosphorylation and activity of glycogen synthase kinase 3. Fertil Steril 2008;90,6:2291-2297

[928] Wu XK, Zhou SY, Liu JX, *et al.* Selective ovary resistance to insulin signaling in women with polycystic ovary syndrome. Fertil Steril 2003;80:954-956

[929] Liberman Z, Eldar-Finkelman H. Serine 332 phosphorylation of insulin receptor substrate-1 by glycogen synthase kinase-3 attenuates insulin signaling. J Biol Chem 2005;280:4422-4428

[930] Nikoulina SE, Ciaraldi TP, Mudaliar, Mohideen P, Carter L, Henry RR. Potential role of glycogen synthase kinase-3 in skeletal muscle insulin resistance of type 2 diabetes. Diabetes 2000;49:263-271

[931] Eldar-Finkelman H. Glycogen synthase kinase 3: an emerging therapeutic target. Trends Mol Med 2002;8:126-132

[932] Dunaif A, Xia J, Book CB, Schenker E, Tang Z. Excessive insulin receptor serine phosphorylation in cultured fibroblasts and in skeletal muscle. A potential mechanism for insulin resistance in polycystic ovarian syndrome. J Clin Invest 1995;96:801-810

[933] Venkatesan AM, Dunaif A, Corbould A. Insulin resistance in polycystic ovary syndrome: progress and paradoxes. Recent Progr Horm Res 2001;56:295-308

[934] Fornes R, Ormazabal P, Rosas C, *et al.* Changes in the expression of insulin signaling pathway molecules in endometria from polycystic ovary syndrome women with or without hyperinsulinemia. Mol Med 2010;16,3-4:129-136

[935] Mioni R, Chiarelli S, Xamin N, *et al.* Evidence for the presence of glucose transporter 4 in the endometrium and its regulation in polycystic ovary syndrome patients. J Clin Endocrinol Metab 2004;89:4089-4096

[936] Mozzanega B, Mioni R, Granzotto M, *et al.* Obesity reduces the expression of GLUT-4 in the endometrium of normoinsulinemic women affected by the polycystic ovary syndrome. NY Acad Sci 2004;1034:364-374

[937] Pang TTL, Narendran P. Addressing insulin resistance in Type 1 diabetes. Diabet Med 2008;25:1015-1024

[938] Moran A, Jacobs D, Steinberger J, *et al.* Insulin resistance during puberty: results from clamp studies in 357 children. Diabetes 1999;48:2039-2044

[939] Perseghin G, Lattuada G, Danna M, *et al.* insulin resistance, intramyocellular lipid content, and plasma adiponectin in patients with type 1 diabetes. Am J Physiol Endocrinol Metab 2003;285:E1174-E1181

[940] DeFronzo RA, Hendler R, Simson D. Insulin resistance is a prominent feature of insulin-dependent diabetes. Diabetes 1982;31:795-801

[941] Dabalea D, Kinney G, Snell-Bergeon JK, *et al.* Effect of type 1 diabetes on the gender difference in coronary artery calcification: a role for insulin resistance? The Coronary Artery Calcification in Type 1 Diabetes (CACT1) Study. Diabetes 2003;52:2833-2839

[942] Heptulla RA, Stewart A, Enocksson S, *et al.* In situ evidence that peripheral insulin resistance in adolescent with poorly controlled type 1 diabetes is associated with impaired suppression of lipolysis: a microdialysis study. Pediatr Res 2003;53:830-838

[943] Hallodin MU, Brismar K, Tuvemo T, Gustafsson J. Insulin sensitivity and lipolysis in adolescent girls with poorly controlled type 1 diabetes: effect of anticholinergic treatment. Clin Endocrinol (Oxf) 2002;57:735-743

[944] Amiel SA, Sherwin RS, Simonson DC, Lauritano AA, Tamborlance WV. Impaired insulin action in puberty. A contributing factor to poor glycemic control in adolescent with diabetes. N Engl J Med 1986;315:215-219

[945] Arslanian S, Nixon PA, Becker D, Drash AL. Impact of physical fitness and glycemic control on *in vivo* insulin action in adolescent with IDDM. Diabetes Care 1990;13:9-15

[946] Himsworth H. Diabetes mellitus: a differentiation into insulin-sensitive and insulin-insensitive types. Lancet 1936;1:127-130

[947] Hirsch IB, D'Alessio D, Eng L, Davis C, Lernmark Å, Chait A. Severe insulin resistance in patient with type 1 diabetes and stiff-man syndrome treated with insulin lispro. Diabetes Res Clin Pract 1998;41:197-202

[948] Nadeau KJ, Regensteiner JG, Bauer TA, *et al.* Insulin resistance in adolescent with type 1 diabetes and its relationship to cardiovascular function. J Clin Endocrinol Metab 2010;95:513-521

[949] Greenfield JR, Samaras K, Chisholm DJ. Insulin resistance, intra-abdominal fat, cardiovascular risk factors, and androgens in healthy young women with type 1 diabetes mellitus. J Clin Endocrinol Metab 2002;87:1036-1040

[950] Perseghin G, Lattuada G, De Cobelli F, *et al.* Reduced intrahepatic fat content is associated with increased whole-body lipid oxidation in patients with type 1 diabetes. Diabetologia 2005;48:2615-2621

[951] Kahn SE, Hull RL, Utzschneider KM. Mechanisms linking obesity to insulin resistance and Type 2 diabetes. Nature 2006;444:840-846

[952] Ginsberg HN. Investigation of insulin sensitivity in treated subjects with ketosis-prone diabetes mellitus. Diabetes 1977;26:278-283

[953] Leslie RD, Taylor R, Pozzili P. The role of insulin resistance in the natural history of type 1 diabetes. Diabet Med 1997;14:327-331

[954] Pedrini MT, Kranebitter M, Niederwanger A, *et al.* Human triglyceride-rich lipoproteins impair glucose metabolism and insulin signalling in L6 skeletal muscle cells independently of non-esterifdied fatty acid levels. Diabetologia 2005;48:756-766

[955] Celi F, Bini V, Santilli E, *et al.* Circulating adipocytokines in non-diabetic and Type 1 diabetic children: relationship to insulin therapy, glycaemic control and pubertal development. Diabet Med 2006;23:660-665

[956] Luna R, Garcia-Mayor RV, Lage M, *et al.* High serum leptin levels in children with Type 1 diabetes mellitus: contribution of age, BMI, pubertal development and metabolic status. Clin Endocrinol (Oxf) 1999;51:603-610

[957] Baron AD, Laakso M, Brechtel G, Edelman SV. Mechanism of insulin resistance in insulin-dependent diabetes mellitus: a major role for reduced skeletal muscle blood flow. J Clin Endocrinol Metab 1991;73:637-643

[958] Makimattila S, Virkamaki A, Groop P, *et al.* Chronic hyperglycemia impairs endothelial function and insulin sensitivity via different mechanisms in insulin-dependent diabetes mellitus. Circulation 1996;94:1276-1282

[959] Orchard TJ, Chang Y-F, Ferrell RE, Petro N, Ellis DE. Nephropathy in type 1 diabetes: A manifestation of insulin resistance and multiple genetic susceptibilities? Further evidence from the Pittsburg Epidemiology of Diabetes Complication Study. Kidney Intern 2002;62:963-970

[960] Yki-Järvinen H, Taskinen MR, Kiviluoto T, *et al.* Site of insulin resistance in Type 1 diabetes: insulin-mediated glucose disposal *in vivo* in relation to insulin binding and action in adipocytes *in vitro*. J Clin Endocrinol Metab 1984;59:1183-1192

[961] Kahn B, Rosen A, Bak J, *et al.* Expression of GLUT1 and GLUT4 glucose transporters in skeletal muscle of humans with insulin-dependent diabetes mellitus: regulatory effects of metabolic factors. J Clin Endocrinol Metab 1992;74:1101-1109

[962] Fourlanos S, Naredran P, Byrnes GB, Colman PG, Harrison LC. Insulin resistance is a risk factor for progression to Type 1 diabetes. Diabetologia 2004;47:1661-1667

[963] Bingley PJ, Mahon JL, Gale EAM. Insulin resistance and progression of type 1 diabetes in the European Nicotinamide Diabetes Intervention Trial (ENDIT). Diabetes Care 2008;31,1:146-150

[964] Acerini CL, Cheetham TD, Edge JA, Dunger DB. Both insulin sensitivity and insulin clearance in children and young adults with type 1 (insulin-dependent) diabetes vary with growth hormone concentrations and with age. Diabetologia 2000;43:61-68

[965] Sharp PS, Mohan V, Vitelli F, Maneschi F, Kohner EM. Changes in insulin resistance with long-term insulin therapy. Diabetes Care 1987;10:56-61

[966] Greenbaum CJ. Insulin resistance in type 1 diabetes. Diabetes Metab Res Rev. 2002;18:192-200

[967] Tilg H, Moschen AR. Adipocytokines: mediators linking adipose tissue, inflammation and immunity. Nat Rev Immunol 2006;6:772-783

[968] Matarese G, Sanna V, Lechler RI, *et al.* Leptin accelerates autoimmune diabetes in female NOD mice. Diabetes 2002;51:1356-1361

[969] Maedler K, Sergeev P, Ris F, *et al.* Glucose-induced B-cell production of IL-1β contributes to Glucotoxicity in human pancreatic islets. J Clin Invest 2002;110:851-860

[970] Bjork E, Kampe O, Karlsson F, *et al.* Glucose regulation of the autoantigen GAD65 in human pancreatic islets. J Clin Endocrinol Metab 1992;75:1574-1576

CHAPTER 5

Therapies and Emerging Targets for the Treatment of Diabetes

Abstract: Current therapeutic approaches were largely developed in the absence of defined molecular targets or a solid understanding of disease pathogenesis. Within the past few years, our understanding of biochemical pathways related to the development of type 2 diabetes mellitus has expanded. The worldwide epidemic of type 2 diabetes has been stimulating the search for new concepts and targets for the treatment of this incurable disease. Studies using transgenic animals, gene transfer and pharmacological agents have yielded many data that have helped understand the molecular alterations characteristic of non-insulin dependent diabetes mellitus. This has opened the possibility for the development of potentially more-effective therapies, mainly focused on attenuating hepatic glucose production, enhancing glucose-dependent insulin secretion, enhancing the insulin signal transduction etc. Increasing knowledge on the biochemical and cellular alterations occurring in type 2 diabetes mellitus has led to the development of novel and potentially more effective therapeutic approaches to treat the disease.

INTRODUCTION

Currently, only limited treatments are available for insulin resistance. Combined innovative pharmaceutical and non-pharmaceutical strategies are needed. Several studies have been carried out covering different aspects of pharmacological interventions along with the effects of weight loss, diet and exercise.

Currently, there are two classes of drugs used for the treatment of diabetes mellitus: insulin and oral agents. Current recommendations of the American Diabetes Association include a trial of diet and exercise as first line therapy for the treatment of type 2 diabetes mellitus [1]. Current strategies to treat diabetes include reducing insulin resistance, supplementing insulin supplies, increasing endogenous insulin production and limiting postprandial glucose absorption [2].

PHARMACEUTICAL THERAPY

Insulin or Insulin Analogues

Insulin therapy started in 1922 using regular insulin before each main meal and one injection in the night, usually at 1 a.m. With the development of intermediate- and long-acting insulin, most patients moved to one or two injections per day after 1935 [3]. Insulin is typically injected 30 to 60 minutes after a meal, but the regimens vary from country to country [2].

Insulin is a pleiotropic hormone, regulating metabolism as well as aspects of growth and development through activation of divergent signaling pathways [4]. Insulin action is mediated mainly by the propagation of insulin signaling through intracellular pathways involving a cascade of phosphorylation and dephosphorylation events [5]. Insulin often activates protein phosphatases and initiates dephosphorylation of enzymes involved in energy metabolism. Some of these are activated by phosphorylation, while others are inactivated through the same mechanism.

Phosphorylated substrates engage, in turn, in the formation of signaling complexes via phosphotyrosine-containing binding motifs with Src homology 2 (SH2) found in different molecules. Phosphorylation of substrates and activation of downstream signaling molecules constitute the basic mechanism of insulin action. IRS proteins are coupled to several additional protein kinase signal systems: pathways signaling through phosphoinositide 3-kinase (PI 3-kinase) and mitogen-activated protein kinases (MAPKinases). The studies in transfected cells suggested that the carcinoembryonic antigen-related cell adhesion molecule 1 (CEACAM1) is also a substrate of the insulin receptor tyrosine kinase in rat hepatocytes, but not in muscle cells or adipose tissues [48, 49]. CEACAM1 is a transmembrane glycoprotein in an alternative insulin-signaling pathway regulating insulin clearance in liver. In contrast to IRS-1 and Shc, CEACAM1 regulates receptor-mediated insulin endocytosis [50].

Glycogen metabolism is under the control of two enzymes, glycogen synthase and glycogen phosphorylase. Insulin stimulates the dephosphorylation of both glycogen synthase and glycogen phosphorylase, resulting in maximal stimulation of glycogen synthesis and inhibition of glycogenolysis [6, 7]. Insulin also stimulates uptake of amino acids, activates protein synthesis from amino acids and glycogen and triglyceride synthesis from glucose. On the other hand, insulin inhibits break-down of triglycerides in adipose tissue and gluconeogenesis in the liver. Insulin has been shown to have a great anti-apoptotic action in a β-cell line [8, 9]. It stimulates mitogen-activated protein kinases pathway – a mitogenic signaling.

In summary: in liver – insulin inhibits gluconeogenesis and glycogenolysis, and stimulates glycogenesis; in muscle – it stimulates glucose transport, glycogenesis and protein synthesis; in pancreas – insulin stimulates β-cell growth, and inhibits β-cell apoptosis; in adipocyte – hormone stimulates glucose transport, protein synthesis and lipogenesis, and inhibits lipolysis. For details see Chapter 2, parts "Insulin actions on the liver" and "Insulin stimulation of GLUT 4 translocation".

In many patients with type 2 diabetes, insulin therapy is necessary for achieving glycemic goals. Despite the presence of multiple treatment modalities, insulin remains an important therapy for patients with type 2 diabetes. This is because the natural history of type 2 diabetes is characterized by progressive loss of β-cell function [10]. Insulin therapy often becomes necessary to achieve adequate glycemic control [11] and is most always effective in achieving glycemic control in type 2 diabetes, even after other agents have failed [12]. Thus, insulin therapy is important in the treatment of type 2 diabetes mellitus [13].

Ideally, insulin delivery should mimic physiological conditions in which the secretion by the pancreas peaks over basal after every snack or meal. There are many forms of insulin available, but they mainly fall into two categories: short-acting and long-acting [2].

The initial insulin preparations available had a short duration of action. Therefore, the initial efforts were directed towards prolongation of duration of its action [14]. This involved modification in the structure of the insulin the addition of zinc for complexing it with neutral protamine. In recent times alteration in the amino acid sequence has also been made.

The insulin molecule consists of two polypeptide chains, the A chain (21 amino acids) and B chain (30 amino acids). It exists as monomers in dilute solutions such as circulation but as hexamers in crystals and in β-cell secretory granule [15]. Human insulin differs from porcine insulin at position B30 (threonine in man versus alanine in pig), and from bovine insulin, at positions A8 and A10 (respectively theronine and isoleucine in man versus alanine and valine in the ox) [15]. The animal's insulin has slower absorption and longer duration of action than purified preparation and human insulin. Increased local temperature leads to rapid absorption of insulin from local site [14].

Short Acting Insulins

Regular insulin (usually identical to human insulin) is still used as an essential component of most daily replacement regimens in many parts of the world. It is combined with intermediate-acting insulin in twice daily regimen or as pre-meal bolus injections in basal-bolus regimens together with intermediate-acting insulin twice daily or a basal analog given once or twice daily [3]. Human regular insulin has an onset of action 30 – 60 minutes, peak of action 2 – 4 hours and duration of action 6 – 8 hours [3, 14, and 16].

Biphasic human insulin 70/30 has been in use for many years. It is a mixture of human neutral protamine (NPH) insulin and soluble human (Regular) insulin. The soluble human insulin has a delayed onset of action and prolonged duration [13]. When soluble human insulin is administered subcutaneously, as a biphasic insulinin combination with NPH, it peaks in about 2 – 3 hours and remains in thecirculation for up to 6 hours [43]. Biphasic human insulin can result in early post-prandial hyperglycemia followed by subsequent hypoglycemia, therefore, biphasic human insulin should be administered 30 minutes before a meal [13].

Rapid Acting Insulin Analogs

Insulin hexamer formation is an obstacle to mimicking physiological insulin profiles after subcutaneous injection. Therefore, several novel insulin analogs have been developed. The first rapid-acting insulin analog became available in 1996 and other rapid-acting analogs have been developed since then. Insulin analogs have been created by human insulin engineering; by a variety of modifications to the chemical structure of the protein or alteration of selected amino acids in different positions [17]. They are absorbed 2 – 3 times faster, after injection into subcutaneous tissues, than the regular hexameric insulins [17, 18]. Rapid-acting insulin analogs have this effect because, after subcutaneous injection, the proportion that is bound in the form of dimers and hexamers is lower, which means that the monomeric analog molecule can be absorbed at the point of injection more quickly.

Three rapid-acting types are currently available; insulin lispro and insulin aspart were the first to be used. More recently, a third rapid-acting analog, insulin glulisine, was cleared for use in the United States. Rapid-acting insulin analogs have onset of action 10 – 15 minutes, peak of action 1 – 2 ours and duration of action 3 – 5 hours [3, 16, and 19].

Insulin lispro, introduced in 1996, the first insulin analog to be used clinically, differs from human insulin by a switch at lysine B28 and proline B29, resulting in reduced self-association [18, 20]. In the vial, the insulin lispro exists as a hexameric formulation. After subcutaneous injecting, it dissociates into a monomeric formulation, leading to a more rapid absorption and shorter duration of action [21 – 23]. Its efficacy, antigenicity (immunogenicity), receptor binding and metabolic effects are comparable to that of human insulin [24 – 26]. Insulin lispro is indicated in postprandial hyperglycemia, in children where food intake may be unpredictable, and in patients with end-stage renal disease [14, 21]. It can also be used safely in pregnant women with type 1, type 2 and gestational diabetes [27]. Although optimal time for injecting insulin lispro is immediately before the meal, it can be injected up to 15 minutes after a meal [15, 28].

Biphasic insulin lispro 75/25 is an admixture consisting 75% protaminated lispro and 25% soluble lispro [13]. It has a more rapid onset of action and shorter duration of action as compared to biphasic human insulin. Biphasic insulin analogs reduce post-prandial glucose more effectively and are more physiologic than biphasic human insulin [13].

Insulin aspart was created through recombinant DNA technology so that the amino acid, B28, which is proline, is substituted with an aspartic acid residue. This substitution results in reduced self-association of the insulin molecule. After subcutaneous injection, insulin aspart, which initially exists as hexamers, rapidly dissociates into dimers and monomers [22]. It is absorbed faster than regular human insulin, with higher peak insulin concentrations and a reduced duration of action [29, 30]. The time of maximum concentration is 52 minutes versus 145 minutes with human regular insulin. Insulin aspart shows better post-prandial glucose control compared with regular insulin [31]. It improves glycemic control compared to regular insulin in patients with type 1 diabetes [31, 32]. Insulin aspart can be administered immediately prior to a meal or postprandially. A study comparing insulin aspart and insulin lispro demonstrated them to be very similar; however, insulin lispro peaked approximately 10 minutes earlier [21].

Biphasic insulin aspart 70/30, is an admixture consisting of 70% intermediate-acting protamine-crystallized insulin aspart, and 30% rapid-acting non-protaminated (soluble) insulin aspart. In comparison to biphasic human insulin 70/30 (Neutral Protamine Hagedron/Regular), biphasic insulin aspart 70/30 has a more rapid and higher peak for more effective mealtime coverage [33, 34]. Biphasic insulin aspart 70/30 is the most well studied biphasic insulin analog, even more extensively studied than biphasic insulin lispro 75/25 [13]. Biphasic insulin aspart more effectively reduces post-prandial glucose compared to other biphasic insulins [13].

Insulin glulisine is the newest human insulin analog produced by recombinant DNA technology. It differs from human insulin by two amino acid substitutions on the B chain of the protein, which prevents the formation of inactive hexamers when injected. Insulin glulisine is created by substitution of asparagines at position B3 by lysine and lysine at position B29 by glutamine in the human insulin [35, 36]. Insulin glulisine has more rapid onset of action and shorter duration of action compared to regular human insulin. Pharmacokinetic studies with insulin glulisine have shown an absorption profile with a peak insulin concentration approximately twice that of regular human insulin [35]. Insulin glulisine has similar binding properties, and is associated with a faster onset but similar level of glucose disposal, to regular human insulin. Insulin glulisine and insulin lispro have similar effects on glucose levels [37]. It is effective when compared to other short- and rapid-acting insulins. The potencies of insulin glulisine for metabolic and mitogenic response are comparable to those of insulin [8, 38 – 39]. Insulin glulisine and regular human insulin show similar insulin receptor-mediated phosphorylation, IRS-2 activation and stimulation of DNA synthesis [40]. Meal studies in patients with type 1 diabetes show that insulin glulisine provides better postprandial blood glucose control than regular human insulin when administered immediately pre-meal. In patients with type 2 diabetes, the overall post-prandial blood glucose excursions were lower with insulin glulisine than with insulin lispro [35].

Insulin glulisine mimics endogenous insulin secretion more closely than recombinant human insulin. Due to its rapid action, insulin glulisine can be administered just before or after meal, to avoid risk of hypoglycemia.

Long Acting Insulins

The first successful insulin preparation with a prolonged action was protamine insulin followed by the lente crystalline zinc-insulin series. To obtain prolongation of insulin action, several preparations e.g. isophane insulin, lente insulin, ultralente and extended acting insulin preparations were introduced. Classically long-acting insulins have been obtained by the addition of small amounts of zinc that at high insulin concentrations and neutral pH increase self dissociation into dimers and hexamers [14]. The resulting insulin is absorbed slowly from the injected depot [15]. Long-acting insulins were designed to have a duration of more than 24 hours to meet basal insulin requirements, and therefore could be used in basal-bolus injection regimens [3].

Isophane insulin, also known as NPH (Neutral Protamine Hagedron) insulin, is prepared by addition, in stoichiometric proportion, of protamine to insulin. A small amount of zinc is added for better stabilization of insulin [41]. Isophane insulin is usually too short-acting for a once a day dosing [42]. It has an onset of action 1 – 3 hours, peak of action 5 – 7 hours, and duration of action 13 – 18 hours [14, 15].

Ultralente (Ultratard) insulin is the longest acting human insulin-zinc crystalline suspension. Prolongation of duration of action is due to its slow absorption from the subcutaneous tissues. Ultralente insulin has onset of action 2 – 4 hours, peak of action 8 – 14 hours and duration of action 18 – 30 hours [14, 15].

Lente insulin, an intermediate acting insulin, is a mixture of ultralente and semilente insulin (70/30). Pharmacokinetic parameters of lente insulin after subcutaneous injection are: onset of action 1 – 3 hours, peak of action 4 – 8 hours and duration of action 13 – 20 hours [14, 15].

Long Acting Insulin Analogs

The principle employed in the development of long acting analog is to reduce solubility at the pH of subcutaneous tissue fluid. This is done by the addition of arginine residue to the CV-terminus of the B-chain, by the addition of a fatty acid chain or by the substitution of hydrophobic amino acids within the insulin monomer. Two long-acting insulin analogs are available; insulin glargine and insulin detemir.

Insulin glargine (A21 Gly, B31 Arg, B32 Arg) is a long-acting human insulin analog. Insulin glargine is clear insulin that precipitates in the subcutaneous tissues. It became available in 2000 [19]. It has a near peakles action for at least 24 hours with reduced incidence of hypoglycemia [44].

The majority of studies using insulin glargine found reductions in hypoglycaemic episodes, particularly of nocturnal hypoglycaemia [45]. Insulin glargine has an onset of action 1 – 2 hours, no peak of action and duration of action 24 hours [19].

Insulin detemir is the newest long-acting analog, with an action that last approximately 6 – 23 hours [46]. It is soluble analogue with a fatty acyl chain attached to B29 Lys. Acylation of detemir allows the insulin to bind to non-esterified binding on albumin. It dissociates slowly from albumin and favours the hexameric state the resultant absorption and duration of action are longer. Pharmacokinetic and pharmacodynamic parameters of insulin detemir are similar to insulin glargine [19]; however, insulin detemir is characterized by a more reproducible pharmacokinetic profile than glargine in children and adolescents with type 1 diabetes [47]. It appears to produce a more predictable glycemic control, a smoother plasma glucose profile with a significant reduction in hypoglycemia [15], and is, therefore, a promising new option for basal insulin therapy.

Enhancers of Insulin Release (Insulin Secretagogues)

Sulfonylureas

Sulfonylureas were among the first oral medicines available for the treatment of type 2 diabetes. The hypoglycemic effect of sulfonamides was first discovered in 1942 by Marcel Jambon and colleagues, who studied sulfonamide antibiotics and discovered that the compound sulfonylurea induced hypoglycemia in experimental animals and in patients treated with sulfonamides for typhoid fever. The first sulfonylurea became available in 1955. The oldest class of oral antidiabetic agents has dominated the market for many years. Despite the many new diabetes therapies that have been discovered over the past 50 years, metformin and sulfonylureas are still two of the initial choices for treatment. On the other hand, presently, sulfonylureas are no longer recommended as first line therapy in the majority of type 2 diabetic patients, but they remain indispensable in the later stages of the disease [51].

Sulfonylureas are insulin secretagogues widely used to stimulate insulin secretion in the treatment of non-insulin dependent diabetes mellitus. Sulfonylureas stimulate the pancreatic β-cells to produce more insulin. Since sulfonylureas work by stimulating the pancreas to release insulin, they are only useful in people with type 2 diabetes whose β-cells still produce insulin. Sulfonylureas do not work in those with type 1 diabetes nor in any one with type 2 diabetes whose β-cells no longer produce insulin, as for example in people with type 2 diabetes for more than 6 to 15 years. The sulfonylureas influence insulin secretion in direct proportion to plasma glucose levels from 3,3 – 10 mmol/L. They do not stimulate insulin secretion when the plasma glucose is lower than 3,3 mmol/L [57, 58]. Sulfonylureas do not promote the synthesis of proinsulin [51]. They do not have a significant effect on lipids. Additionally, they do not reduce insulin resistance, a common feature of the type 2 diabetes [52].

However, the effect of sulfonylureas on insulin secretion is not rapidly reversible, and therefore this treatment is associated with an increased risk of hypoglycemia [53, 54]. Mild hypoglycemia is the most commonly occurring adverse event of sulfonylurea therapy, affecting ~ 2% to 4% of the patients, and although hypoglycemia is rarely severe enough to warrant hospitalization, severe hypoglycemia occurs at a rate of 0,02% to 0,04% per year [55, 56]. Severe low blood sugar occurs about 500 times more often with insulin than with sulfonylureas.

Sulfonylureas are divided into generations based on their receptor selectivity and potency. Sulfonylureas have gone through several steps of development and are categorized as first-, second- or third-generation drugs. The main difference between the generations is how well they bind to the sulfonylurea receptor, with each progressive generation binding more tightly and thus requiring a lower dose to bring about the same amount of insulin secretion [52].

The first generation-agents, drugs that were introduced long ago, include acetohexamide (Dymelor), chlorpropamide (Diabinese), tolazamide (Tolinase) and tolbutamide (Orinase) [21, 56]. These drugs work well in lowering the blood sugar, but they have a major drawback. Because they bind to proteins in the blood, they can be dislodged by other medications that bind to these same proteins. Once dislodged, their activity can increase rapidly and lead to low blood sugars. Orinase acts over 6 – 10 hours, Diabinese lasts longer in the blood (24 – 72 hours) and on rare occasions can cause a severe long-lasting form of hypoglycemia. Hypoglycemia is especially a problem with the first-generation agents because of their long half-lives. Other adverse effects like immune-allergic accidents, digestive intolerance, dilution hyponatremia or alcohol flushing are very rare and drug dependent [51]. Because sulfonylureas are eliminated from the body by the kidneys, decreased kidney function may lead to increased blood levels of the medicine, with a subsequent increased risk of side effects.

The second-generation agents differ in potency, safety, and pharmaceutics. The second-generation agents are more potent, have better pharmacokinetics and safety profiles, and are stronger than the first-generation sulfonylureas and require lower dosage. The second-generation agents include glipizide (Glucotrol), glyburide (DiaBeta, Glynase, Micronase) and gliclazide [1, 60 – 62].

Clinical trials have shown that glipizide and glyburide are associated with similar reductions in fasting blood glucose levels and HbA$_{1C}$ [61]. Glipizide acts over 12 hours, glipizide extended-release acts over 24 hours, and glyburide acts over 18 – 24 hours [59]. Many studies suggest that sulfonylureas have direct extrapancreatic actions. Gliclazide and glyburide increased 2-deoxy-D-glucose uptake in a time- and dose-dependent fashion in L6 myotubes, a model of skeletal muscle. Gliclazide stimulates glucose transport activity by the induction of GLUT 1 gene expression through protein kinase A [62]. The obtained results suggest an action of gliclazide and glyburide to stabilize GLUT 1 protein at the plasma membrane [61]. On the other hand, gliclazide therapy is not associated with any change in DNA or protein content per g muscle or any alteration in GLUT 4 levels expressed either per μg membrane protein or per DNA [60].

Less than 4% of patients taking second-generation agents experience adverse effects. The main side effect of glyburide is hypoglycemia with the severity of the symptoms being dose related. Older diabetic patients are at greater risk for a hypoglycemic episode than the young [58].

Glimeperide (Amaryl) is a new sulfonylurea drug. It represents the latest, third generation of this class of anti-diabetes medications. Glimeperide has 2,5 – 3 fold faster rate of association and 8 – 9 fold faster rate of dissociation from the β-cells sulfonylurea binding site in comparison with a second-generation agent, glyburide.

This results in a more rapid release and a shorter duration of insulin secretion.Glimeperide significantly increases second-phase insulin secretion, whole body glucose uptake and insulin sensitivity [63]. It has been shown to cause a more rapid reduction in fasting blood glucose levels than glipizide [56, 64]. Glimeperide acts over 16 – 24 hours [55, 59].

Although the sulfonylureas are often capable of restoring insulin secretion initially, they unfortunately become ineffective after a few years of therapy (secondary failure). After a good initial response to sulfonylurea therapy, the secondary failure rate is about 5% to 7% per year, and after 10 years, most sulfonylurea-treated patients require a second oral agent [55].

Mechanism of Action

Insulin is released in a biphasic fashion consisting of a first phase followed by a sustained second phase [65]. It is now well established that increasing the closed probability of the β-cell ATP-dependent potassium channel (K_{ATP}) is the major mechanism through which sulfonylureas, as well as glucose, stimulate insulin release from pancreatic β-cells [66].

Sulfonylureas act by binding to the sulfonylurea receptor (SUR1) associated with the proteic units of the K^+ channel of the β-cell (Kir6.2) [67]. The K_{ATP} channel is a hetero-octameric complex of two different types of protein subunits: an inwardly rectifying K^+ channel, Kir6.x, and a sulfonylurea receptor [69]. Kir6.x belongs to the family of inwardly rectifying K^+ channels. Binding of ATP to the intracellular domains of this subunit produces channel inhibition [70]. Sulfonylurea receptor is a member of ABC (ATP-binding cassette proteins) transporter family, with 17 transmembrane helices, arranged as one group of 5 transmembrane helices, and two repeats each of 6 transmembrane helices followed by a large cytosolic loop [68].

More than one isoform exists for both Kir6.x (Kir6.1 and Kir6.2) and sulfonylurea receptor (SUR1, SUR2A and SUR2B). Kir6.2 serves as the pore-forming subunit and associates with SUR1 in the pancreas [71, 72 and 75]. All drugs that block K_{ATP} channels stimulate insulin secretion, but only those that interact with the SUR subunit are used therapeutically to treat type 2 diabetes.

Binding of sulfonylureas to the cytoplasmic domains of SUR1 ultimately results in closure of the pore formed by Kir6.2, an effect, which is physiologically induced by the increase of the ATP/ADP ration resulting from the metabolism of glucose in the β-cell. The resulting reduction in potassium ion efflux causes depolarization of the β-cell plasma membrane, which in turn leads to opening of voltage-sensitive Ca^{2+} channels of the L-type. The increased influx of Ca^{2+} and, thus, the elevated cytosolic Ca^{2+} levels trigger the fusion of insulin-containing secretory granules withthe plasma membrane [73, 74].

Non-Sulfonylurea Secretagogues

The non-sulfonylureas secretagogues are the meglitinide analogs, including nateglinide (Starlix), a derivative of the amino acid D-phenylalanine, and repaglinide (Prandin), a benzoic acid derivative, that are available since 2000.

These agents bind to K_{ATP} channels, albeit at a different site than traditional sulfonylureas. The meglitinide analogs stimulate the release of insulin from pancreatic β-cells if glucose is present, and have no effect on lipids. These analogs have much shorter half-lives than do sulfonylureas [21].

Nateglinide mimics physiologic insulin secretion dynamics seen in healthy individuals by increasing early phase insulin secretion into the portal vein. It rapidly acts at the same pancreatic β-cell K^+ ATPase channel as sulfonylureas and repaglinide but dissociates from the receptor within seconds. Therefore, delayed hyperinsulinemia and an increased risk of hypoglycemia are unlikely with nateglinide [21].

Incretins

The term "incretins" refers to secretory products of the intestine that influence pancreatic β-cell function, and the "incretin effect" designates the amplification of insulin secretion elicited by hormones secreted from the gastrointestinal tract [21, 76]. In the most strict sense "it is quantified by comparing insulin responses to oral and intravenous administration, where the intravenous infusion is adjusted so as to result in the same (isoglycemic) peripheral (preferably arterialized) plasma glucose concentrations" [77, 78].

The insulin secretory response of incretins, the incretin effect, accounts for at least 50% of the total insulin secreted after oral glucose intake. Many hormones have been suspected to be responsible for the incretin effect [79 – 83], but today there is ample evidence to suggest that the two most important incretins are GIP (glucose-dependent insulinotropic peptide) and GLP-1 (glucagon-like peptide-1) [84, 85].

The incretin-based therapies represent a new potential goal-oriented treatment approach [86]. These drugs have a peculiar mechanism of action that can impact on several possible causes of clinical inertia [87]. A mechanism of action is associated with lack of hypoglycemia and weight loss or neutrality [88]. Both GLP-1 and GIP produce a similar early insulin release, while later-phase insulin levels are much higher with GLP-1 than GIP infusion [89]. Glucagon-like peptide-1 is the major relevant incretin in type 2 diabetes. Glucose-dependent insulinotropic peptide has little stimulatory capacity, and GIP circulates up to 10-fold higher concentrationsthan GLP-1 after meal. Since GIP has little effect on insulin production in type 2 diabetes, the focus shifted to GLP-1, and GLP-1 appeared to have potential clinical benefit in type 2 diabetes mellitus [87]. From the two major incretins, GLP-1 and GIP, only the first one or its mimetics or enhancers can be used for treatment because the diabetic β-cell is resistant to GIP action [90].

Within some minutes of release from their intestinal sites, GIP and GLP-1 undergo rapid metabolism to inactive metabolites by the enzyme dipeptidyl peptidase-IV (DPP-IV). A number of pharmacological strategies have been developed to provide continuous delivery of GLP-1 and to prevent degradation of GLP-1, including continuous administration of GLP-1, DPP-IV resistant GLP-1 analogs and DPP-IV inhibitors [91].

Glucagon-Like Peptide-1 (GLP-1)

The human proglucagon gene located on the long arm of chromosome 2 has six exons, of which exons 2 to 5 encode distinct functional domains, and five introns [92]. Glucagon is encoded in exon 3, and GLP-1 is encoded in exon 4 [93]. A single size structurally identical mRNA transcript is produced in all tissues that contain proglucagon [94, 95].

GLP-1 is produced as an inactive 37-amino-acid peptide whose C-terminal end contains glycine. The active form is produced by post-translational cleavage of six amino acids from the N-terminal end of GLP-1 (1-37). GLP-1 is a 30- or 31-amino-acid peptide synthesized and secreted by L cells mainly within the distal small intestine (ileum) and colon in response to meal intake. GLP-1 exists in two circulating equipotent molecular forms, GLP-1 (7-37) and GLP-1 (7-36) amide, although GLP-1 (7-36) amide is more abundant in the circulation after eating.

Circulating GLP-1 concentrations are low in the fasting stage. It is released 5 – 30 minutes after food ingestion in proportion to energy content. The primary physiological stimuli for the secretion of GLP-1 are fat- and carbohydrate-rich meals, but mixed meals or individual nutrients, including glucose and other sugars, fatty acids, amino acids etc, also can stimulate GLP-1 secretion [96]. Plasma concentrations of GLP-1 increase six- to eight-fold after a carbohydrate meal [98]. Meal ingestion results in a biphasic pattern of GLP-1 secretion, with an early phase beginning within 5 to 15 minutes and a prolonged second phase, following within 30 to 60 minutes [79, 97].

GLP-1 stimulates insulin secretion in a glucose-dependent manner, i.e. only in the presence of raised blood glucose. It inhibits glucagon secretion, lower plasma glucose and HbA_{1C}, inhibits gastric emptying and decreases appetite and energy intake, and slows the rate of endogenous glucose production [99 – 102], all of which should help to lower blood glucose, in patients with type 2 diabetes. It has also been shown to protect β-cells from apoptosis [103] and to stimulate β-cell proliferation [104, 105].

The effects of GLP-1 on glycemic regulation are transduced via widely distributed specific G-protein-coupled receptors, which can increase intracellular cyclic adenosine monophosphate (cAMP) and calcium concentrations of signal transduction [88].

The secretion of GLP-1 in patients with type 2 diabetes has been largely studied [106]. Plasma levels of GLP-1 are reduced in type 2 diabetic patients or in patients with impaired glucose tolerance, as compared to healthy subjects. The mechanism of the impaired secretion of GLP-1 is unknown [91].

The promising therapeutic potential of GLP-1 as a pharmacologic tool for treating type 2 diabetes was proposed in the 1990s [107]. The insulinotropic effect of GLP-1 depends even more closely on the actual glucose concentration providing the possibility of glucose normalization without the risk of hypoglycemia. GLP-1 is effective in patients with type 2 diabetes, increasing insulin secretion and normalizing both fasting and postprandial blood glucose when given as a continuous intravenous infusion, even in subjects with advanced type 2 diabetes long after sulfonylurea secondary failure [108]. The preliminary experiences with GLP-1 were encouraging and confirmed the potential for incretin-based therapies in the treatment of diabetes [100].

As a peptide, GLP-1 cannot be administered orally because it is immediately denatured and inactivated by gastric acid. Subcutaneous or intravenous administration is required for GLP-1 to reach the circulation. Nevertheless, glucagon-like peptide-1 cannot be immediately employed because of its extensive and rapid degradation by the enzyme dipeptidyl peptidase-IV [91].

It was clear from the beginning that GLP-1 itself was unsuitable for therapeutic use due to its very short half-life. While GLP-1 has marked benefits in patients with type 2 diabetes, native GLP-1 administration, as a treatment strategy, is severely limited by a short half-life *in vivo* ($T_{1/2}$ = 1 – 2 minutes) due to inactivation by DPP-IV and the impracticality of continuous infusion. The continuous subcutaneous infusion of GLP-1 via a portable minipump has been proven to provide stable plasma concentrations. But this method is associated with an increased risk of catheter infection [91]. Two approaches have been pursued to develop incretin-based anti-diabetic agents: injectable GLP-1 mimetics or analogs, consisting of molecules modified from the native GLP-1 (resistant to the effects of DPP-IV) and inhibitors of DPP-IV [91, 109 and 110].

Exenatide

Exenatide (Byetta) is the first agent in the class of incretin mimetics. It is indicated for the treatment of type 2 diabetes in combination with other oral therapies. As a GLP-1 receptor agonist, exenatide mimics the action of naturally occurring GLP-1 and is therefore classified as an incretin mimetic.

Exenatide is the synthetic version of exendin-4, a natural of 39 amino acid peptide originally isolated from the lizard *Heloderma suspectum* (Gila monster), a large lizard living in Arizona desert [111]. Exendin-4 is coded by a gene distinct from that of GLP-1, but shows a 52% amino acid identity to full length human GLP-1 [112]. It binds with greater affinity than GLP-1 to the GLP-1 receptor in GLP-1 receptor expressing cells [113, 114]. Exenatide is a not substrate for dipeptidyl peptidase-IV because it has a Gly^8 in place of an Ala^8 [79]. This GLP-1 receptor agonist is longer lived and the half-life ranges from 3,3 to 4,0 h [115], and its biological effect remains for up to at least 8 h after dosing. It is detected in the plasma up to 15 h after subcutaneous injection [115]. It has ~ 5000-fold greater potency in lowering blood glucose than GLP-1 [116] and it has all of the same effects in the pancreas [79].

Exenatide, a peptide, must be injected subcutaneously and is twice daily administered within 60 minutes before breakfast and dinner [87]. Studies of exenatide in both healthy volunteers and patients with type 2 diabetes found that it enhanced insulin release only in the presence of hyperglycemia [117 – 119].

Exenatide has been shown to restore first-phase insulin secretion in patients with type 2 diabetes. Compared with placebo, exenatide induced reductions of HbA_{1C}, fasting glucose and body weight [88, 120 – 123]. The risk of hypoglycemia was increased only when exenatide was associated with sulfonylurea [120, 122]. The effect of exenatide on lipids was substantially neutral. In studies comparing exenatide with insulin glargine [124] and biphasic aspart [125], no differences were observed with regard to HbA_{1C} and fasting glucose, with significant reduction of postprandial glycemia and body weight in patients treated with exenatide.

The commonest adverse events with exenatide were gastrointestinal. Mild-to-moderate nausea occurs in about 40% of patients receiving twice-daily exenatide, with diarrhea and vomiting in less than 15% [87]. However, exenatide was rarely discontinued because of side-effects, and the occurrence of nausea lessened the longer the duration of therapy. Nausea disappears within 4 weeks in most of the patients. Formation of antibodies to exenatide has been reported in up to 50% of the treated patients [87]. Antibody formation has not been associated with impaired antidiabetic effectiveness of exenatide in most of those patients [88].

Liraglutide

Liraglutide (Victoza) is a long-acting GLP-1 analogue with a 97% homology with the human native hormone. It contains a Arg 34 Lys substitution and glutamic acid and 16-C free-fatty-acid addition to Lys26 [126]. Acetylating the peptide with a free fatty acid chain improves binding to albumin, makes it less accessible to DPP-IV and inhibits renal filtration. Also the binding to albumin induces a slower resorption from the place of injection. Thanks to these characteristics, liraglutide has a half-life of about 12 hours. Due to its prolonged action it is suitable for once-daily injection.

Animal and human studies have demonstrated blood glucose-lowering effects. In patients with type 2 diabetes, liraglutide provided effective glycemic control, i.e. HbA_{1C} and fasting serum glucose being significantly lower than with placebo, and was not associated with weight gain [127]. Animal studies have shown that liraglutide increases insulin secretion, inhibits gastric emptying and appetite and increased β-cell mass [128].

Frequently reported side effects were nausea, vomiting and diarrhea as with all GLP-1-like drugs. Nausea occurred in some patients at the beginning of therapy, but it was usually mild or moderate and did not lead to a discontinuation of treatment. Vomiting and diarrhea were generally mild, transient, and rarely caused discontinuation of liraglutide treatment [129, 130]. As with exenatide, gastrointestinal symptoms were the chief adverse effects and led to discontinuation in ~ 3% of liraglutide patients in the European study [131]. No patient experienced hypoglycemic episodes, and there was no treatment-related anti-liraglutide antibody induction [131].

Dipeptidyl Peptidase-IV Inhibitors

The therapeutic principle of GLP-1 can also be implemented by inhibiting GLP-1 degradation. The observation that GLP-1 is rapidly degraded by dipeptidyl peptidase-IV has fostered the development of specific protease inhibitors that prevent the rapid fall of GLP-1 in circulating plasma after eating. Dipeptidyl peptidase-IV is a membrane-spanning cell-surface aminopeptidase widely expressed in many tissues. Many gastrointestinal hormones are substrates for DPP-IV, among them being both GIP and GLP-1.

DPP-IV inhibitors mimic many of the actions ascribed to agonists of glucagon-like receptor. DPP-IV inhibitors stimulate insulin secretion, β-cell proliferation, inhibit glucagon secretion, and β-cell apoptosis [81, 132]. The inhibitors of dipeptidyl peptidase-IV are generally not associated with a deceleration of gastric emptying or weight loss.

A number of DPP-IV inhibitors are undergoing clinical development for diabetes therapy. They have been shown to prevent the degradation of endogenous incretins. DPP-IV inhibitors offer the advantage of an oral administration. Their potential limitation is that dipeptidyl peptidase-IV is a ubiquitous enzyme. Thus, nonspecific inhibition may result in increased levels of other peptides that are also cleaved by DPP-IV, such as neuropeptide Y, GH-RH, GLP-2, with potential unknown adverse effects [91]. Because DPP-IV is involved in the degradation of many peptide hormones, the action of DPP-IV is less specific than "incretin mimetics" [108]. Along with this, the long-term immunological effects of DPP-IV inhibitors in humans are not yet known, since DPP-IV is also expressed on lymphocytes as CD26 [133, 134].

Many small-molecule DPP-IV inhibitors have been developed that specifically inhibit DPP-IV activity after oral administration. These agents reduce serum DPP-IV activity by more than 80%, with some inhibition maintained for 24 h after one dose or with once daily treatment. DPP-IV inhibition is accompanied by a rise in postprandial levels of intact GLP-1 [135, 136]. Because these agents rely on endogenous incretin secretion, they may best be employed in early disease [137, 138]. Currently, vildagliptin and sitagliptin are approved in Europe. For both compounds, efficacy and safety have been shown both as monotherapy and in combination therapy.

Vildagliptin

Vildagliptin (Glavus) is a very selective, reversible, orally competitive inhibitor of dipeptidyl peptidase-IV [133]. It is rapidly absorbed and achieves peak plasma levels in 1 to 2 h [139]. Its half-life is 2 h, bioavailability is approximately 85% [140], and pharmacokinetics seems unaffected by food [141]. Approximately 69% of vildagliptin is hydrolyzed in the liver to an inactive metabolite, and it, in addition to vildagliptin, is then excreted by liver [79].

Monotherapy with vildagliptin during 12 weeks improves HbA_{1C} in patients with type 2 diabetes [142]. It was shown that DPP-IV inhibition resulted in statistically significant lower mean 24-hour glucose levels, lower fasting glucose levels, lower mean 4-hour post-breakfast glucose levels and lower peak post-breakfast glucose levels, without changes in fasting or mean 24-hour insulin levels [135, 143]. Plasma glucagon concentrations were suppressed after vildagliptin treatment, together with an increase in the ratio of insulin to glucose [135].

Vildagliptin is well-tolerated; no characteristic pattern of adverse events has been associated with the use of vildagliptin [144]. Headache, dizziness and nosopharyngitis have been the adverse events most commonly reported in clinical trials. With an incidence similar to placebo [145 – 148] hypoglycemia occurred in less than 1% of patients treated with vildagliptin [147].

Sitagliptin

Sitagliptin (Januvia) is the sole DPP-IV inhibitor in use for the treatment of type 2 diabetes, though there are others in the pipeline. It is a small non-peptide-based orally active molecule that seems to be selective for dipeptidyl peptidase-IV. Sitagliptin not interacts with other closely related proteases [79]. Sitagliptin is rapidly absorbed and achieves peak plasma levels in 1 to 6 h, and its half-life is 8 to 14 h [149]. Approximately 80% of the dose is excreted unchanged by the kidney [79]. The administration is independent of meals.

Sitagliptin is indicated for the treatment of type 2 diabetes mellitus either as monotherapy or in combination with metformin and/or sulfonylureas in patients poorly controlled on maximum doses of these drugs [87].

Clinical studies with sitagliptin indicated that sitagliptin is well tolerated and effective in both monotherapy and in combination with metformin or pioglitazone. The effect on weight and hypoglycemia is not given [149, 150]. Sitagliptin monotherapy in combination with other anti-hyperglycemic agents, has been shown to reduce the HbA_{1C} and fasting plasma levels [151]. An indirect assessment of β-cell function using HOMA-B showed improved function. However, no data on glucagon were provided [143].

Nosopharyngitis, upper respiratory infections, and headache occur in less than 3% of sitagliptin-treated patients [152]. Gastrointestinal disturbances are uncommon and occur in 9% to 16% of patients compared with 6% to 14% for placebo. Hypoglycemia, which is usually mild to moderate, occurs in 0% to 4% and 0% to 2%, respectively [153 – 155]. There have been reports of serious hypersensitivity reactions occurring within three months of initiating sitagliptin therapy. These reactions sometimes occur after the first dose [145].

INHIBITORS OF HEPATIC GLUCOSE PRODUCTION

The liver has a critical role in regulating endogenous glucose production from *de novo* synthesis (gluconeogenesis) or the catabolism of glycogen (glycogenolysis). Increased rates of hepatic glucose production are largely responsible for the development of overt hyperglycemia in patients with diabetes [156]. Several drug targets in the liver offer new ways of attenuating excessive hepatic glucose production [1, 157].

Metformin

Metformin (Glucophage) is a biguanide oral hypoglycemic agent, which was introduced in clinical practice in the 1950s. It is an oral anti-hyperglycemic agent that is chemically and pharmacologically unrelated to the sulfonylureas. It is a synthetic analog (dimethylbiguanide) of the natural product guanidine.

Metformin is a drug that works independently of the pancreas, sparing insulin [10]. Its primary effect is to inhibit the liver's production of glucose. The primary site of action appears to be the hepatocyte mitochondria, where metformin disrupts respiratory chain oxidation [158]. The mechanism of action of metformin, a widely used agent for treating type 2 diabetes mellitus, is poorly understood. Metformin inhibits hepatic gluconeogenesis both *in vitro* [159] and *in vivo* [160]. It also has an inhibitory effect on hepatic glycogenolysis [161]. One theory is that the decrease in hepatic glucose production is predominantly due to attenuation of gluconeogenesis rather than to glycogenolysis [162]. Metformin decreases gluconeogenesis through inhibition of hepatic lactate uptake [163]. It phosphorylates the transcriptional co-activator CBP via $PKC_{1/\lambda}$ and this event triggers the dissociation of the CREB-CBP-TORC2 transcription complex and reduces gluconeogenic enzyme gene expression [164]. In rat hepatocytes, metformin lowers intracellular concentration of ATP, an allosteric inhibitor of pyruvate kinase [165], inhibits pyruvate carboxylase-phosphoenolpyruvate carboxykinase (PEPCK) activity and activates the pyruvate to alanine conversion [166]. The mechanism of action of metformin in liver involves insulin receptor activation (it increases insulin receptor tyrosine phosphorylation), followed by selective IRS-2 activation (but not IRS-1), and increased GLUT 1 translocation from the microsomal fraction to the plasma membrane of hepatic cells [167].

Metformin, as described above, lowers glucose production by suppressing hepatic glucose production [168] and diminished hepatic glucose output [169]. There is some data to suggest that it may slightly improve peripheral insulin sensitivity. Metformin often is reviewed as an insulin sensitizer because it reduces the hyperinsulinemia associated with insulin resistance [170]. The *in vivo* studies are supported by *in vitro* data. Metformin enhances muscle insulin sensitivity [160] and stimulates the process of transporting glucose into muscle [21]. Metformin increases glucose uptake in cultured muscle cells and this effect is associated with multiple actions, including increased insulin receptor tyrosine kinase activity [171], enhanced glycogen synthesis [161] and augmented GLUT 4 transporter number and activity [172]. The drug acts by causing the translocation of GLUT 4 to the plasma membrane in muscle cells and adipocytes. Metformin activates the AMP-activated protein kinase, a major cellular regulator of lipid and glucose metabolism [173]. It up-regulates adenosine monophosphate kinase (AMPK) activity in muscle cells by stimulating AMPK phosphorylation in a dose-dependent manner. On the other hand, metformin did not alter IRS-1-associated PI3-kinase or AKT activity in skeletal muscle [174].

There is no effect of metformin on insulin receptor kinase activity in any studies of adipocytes [175]. The reason for this is unclear, because there was a significant effect of kinase activity in other systems [167]. Metformin did not have a significant additional effect on insulin receptor phosphorylation in the presence of insulin, either at low or high dose. Metformin is also as capable as the sulfonylureas in reducing HbA_{1C}. Other effects include a reduction in plasma triglyceride levels and low-density lipoprotein (LDL, the "bad") cholesterol levels by about 10% and lowers fatty acids. Metformin's mechanism of action includes decreased intestinal absorption of glucose.

Metformin is the only oral agent that when used as a monotherapy, has been reported to reduce the risk of developing macrovascular complications. Most patients treated with metformin lose weight or fail to gain weight. Metformin therapy is effective as a combination therapy with sulfonylurea [55]. Metformin has no direct effect on β-cell function. It also has no significant effect on the secretion of glucagon, cortisol, growth hormone, or somatostatin.

The peak plasma level of metformin when given as a single agent occurs within 4 hours, and the plasma elimination half-life approximates 6 hours. Absorption is reduced by food intake. Metformin is not metabolized, and is eliminated unchanged in the urine [58]. One attractive aspect of metformin during pregnancy is that it does not stimulate the fetal pancreas to secrete insulin [58].

Side effect can be a problem with metformin. Up to 30% of patients develop gastrointestinal complaints. Bloating, flatulence, diarrhea and abdominal discomfort and pain are major complications [21]. Although uncommon, lactic acidosis has been reported, with a frequency of 0,003% annually [55]. Less than 4% to 5% of patients cannot tolerate metformin therapy [176]. Because metformin does not increase secretion of insulin, hypoglycemia is rare in diabetic patients treated with metformin alone [176].

Contraindications for metformin include evidence of kidney disease, significant liver disease, chronic alcoholism or congestive heart failure. In elderly patients, an age-related decrease in glomerular filtration rate is often seen [55]. Weight gain does not occur in patients with type 2 diabetes who receive metformin alone or in combination with other oral agents or insulin [55].

Other Drugs

New drugs are in development, as for example: glucagon receptor antagonists and inhibitors of glycogen phosphorylase, pyruvate dehydrogenase kinase, fructose-1,6-bisphosphatase and glucose-6-phosphatase [2, 53 and 177].

INHIBITORS OF GLUCOSE UPTAKE

α-Glucosidase Inhibitors

Inhibition of α-glucosidases in the upper gastrointestinal tract limits the degradation of fructose to glucose and delays the breakdown oligosaccharides and disaccharides into monosaccharides [178, 179]. These drugs act as competitive, reversible inhibitors of pancreatic α-glucosidase and pancreatic α-amylase, which convert non adsorbable dietary starch and sucrose into absorbable glucose and hydrolyze complex starches, respectively [21]. The α-glucosidase inhibitors bind competitively to the oligosaccharide binding site of the α-glucosidase enzymes, thereby preventing enzymatic hydrolysis. By delaying digestion of carbohydrates, the absorption is shifted to more distal parts of the small intestine and colon. These inhibitors slow down the rate of carbohydrate absorption in the small intestine, which results primarily in a reduction in postprandial plasma glucose levels. Each drug is approved for use as monotherapy, which results in a significant reduction in fasting plasma glucose, postprandial glucose and HbA$_{1C}$, however clinical trials have shown that the hypoglycemic potency of α-glucosidase inhibitors is less than 50% than that of either sulfonylurea or metformin [178, 179]. By slowing down the digestive and absorptive process, α-glucosidase inhibitors retard glucose entry into the systemic circulation, allowing, the β-cell ample time to augment insulin secretion in response to the blunted increase in plasma glucose level.

These inhibitors do not affect insulin levels, so they do not cause hypoglycemia when used alone. Some but not all studies have reported small decreases in plasma triglyceride levels [180, 181] without a change in LDL or HDL cholesterol level with α-glucosidase inhibitors. It does not cause weight gain and does not significantly affect plasma lipid levels [55]. α-glucosidase inhibitors do not cause malabsorption. Acarbose must be ingested with the first bite of food because the drug must be present in small bowel with food to be effective [55]. α-glucosidase inhibitor is most useful in patients with new-onset type 2 diabetes who have mild fasting hyperglycemia. These medicines are not usually used for primary therapy unless a patient appears to have large increases blood glucose levels after meals [21]. The drugs in this group may be useful as monotherapy, but are typically used in combination with other oral antidiabetic agents (as for example sulfonylurea or metformin) and/or insulin.

Gastrointestinal side effects are common, affecting up to 30% of patients [21, 55]. Bloating, flatulence, diarrhea, abdominal discomfort and pain are major complaints. These side effects tend to diminish with continued drug use [55] and can be reduced due to eating less carbohydrate in the diet [21]. The α-glucosidase inhibitors have been available since 1996 and include acarbose and miglitol. The mechanism of action of these inhibitors is similar but not identical.

Acarbose

Acarbose (Precose), the first α-glucosidase inhibitor discovered, is a nitrogen-containing pseudotetrasaccharide. Its binding affinity for the α-glucosidase enzymes is: glycoamylase, sucrase, maltase, and dextranase [55]. Acarbose has little affinity for isomaltase and no affinity for lactase.

Miglitol

Miglitol (Glyset) is a synthetic analog of 1-deoxynojirimycin. It is a more potent inhibitor of sucrase and maltase that acarbose, has no effect on α-amylase, but does inhibit intestinal isomaltase. Miglitol does not seem to have any significant advantages over acarbose.

Other Drugs

New drugs are in development, as for example inhibitors of Na$^+$/glucose cotransporters. The low-affinity sodium glucose cotransporter (SGLT 2), which is expressed specifically in the kidney, plays a major role in renal glucose reabsorption. The inhibition of renal glucose reabsorption is a novel approach to the treatment of diabetes. Inhibition of the SGLTs is complicated by differences in two isoforms: SGLT 1 and SGLT 2. The high-affinity sodium glucose cotransporter SGLT 1 is highly expressed in the gastrointestinal tract. Several mutations in the human *SLC5A2* gene can cause renal glucosuria [194, 195] and mutations in the *SLC5A1* gene leading to a functional defect in SGLT 1 are responsible for glucose/galactose malabsorption [196, 197].

Sergliflozin

Katsuno and colleagues [198] have discovered sergliflozin, a prodrug of a novel selective DGLT 2 inhibitor, based on benzylphenol glucoside. In structure, it belongs to a new category of SGLT 2 inhibitors and differs from the phlorizin, a nonselective SGLT inhibitor. Sergliflozin-A (active form) is a highly selective and potent inhibitor of human SGLT 2. At pharmacological doses, sergliflozin and sergliflozin-A had no effects on facilitative glucose transporter 1 (GLUT 1). The obtained results indicate that selective inhibition of SGLT 2 increases urinary glucose excretion by inhibiting renal glucose reabsorption. Sergliflozin may provide a new and unique approach to the treatment of diabetes mellitus [198].

Dapagliflozin

Han and colleagues have identified dapagliflozin as a potent and selective inhibitor of the renal SGLT 2 [199]. *In vivo*, dapagliflozin reduces hyperglycemia in Zucker diabetic fatty rats after single oral doses. Once-daily dapagliflozin treatment over 2 weeks significantly lowered fasting and fed glucose levels. These data suggest that dapagliflozin has the potential to be an efficacious treatment for type 2 diabetes.

ENHANCERS OF INSULIN ACTION

Reduction of insulin resistance is necessary to improve the blood level in type 2 diabetic patients with obesity and insulin resistance.

The thiazolidinediones (TZDs) enhance insulin action in muscle, fat, and other tissues and are known as insulin sensitizers or as peroxisome proliferators-activated receptor γ (PPAR γ) agonists. They require the presence of insulin in order to work. Thiazolidinediones insulin sensitivity by activating certain genes is involved in fat synthesis and carbohydrate metabolism. These agents have a notable effect on improving insulin resistance, but have no effect on insulin secretion. TZDs cause a significant decrease in the release of free fatty acids from adipose tissue. This result is a significant decline in plasma levels of free fatty acids [183]. Hepatic glucose production is decreased although perhaps only at the highest doses [184]. Thiazolidinediones enhance the responsiveness and efficiency of β-cells; however they do not stimulate pancreatic islet cells to secrete more insulin, presumably by decreasing glucose and free fatty acid levels, both of which have deleterious effects on insulin secretion [185]. Obtained results suggest that thiazolidinediones may actually prolong β-cell survival [186].

Tumor necrosis factor-α (TNF-α) has been shown to be an important mediator of insulin resistance linked to obesity. This cytokine induces insulin resistance through inhibition of the tyrosine kinase activity of the insulin receptor. Thiazolidinediones have been shown to improve insulin resistance in obesity and non-insulin-dependent diabetes mellitus in both rodents and man. Thiazolidinediones essentially eliminate the reduction in tyrosine phosphorylation of insulin receptor and IRS-1 caused by TNF-α in fat cells. TZDs can specifically block certain actions of TNF-α related to insulin resistance [200]. Thiazolidinediones are strongly protein bound in circulation, predominantly to albumin [189, 190].

Adverse effects of TZDs include weight gain, which can be as great as or greater than that with sulfonylureas, and edema. Both weight gain and edema are more common in patients who receive thiazolidinediones with insulin. The weight gain may be due to a change in fat distribution with an increase in subcutaneous adipose fat and decrease in visceral fat, and mild to moderate edema (5% to 7% of patients treated with TZDs) is thought to be due to a decrease in renal excretion of sodium and an increase in sodium and free water retention [21]. Other adverse effects that may be expected when using the thiazolidinediones include upper respiratory tract infections, headaches and dilutional anemia due to an increase in plasma volume [191]. These drugs have also been linked to increased risk for bone fracture, especially in postmenopausal women [192].

Thiazolidinediones have been associated with an increase in aspartate aminotransferase and alanine aminotransferase greater than 3 times the upper limit of normal. TZDs should be used with caution in patients with already established liver diseases [187], and with peripheral edema [191]. Use of thiazolidinediones is contraindicated in pregnancy and lactation [193].

In 1997, troglitazone, a TZD, was introduced in the United States. It was withdrawn from US, European, and Japanese markets in March 2000 due to idiosyncratic hepatic reaction leading to hepatic failure [188].

No significant drug interactions have been reported with the thiazolidinediones [190]. They can be prescribed as monotherapy or in combination with metformin or sulfonylureas. Thiazolidinediones currently available include pioglitazone and rosiglitazone.

Pioglitazone

Pioglitazone (Actos) has a neutral effect on LDL-cholesterol, decreases triglycerides and increases HDL-cholesterol [187]. This agent reduces fasting plasma glucose levels and significantly decreases HbA_{1C}. GLUT 5 dramaticallyincreases in diabetic patients muscles. Pioglitazone treatment reverses this overexpression. The role of this fructose transporter expression in the insulin-enhancing effect of pioglitazone in muscle is unclear [201]. Pioglitazone is metabolized by CYP3A4 (190].

Rosiglitazone

This agent increases LDL-cholesterol, has no effect on triglycerides, and increases HDL-cholesterol [187]. Patients with type 2 diabetes treated with rosiglitazone had significant mean decreases in HbA_{1C} and fasting plasma glucose. Rosiglitazone was shown to significantly improve insulin sensitivity and reduce the rate of loss of β-cell function versus the metformin and glyburide [187]. It is metabolized by cytochrome P450 2 C8 [187].

NON-PHARMACEUTICAL THERAPY

Exercise, diet, and weight loss are the center of any therapeutic program. A controlled-energy diet and regular exercise are recommended for the majority of patients with type 2 diabetes mellitus, which are usually overweight.

EXERCISE AS A MODE OF THERAPY

Physical exercise is a non-pharmacological treatment for diabetes mellitus that can improve whole-body insulin sensitivity and glucose tolerance. Exercise training can positively moderate glucose homeostasis in patients with type 2 diabetes. Physical exercise enhances glucose transport and insulin action in the working skeletal muscle [202]. The increased skeletal glucose transport and insulin sensitivity may be a mechanism to explain evidence that regular exercise prevents or delays the onset of type 2 diabetes [203]. The molecular mechanisms of this important phenomenon are still not fully understood [204].

Skeletal muscle is a tissue that has a remarkable ability to adapt to external demands, such as exercise. During physical exercise, as an acute effect, the glucose uptake by the working muscles rises 7 to 20 times over the basal level [205]. Long-lasting physical training improves reduced peripheral tissue sensitivity to insulin in impaired glucose tolerance and type 2 diabetes [206]. Aerobic exercise such as walking is more effective than anaerobic exercise such as weight-lifting in increasing *in vivo* insulin sensitivity [207]. Plasma glucose levels can be lowered during aerobic exercise due to increased contraction-mediated glucose uptake [208, 209]. A single bout of exercise is sufficient to induce the expression of some metabolic genes [210] and in humans with diabetes mellitus can reduce hepatic glucose production [211]. Short-term aerobic exercise training in obese diabetic patients improves whole-body insulin sensitivity [212].

Numerous factors can contribute to the improvements in glucose homeostasis that are seen after physical exercise in patients with insulin resistance, as for example in patients with type 2 diabetes mellitus. These adaptive responses include enhanced glucose transport system, reduced hormone stimulation of hepatic glucose production, improved blood flow to skeletal muscle, and normalization of abnormal blood lipid profile [213].

Glucose transport into the skeletal muscle is regulated by insulin and insulin-like factors through the activation of an intracellular signaling pathway. Glucose transport into the myocyte is also stimulated by an insulin-independent mechanism that is activated by contractions [214, 215]. Exercise can cause potent systemic responses (e.g., hormones, catecholamines), which in turn could result in the activation of specific cell surface receptors [216, 217]. Strength training increases protein kinase B – α/β, and glycogen synthase in skeletal muscle in patients with type 2 diabetes. *SLC2A4* expression is increased also immediately following a single bout of exercise [210]. After 2 weeks of one-legged low-intensity training, a 26% increase was observed in total skeletal muscle crude membrane GLUT 4 content [219]. Stimulation of glucose transport by muscle contraction is largely mediated by translocation of the GLUT 4 from intracellular space to the plasma membrane (Fig. **1**). The increase in membrane permeability following exercise most likely reflects an increase in GLUT 4 protein associated with the plasma membrane [220]. Leg blood flow is higher in trained versus untrained legs [218].

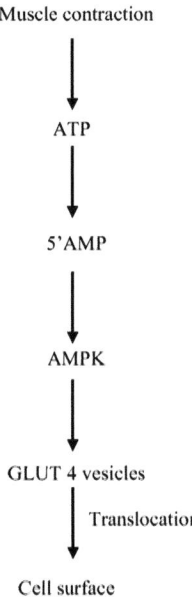

Figure 1: Intracellular signaling pathway involved in translocation of GLUT 4 to the cell surface in skeletal muscle [303, modified].

Stimulation of glucose transport by muscle contraction as well as insulin is largely mediated by translocation of the glucose transporter GLUT 4 from intracellular sites to the plasma membrane. The increase in membrane permeability to glucose following exercise most likely reflects an increase in GLUT 4 protein associated with the plasma membrane. This insulin-like effect on muscle glucose transport induced by muscle contraction, however, reverses rapidly after exercise is stopped [220]. The short-term (5 – 10 days) exercise training increases GLUT 4 expression in human skeletal muscle [221 – 223]. In rat, exercise has been show to increase transcription of the *Slc2a4* gene in skeletal muscle 1,8 fold when measured 3 h after exercise [224]. The GLUT 4 mRNA levels are increased in human skeletal muscle immediately and 3 h after a single exercise about at 70 – 75% [225], suggesting increased GLUT 4 transcription and/or enhanced mRNA stability [226]. In human skeletal muscle GLUT 4 was increased after 7 days of exercise training [216]. The exercise bouts at ~ 40% and ~ 80% increased GLUT 4 mRNA and GLUT 4 protein in human skeletal muscle to a similar extent, despite differences in exercise intensity and duration [227].

The molecular mechanism responsible for increased GLUT 4 transcription after exercise have been fully elucidated, but increased sarcoplasmic calcium and altered energy status play important roles, with the Ca^{2+}/calmodulin dependent kinase (CaMK) and AMP-activated protein kinase (AMPK) being key links between these stimuli and GLUT 4 transcriptional activation [228]. Increases in GLUT 4 protein have been also observed during recovery from a single exercise bout, suggesting activation of posttranscriptional processes [229].

From transgenic studies, it has been established that two conserved regions on the *Slc2A4* gene promoter are required for normal Glut 4 expression in the skeletal muscle. The first proximal region contains a binding site for the myocyte enhancer factor 2 (MEF2) [230]. The second region, termed domain 1, contains a binding domain for the Glut-4 enhancer factor (GEF) [231]. The MEF2 and GEF physically interact to regulate the *SLC2A4* gene [232]. The MEF2 appears to be important, since the elevated Glut 4 levels in response to increased calcium and AMPK activation were associated with increased expression of MEF2 [228]. Given that MEF2 is a transcription factor required for many exercise responsive genes, it is possible that these mechanisms are responsible for regulating the expression of a variety of metabolic genes during exercise [210].

The MEF2 family of transcription factors consists of four isoforms termed A, B, C and D, with the exception of MEF2B, being highly expressed in mature skeletal muscle. A number of MEF2 isoforms are expressed in skeletal muscle (MEF2A, MEF2C, and MEF2D) and all members of the MyoD family have the capacity to participate in the activity of the Glut 4 enhancer. The muscle-specific enhancer of Glut 4 is fibre-type-dependent and innervation-independent [224, 233].

In the basal state, MEF2 is associated with the class II histone deacetylase (HDAC) transcriptional repressor, which includes isoforms 4, 5, 7 and 9 [210, 234]. During exercise, phosphorylation of HDAC5 by adenosine monophosphate-activated protein kinase results in the dissociation from MEF2 and nuclear export. Therefore, the exercise reduces MEF2 association with the transcriptional repressor histone deacetylase 5 and increases MEF2-DNA binding [210, 235]. These molecular events contribute to enhanced Glut 4 transcription.

Another potential transcriptional coactivator expressed in skeletal muscle that could play a role in MEF2 regulation is the peroxisome proliferators-activated receptor gamma coactivator 1 α (PGC-1α), which is thought to be involved in the transcriptional response to exercise [210]. PGC-1α associates with MEF2 presumably to recruit cofactors with HAT (histone acetyl transferase) activity to MEF2. Exercise increases p38 mitogen-protein kinase (MAPK) phosphorylation and association with MEF2. The p38 MAPK phosphorylates MEF2 on threonine residues. These events result in enhanced MEF2 transcriptional activity [210]. Acute exercise induces glucose transport also through GLUT 4 translocation, in an additive manner to insulin action in skeletal muscle [236]. Exercise training leads to enhanced insulin sensitivity, which appears to be mediated by increased post-receptor insulin signaling, specifically at the distal steps of the insulin/PI 3-kinase signaling cascade. Studies in human skeletal muscle do not support at paradigm that exercise training increases expression of the proteins that comprise the pathway, but exercise training does enhance insulin-mediated phosphorylation and protein activation. Although exercise generally exerts a positive effect on insulin sensitivity, it may paradoxically promote insulin resistance if it causes disruption of muscle-cell integrity. The cellular mechanism associated with exercise-induced insulin resistance appears to be related to the acute-phase response and increased TNF-α secretion [237].

After an exercise bout, a decrease in the circulating insulin level is observed. This result together with the observation that acute exercise induces glucose transport through GLUT 4 translocation suggests that exercise induces an insulin-insensitive stimulation of glucose uptake in skeletal muscle. It persists 3 – 6 h after the exercise session [238].

Two elements have been proposed as contributors to the contraction-induced glucose uptake [224]. The first one is the metabolite AMP, produced as a result of ATP hydrolysis during muscle contraction and the second one is Ca^{2+} release from sarcoplasmatic reticulum stores upon depolarization of membranes at the transverse tubules. AMP induces AMPK, while Ca^{2+} is involved in the activation of some PKC isoforms [224].

The exercise and muscle contraction induce the activity of AMPK and numerous additional results indicate that AMPK could be partially involved in exercise-induced glucose uptake in skeletal muscle (discussed in [224]). The increase in cytoplasmic Ca^{2+} has been considered the mediator or initiator of contraction-stimulated glucose transport in skeletal muscle [239]. Recent studies indicate that both acute exercise [240] and endurance exercise [241] activate calcium-independent PKC isoforms (PKC ζ /λ) in human skeletal muscle. The activation of atypical forms of PKC has been implicated in the stimulation of muscle glucose transport by exercise, independently of PI 3-kinase activity [224].

McGee and Hargreaves [210] suggest that increasing GLUT 4 in skeletal muscle could be an effective therapy in the treatment and management of disease states such as insulin resistance and type 2 diabetes mellitus.

The diabetic heart exhibits enhanced sensitivity to ischemic-reperfusion injury [242, 243]. Studies have shown that diabetes is associated with a decrease in the number of sarcolemmal glucose transporters [244]. Exercise training of diabetic subjects has been shown to improve the recovery of contractive function after a period of ischemia and reperfusion [245]. In nondiabetic animals, the myocardial glucose uptake during rest and exercise is significantly increased after exercise training [246]. Exercise training of diabetic rats enhances glucose oxidation rates of diabetic hearts [247], attenuates the reduction in whole heart GLUT 4 levels [248] and increases sarcolemmal GLUT 4 and mRNA content [249]. By Osborn and colleagues [249] enhanced ability of the exercise trained heart to utilize glucose may exert a protective effect in the event of an ischemic episode.

Exercise training of animals with normal signaling leads to an enhancement of specific steps in the insulin signaling cascade, including increased mRNA, protein expression and GLUT 4 translocation. Insulin signaling involves rapid phosphorylation of insulin receptor (IR), insulin receptor substrate-1 and -2 (IRS-1and IRS-2) and the activation of phosphatidylinositol 3-kinase (PI3-kinase) [250]. Exercise and contraction of hindlimb muscles have no effect on tyrosine phosphorylation of the insulin receptor and IRS-1 or PI3-kinase activity [251].

There are different signals leading to glucose transport by insulin and exercise in skeletal muscle [204]. Numerous studies have investigated the hypothesis that MAP kinase (AMP-activated protein kinase) signal transduction pathways play an important role in exercise signaling.

MAP kinase is a member of a protein kinase family consisting of 12 molecules expressed in all eukaryotic cells and include the extracellular signal-regulated kinase 1 and 2 (ERK 1/2), the c-Jun NH_2-terminal kinase (JNK), p38 and extracellular signal-regulated kinase 5 (ERK 5) [217]. Signaling within the MAP kinase pathway involves the sequential phosphorylation and activation of a MAP kinase kinase kinase (MAPKKK), a MAP kinase kinase (MAPKK) and a MAP kinase.

Upstream signaling to ERK 1 /2, is the first MAP kinase signaling pathway to be characterized in mammalian cells, including Raff, the most well-defined MAPKKK for ERK 1/2. ERK 1 and ERK 2 can translocate to the nucleus, where they can phosphorylate a variety of transcription factors [217].

MAP kinase is activated by an increase in the AMP-to-ATP and creatine-to-phosphocreatine ratios via a complex mechanism [252]. When the cell has decreased ATP levels, MAP kinase acts to switch off ATP-consuming pathways and switch on alternative pathways for ATP regeneration [204]. Muscle contractions alter the fuel status of skeletal muscle. There can be significant decreases in both phosphocreatine and ATP concentrations, thus MAP kinase is activated in rat in response to exercise *in vivo* [253]. Muscle contractions lead to activation of ERK 1/2, isoforms of MAP kinase [254]. Moderate-intensity aerobic exercise, as well as high-intensity exercise, increase skeletal muscle MAP kinase activity [255, 256].

Exercise activates ERK 1/2, JNK, and p38 signaling in skeletal muscle [254]. Activation of ERK 1/2 signaling has been reported in rat skeletal muscle in response to *in vivo* and *in situ* contraction [257 – 260], stretch [261], in mouse muscle [262] and in human skeletal muscle in response to physical exercise [263]. Activation of JNK signaling has been reported in rat skeletal muscle to *in vitro* and *in situ* contractions [261, 264]. In human subjects, JNK is activated, for example, in response to cycle ergometer exercise [265] and marathon running [266]. Activation of p38 has been reported in rat skeletal muscle in response to *in vitro* and *in vivo* contractions [267, 268] and mechanical stretch [261]. p38 signaling increases in humans during cycle ergometer exercise [269] and marathon running [266].

Early studies suggested that the ERK 1/2 signaling cascade is involved in the regulation of both glucose transport and glycogen metabolism [270]. Initial evidence in support of a role for MAP kinase in contraction-stimulated glucose transport came from studies using AICAR. AICAR is a compound that is taken up into skeletal muscle and metabolized by adenosine kinase to the monophosphorylated derivative that mimics the effects of AMP on MAP kinase [271]. It can stimulate glucose transport in the absence of insulin, similar to the effects of contraction [271]. Exercise training upregulates GLUT 4 protein expression [210, 272 and 273], and increases GLUT 4 translocation [273] and cell surface [274] after insulin stimulation.

Contraction of skeletal muscle fibers depends on the release of calcium ions from the sarcoplasmic reticulum. The increase in intracellular calcium concentrations has been proposed to be a signal in the initiation of contraction-stimulated glucose transport and GLUT 4 translocation [231, 276]. The mechanism by which calcium might regulate exercise-stimulated glucose transport is unknown. One or more of the calcium-regulated intracellular proteins may lead to GLUT 4 translocation. Potential candidates include calmodulin, the calmodulin-dependent protein kinases (CaMK), and the protein kinase C (PKC) family [204].

DIET AND WEIGHT LOSS AS A MODE OF THERAPY

A diet high in fat and low in carbohydrate reduces the respiratory exchange ratio, indicating increased fat oxidation [277]. In the late 1960s, it was discovered that diets high in carbohydrate increased muscle glycogen concentrations and resulted in glycogen stores up to twice the normal resting level [278]. The results obtained by Coyle and colleagues suggest that dietary fat has an important role to play after exercise, in that it helps to restore intramuscular fat stores [279]. Chronic high fat diets have been shown to result in a shift towards fat metabolism. These diets have been shown to result in increases in β-hydroxy-acyl-CoA dehydrogenase activity, fatty acid-binding protein content in the sarcolemma and decreases in hexokinase activity [280, 281].

Macronutrient content and composition of the diet strongly influence glucose transport into muscle and adipose cells by altering both the expression of the *SLC2A1* and *SLC2A4* genes, and the functional activity of the gene products, GLUT 1 and GLUT 4. Dietary regulation of glucose transporters is tissue specific [282]. Nutrient content has profound effects on *in vivo* glucose disposal and on glucose transport in muscle and fat tissue [283 – 286]. In adipocytes from rats on different diets, there are marked changes in the expression of the *SLC2A4* gene, whereas in skeletal muscle there are smaller changes in *SLC2A4* expression and apparently greater alterations in the functional activity of GLUT 4 [285].

It is known that high fat diet results in insulin resistant glucose uptake *in vivo* [283]. In adipose cells from obese rats (obesity was due to high fat feeding and high calorie feeding), glucose transport after insulin stimulation was reduced only in adipocytes from the high fat fed rats [282]. The changes in glucose transport in adipocytes were associated with alterations in expression of *SLC2A1* and *SLC2A4*. In high fat fed rats, GLUT 4 protein levels were decreased by > 90% and GLUT 1 protein was decreased by 62% [282]. Levels of GLUT 4 protein in skeletal muscle were reduced by 34% in high fat fed rats, and levels of GLUT 1 mRNA were reduced [282]. High fat feeding also impairs insulin-stimulated GLUT 4 recruitment [298]. High fat diet is known to reduce both GLUT 2 and glucokinase expression thereby impairing glucose-stimulated insulin secretion and induces oxidative stress and apoptosis which reduces β-cell mass and comprises β-cell function [299].

By American Diabetes Association (ADA), major nutrient recommendations are [287, 288]:

- Reduce the amount of dietary fat. The current ADA guidelines advise that less than 7% of calories should come from saturated fat. Saturated fat is linked to low density lipoprotein (LDL, "bad") cholesterol. Dietary cholesterol should be less than 200 mg/day. Total fat should be 30% to 35% of total calories. Polyunsaturated fat is limited to 10% and monounsaturated fat to 20% of total calories.

- Protein intake accounts for 15% - 20% of total calories consumed among the general populations as well as those with diabetes.

- Simple sugars are more rapidly digested and absorbed than starches. They are more likely to cause high sugar levels, therefore choices should come from whole-grain breads, fruits, vegetables etc.

- Dietary fiber recommendations for diabetic patients are the same as for healthy subjects; 20 to 30 grams for a wide variety of sources daily.

Obesity is a major risk factor for development of diabetes [289, 300 and 301], because it is characterized by a reduced number of insulin receptors and insulin resistance [290, 291] which is reversible with weight loss [292, 293]. Obesity and weight gain can increase risk for diabetes by greater than ninety fold [294].

Among women of average BMI, 23 – 23, 9 kg/m^2, the relative risk of type 2 diabetes mellitus is 3,6 times than that of women having BMI less than 22 kg/m^2. For an increase of 20 – 35 kg, the relative risk is 11,3, and for an increase more than 35 kg, the relative risk is 17,3 [295].

Very-low-energy diets decrease fasting plasma glucose values by ~ 50% within two weeks. Twelve weeks of energy-restricted diets are associated with these significant decreases of body weight, serum cholesterol and serum triglycerides [294]. Obese patients with type 2 diabetes mellitus, who were advised to lower their carbohydrate intake to 20%, over 6 months achieved significantly better control of hyperglycemia and body weight than a control group of similar patients [296].

Weight management may be the most important therapeutic task for most obese type 2 diabetic individuals [294]. The majority of cases of type 2 diabetes could be prevented by the adoption of a healthier lifestyle [297, 302].

REFERENCES

[1]   Chakrabarti R, Rajagopalan R. Diabetes and insulin resistance associated disorders: Disease and the therapy. Curr Sci 2002;83,12:1533-1538

[2]   Wagman AS, Nuss JM. Current therapies and emerging targets for the treatment of diabetes. Curr Pharm Des 2001;7:417-450

[3]   Bangstad H-J, Danne T, Deeb L, Jarosz-Chobot P, Urakami T, Hanas R. Insulin treatment in children and adolescent with diabetes. Ped Diab 2009;10,Suppl.12:82-99

[4]   Virkamaki A, Ueki K, Kahn CR. Protein-protein interaction in insulin signaling and the molecular mechanisms of insulin resistance. J Clin Invest 1999;103:931-943

[5]   Saltiel AR, Kahn CR. Insulin signaling and the regulation of glucose and lipid metabolism. Nature 2001;414:799-806

[6]   Barthel A, Schmoll D. Novel concepts in insulin regulation of hepatic gluconeogenesis. Am J Physiol Endocrinol Metab 2003;285:E685-E692

[7]   Dentin R, Liu Y, Koo S-H, *et al.* Insulin modulates gluconeogenesis by inhibition of the coactivator TORC2. Nature 2007;449:366-370

[8]   Ciaraldi TP, Phillips SA, Carter L, Aroda V, Mudaliar S, Henry RR. Effects of the rapid-acting insulin analog glulisine on cultured human skeletal muscle cells: comparison with insulin and insulin-like growth factor I. J Clin Endocrinol Metab 2005;90:5551-5558

[9]   Rakatzi I, Seipke G, Eckel J. {LysB3, GluB29} insulin: a novel insulin analog with enhanced β-cell protective action. Biochem Biophys Res Commun 2003;310:852-859

[10]   Stumvoll M, Goldstein BJ, van Haeften TW. Type 2 diabetes: principles of pathogenesis and therapy. Lancet 2005;365:1333-1346

[11]   Tibaldi J, Rakel RE. Why, when and how to initiate insulin therapy in patients with type 2 diabetes. Int J Clin Pract 2007;61:633-644

[12]   Mudaliar S, Edelman SV. Insulin therapy in type 2 diabetes. Endocrinol Metab Clin North Am 2001;30:935-982

[13]   Raja-Khan N, Warehime SS, Gabbay RA. Review of biphasic insulin aspart in the treatment of type 1 and type 2 diabetes. Vasc Health Risk Manag 2007;3,6:919-935

[14]   Agarwal JK, Bhadada SK, Sahay RK, Jyotsna VP. Modulators of insulin action. Int J Diab Dev Countries 2000;20:68-72

[15]   Ahmad B. Pharmacology of insulin. Br J Diab Vasc Dis 2004;4:10-14

[16]   Yadav S, Parakh A. Insulin therapy. Indian Pediatr 2006;43:863-872

[17]   Brange J, Ribel U, Hansen JF, *et al.* Monomeric insulins obtained by protein engineering and their medical implications. Nature 1988;333:679-682

[18]   Brange J, Owens DR, Kang S, Volund A. Monomeric insulins and their experimental and clinical implications. Diabetes Care 1990;13:923-954

[19]   Schmid H. New options in insulin therapy. J Pediatr (Rio J) 2007;83,Suppl.5:S146-S154

[20]   Brens DN, Alter LA, Beckage MJ, *et al.* Altering the association properties of insulin by amino acid replacement. Protein Eng 1992;5:527-533

[21]   Modi P. Diabetes beyond insulin: review of new drugs for treatment of diabetes mellitus. Curr Drug Disc Technol 2007;4:39-47

[22]   Bolli GB, Di Marchi RD, Park GD, Pramming S, Koivisto VA. Insulin analogues and their potential in the management of diabetes mellitus. Diabetologia 1999;42:1151-1167

[23]   Radziuk JM, Davis JC, Pye WS, *et al.* Bioavailability and bioeffectiveness of subcutaneous human insulin and two it's analogues- LysB28, ProB29-human insulin and AspB10, LysB28, ProB29-human insulin-assessed in a conscious pig model. Diabetes 1997;46:548-556

[24]   Fineberg SE, Fineberg NS, Anderson JH, *et al.* Insulin immune response to LYSPRO human insulin therapy in insulin native type 1 and type 2 patients. Diabetologia 1995;38,Suppl.1:A4

[25]   Somwar R, Sweeny G, Ramlal T, Klip A. Stimulation of glucose and amino acid transport and activation of the insulin signaling pathways by insulin lispro in L6 skeletal muscle cells. Clin Ther 1998;20:125-140

[26]   Kurtzhals P, Schaffer L, Sorensen A, *et al.* Correlations of receptor binding and metabolic and mitogenic potencies of insulin analogs designed for clinical use. Diabetes 2000;49,6:999-1005

[27]   Bhattacharyya A, Brown S, Hughes S, Vice PA. Insulin Lispro and regular insulin in pregnancy. QJM 2001;94,5:255-260

[28]   Schernthaner G, Wein W, Sandholzer K, *et al.* Post prandial insulin lispro. A therapeutic option for type 1 diabetic patients. Diabetes Care 1998;21:570-573

[29]   Mudaliar SR, Lindberg FA, Joyce M, *et al.* Insulin aspart (B28 asp-insulin): a fast-acting analog of human insulin: absorption kinetics and action profile compared with regular human insulin in healthy nondiabetic subjects. Diabetes Care 1999;22,9:1501-1506

[30]   Kang S, Brange J, Burch A, Volund A, Owens DR. Absorption kinetics and action profiles of subcutaneously administered insulin analogues (AspB9, GluB27, AspB10, AspB28) in healthy subjects. Diabetes Care 1991;14:1057-1065

[31]   Raskin P, Guthrie RA, Lerter L, Riis A, Jovanovic L. Use of insulin aspart, a fast-acting insulin analog as the mealtime insulin in the management of patients with type 1 diabetes. Diabetes Care 2000;23,5:583-585

[32]   Brunner GA, Hirschberger S, Sendlhofer G, *et al.* Post-prandial administration of the insulin analogue insulin aspart in patients with Type 1 diabetes. Diabet Med 2000;17,5:371-375

[33]   Jacobsen LV, Sogaard B, Riss A. Pharmacokinetics and pharmacodynamics of a premixed formulation of soluble and protamine-retarded insulin aspart. Eur J Clin Pharmacol 2000;56:399-403

[34]   Hermansen K, Colombo M, Storgarrd H, *et al.* Improved postprandial glycemic control with biphasic insulin aspart relative to and biphasic insulin lispro and biphasic human insulin in patients with type 2 diabetes. Diabetes Care 2002;25:883-888

[35]   Becker RHA, Frick AD. Clinical pharmacokinetics and pharmacodynamics of insulin glulisine. Clin Pharmacokinet 2008;46,1:7-20

[36]   Girish C, Manikandan S, Jayanthi M. Newer insulin analogues and inhaled insulin. Indian J Med Sci 2006;60:117-123

[37]   Garnock-Jones KP, Plosker GL. Insulin glulisine: a review of its use in the management of diabetes mellitus. Drugs 2009;69,8:1035-1057

[38]   Hennige AM, Lehmann R, Weigert C, *et al.* Insulin glulisine. Insulin receptor signaling characteristics in vivo. Diabetes 2005;54:361-366

[39]   Hohberg C, Forst T, Larbig T, *et al.* Effect of insulin on microvascular blood flow and endothelial function in the postprandial state. Diabetes Care 2008;31:1021-1025

[40]   Stammberg I, Seipke G, Bartels T. Insulin glulisine – a comprehensive preclinical evaluation. Int J Toxicol 2006;25,1:25-33

[41]   Starke AAR, Heinemann L, Howman A, *et al.* The action profiles of human NPH insulin preparation. Diab Med 1989;6:239-244

[42]   Barnett AH. A review of basal insulins. Diab Med 2003;20:873-885

[43]   Home PD, Barriocanal L, Lindholm A. Comparative pharmacokinetics and pharmacodynamics of the novel rapid-acting insulin analogue, insulin aspart, in healthy volunteers. Eur J Clin Pharmacol 1999;55:199-203

[44]   Lepore M, Pampanelli S, Fanelli C, *et al.* Pharmacokinetics and pharmacodynamics of subcutaneous injection of long-acting human insulin analog glargine, NPH insulin, and ultralente human insulin and continuous subcutaneous infusion of insulin lispro. Diabetes 2000;49,12:2142-2148

[45]   Carielo A. postprandial hyperglycemia and diabetes complications: is it time to treat? Diabetes 2005;54:1-7

[46]   Plank J, Bodenlenz M, Sinner F, *et al.* A double-blind, randomized, dose-response study investigating the pharmacodynamic and pharmacokinetic properties of the long-acting insulin analog detemir. Diabetes Care 2005;28:1107-1112

[47]   Danne T, Datz N, Endahl L, *et al.* Insulin detemir is characterized by a more reproducible pharmacokinetic profile than insulin glargine in children and adolescent with type 1 diabetes: result from a randomized, double-blind, controlled trial. Pediatr Diab 2008;9:554-560

[48]   Rees-Jones RW, Taylor SI. An endogenous substrate for the insulin receptor-associated tyrosine kinase. J Biol Chem 1985;260:4461-4467

[49]   Accili D, Perrotti N, Rees-Jones R, Taylor SI. Tissue distribution and subcellular localization of an endogenous substrate (pp120) for the insulin receptor-associated tyrosine kinase. Endocrinol 1986;119:1274-1280

[50]   Najjar SM. Regulation of insulin action by CEACAM1. TRENDS Endocrinol Metab 2002;13,6:240-245

[51]   Virally M, Blicklé J-F, Girard J, Halimi S, Simon D, Guillausseau P-I. Type 2 diabetes mellitus: epidemiology, pathophysiology, unmet needs the therapeutical perspectives. Diab Metab 2007;33:231-244

[52]   Marion M. Diabetes drugs: sulfonylureas.
http: //www.diabetesselfmanagement.com/blog/mark-marino/diabetes-drugs-sulfonylureas

[53]   Morral N. Novel targets and therapeutic strategies for type 2 diabetes. TRENDS Endocrinol Metab 2003;14,4:169-175

[54]   Raptis SA, Dimitriadis GD. Oral hypoglycemic agents: insulin secretagogues, α-glucosidase inhibitors and insulin sensitizers. Exp Clin Endocrinol Diabetes 2001;109:S265-S287

[55]   DeFronzo RA. Pharmacologic therapy for type 2 diabetes mellitus. Ann Intern Med 1999;131:281-303

[56]   Bell DSH. Practical considerations and guidelines for dosing sulfonylureas as monotherapy or combination therapy. Clin Ther 2004;26:1714-1727

[57]   Mitrakou A, Kelley D, Mokan M, *et al.* Role of reduced suppression of glucose production and early insulin release in impaired glucose tolerance. N Engl J Med 1992;326:22-29

[58]   Yogev Y, Langer O. The use of anti-hyperglycaemic and hypoglycaemic agents in pregnancy. Fetal Mat Med Rev 2004;15,2:133-143

[59]   Medications. Sulfonylureas. http://www.diabetesnet.com/diabetes_treatments/sulfonylureas.php

[60]   Vestergaard H, Weinreb JE, Rosen AS, *et al.* Sulfonylurea therapy improves glucose disposal without changing skeletal muscle GLUT4 levels in noninsulin-dependent diabetes mellitus: A longitudinal study. J Clin Endocrinol Metab 1995;80:270-275

[61]   Tsiani E, Ramlal T, Leiter LA, Klip A, Fantus G. Stimulation of glucose uptake and increased plasma membrane content of glucose transporters in L6 skeletal muscle cells by the sulfonylureas Gliclazide and Glyburide. Endocrinol 1995;136:2505-2512

[62]   Imamura H, Morimota I, Tanaka Y, *et al.* Regulation of glucose transporter expression by gliclazide in rat L6 myoblasts. Diab Nutr Metab 2001;14:308-314

[63]   Lebovitz HE. Insulin secretagogues: old and new. Diabetes Rev 1999;7:139-153

[64]   Clark CM Jr, Goldberg RB. Glimepiride dosing and efficacy: Results of placebo-controlled, dose-regimen, and active controlled trials. Postgrad Med Special Rep 1997;June:45-56

[65]   Rorsman P. Insulin secretion: function and therapy of pancreatic beta-cells in diabetes. Br J Diabetes Vasc Dis 2005;5:187-191

[66]   Ashcroft SJH, Ashcroft FM. The sulfonylurea receptor. Biochim Biophys Acta 1992;1175:45-59

[67]   Philipson LH, Steiner DF. Pas de deux or more: the sulfonylurea receptors and K^+ channels. Science 1995;268:372-373

[68]   Proks P, Reimann F, Green N, Gribble F, Ashcroft F. Sulfonylurea stimulation of insulin secretion. Diabetes 2002;51,Suppl.1:S368-S376

[69]   Ashcroft FM, Gribble FM. ATP-sensitive K^+ channels and insulin secretion: their role in health and disease. Diabetologia 1999;42:903-919

[70]   Trucker SJ, Gribble FM, Zhao C, Trapp S, Ashcroft FM. Truncation of Kir6.2 produces ATP-sensitive K-channels in the absence of the sulfonylurea receptor. Nature 1997;387:179-181

[71]   Inagaki N, Gonoi T, Clement JP, *et al.* A family of sulfonylurea receptors determines the properties of ATP-sensitive K^+ channels. Neuron 1996;16:1011-1017

[72]   Müller G. The molecular mechanism of the insulin-mimetic/sensitizing activity of the antidiabetic sulfonylurea drug Amaryl. Mol Med 2000;6,11:907-934

[73]   Aguilar-Bryan L, Bryan L. Molecular biology of adenosine triphosphate-sensitive potassium channels. Endocr Rev 1999;20:101-135

[74]   Shi H, Moustaid-Moussa N, Wilkinson WO, Zemel MB. Role of the sulfonylurea receptor in regulating human adipocyte metabolism. FASEB J 1999;13:1833-1838

[75]   Winkler M, Stephen D, Bieger S, Kühner P, Wolff F, Quast U. Testing the bipartite model of the sulfonylurea receptor binding site: binding of A-, B-, and A + B-site ligands. J Pharm Exp Ther 2007;322:701-708

[76]   Holst JJ. The physiology of glucagon-like peptide 1. Physiol. Rev 2007;87:1409-1439

[77]   McIntyre N, Holdsworth CD, Turner DS. New interpretation of oral glucose tolerance. Lancet 1964;11:20-21

[78]   Perley M, Kipnis DM. Plasma insulin responses to oral and intravenous glucose: study in normal and diabetic subjects. J Clin Invest 1967;46:1954-1962

[79]   Kim W, Egan JM. The role of incretins in glucose homeostasis and diabetes treatment. Pharmacol Rev 2008;60,4:470-512

[80]   Gagliardino JJ. Physiological endocrine control of energy homeostasis and postprandial blood glucose levels. Europ Rev Med Pharmacol Sc 2005;9:75-92

[81]   Drucker DJ. The biology of incretin hormones. Cell Metab 2006;3:153-165

[82]   Drucker DJ. The role of gut hormones in glucose homeostasis. J Clin Invest 2007;117:24-32

[83]   Neary MT, Batterham RL. Gut hormones: Implications for the treatment of obesity. Pharmacol Therap 2009;124:44-56

[84]   Vilsbøll T, Holst JJ. Incretins, insulin secretion and Type 2 diabetes mellitus. Diabetologia 2004;47:357-366

[85]   Geelhoed-Duijvestijn LM. Incretis: a new treatment option for type 2 diabetes? Netherlands J Med 2007;65,2:60-64

[86]   Triplitt C, McGill JB, Porte D Jr, Conner CS. The changing landscape of type 2 diabetes: the role of incretin-based therapies in managed care outcomes. J Manag Care Pharm 2007;13:S2-S16

[87]   Nicolucci A, Rossi MC. Incretin-based therapies: a new potential treatment approach to overcome clinical inertia in type 2 diabetes. Acta Biomed 2008;79:184-191

[88]   Drucker DJ, Nauck MA. The incretin system: glucagon-like peptide-1 receptor agonists and dipeptidyl peptidase-4 inhibitors in type 2 diabetes. Lancet 2006;368:1696-1705

[89]   Vilsbøll T, Krarup T, Madsbad S, Holst JJ. Defective amplification of the late phase insulin response to glucose by GIP in obese Type 2 diabetic patients. Diabetologia 2002;45:1111-1119

[90]   Wajchenberg BL. β-cell failure in diabetes and preservation by clinical treatment. Endocrine Rev 2007;28:187-218

[91]   Gautier JF, Fetita S, Sobngwi E, Salaün-Martin C. Biological actions of the incretins GIP and GLP-1 and therapeutic perspectives in patients with type 2 diabetes. Diabetes Metab 2005;31:233-242

[92]   Bell GI. The glucagon superfamily: precursors structure and gene organization. Peptides 1986:7:27-36

[93]   White JW, Saunders GF. Structure of the human glucagon gene. Nucleic Acids Rec 1986;14:4719-4730

[94]   Novak U, Wilks A, Buell G, McEwen S. Identical mRNA for preproglucagon in pancreas and gut. Eur J Biochem 1987;164:553-558

[95]   Drucker DJ, Asa S. Glucagon gene expression in vertebrate brain. J Biol Chem 1988;263:13475-13478

[96]   Baggio LL, Drucker DJ. Biology of incretins: GLP-1 and GIP. Gastroenterol 2007;132:2131-2157

[97]   Herrmann C, Göke R, Richter G, Fehmann HC, Arnold R , Göke B. Glucagon-like peptide-1 and glucose-dependent insulin-releasing polypeptide plasma levels in response to nutrients. Digestion 1995;56:117-126

[98]   Kreymann B, Williams G, Ghatei MA, Bloom SR. Glucagon-like peptide-1 7-36: a physiological incretin in man. Lancet 1987;2:1300-1304

[99]   Van Gaal LF, Gutkin SW, Nauck MA. Exploiting the antidiabetic properties of incretins to treat type 2 diabetes mellitus: glucagon-like peptide-1 receptor agonists or insulin for patients with inadequate glycemic control. Eur J Endocrinol 2008;158,6:773-784

[100] Zander M, Madsbad S, Madsen JL, Holst JJ. Effect of 6-week course of glucagon-like peptide 1 on glycaemic control, insulin sensitivity, and beta-cell function in type 2 diabetes: a parallel-group study. Lancet 2002;359:824-830

[101] Toft-Nielsen MB, Madsbad S, Holst JJ. Continuous subcutaneous infusion of glucagon-like peptide-1 lowers plasma glucose and reduces appetite in type 2 diabetic patients. Diabetes Care 1999;22:1137-1143

[102] Willms B, Werner J, Holst JJ, Orskov C, Creutzfeldt W, Nauck MA. Gastric emptying, glucose responses, and insulin secretion after a liquid test meal: effects of exogenous glucagon-like peptide-1 (GLP-1)-(7-36) amide in type 2 (noninsulin-dependent) diabetic patients. J Clin Endocrinol Metab 1996;81:327-332

[103] Farilla L, Hui H, Bertolotto C, *et al.* Glucagon-like peptide-1 promotes islet cell growth and inhibits apoptosis in Zucker diabetic rats. Endocrinol 2002;143:4397-4408

[104] Perfetti R, Zhou J, Doyle ME, Egan JM. Glucagon-like peptide-1 induces cell proliferation and pancreatic-duodenum homeobox-1 expression and increases endocrine cell mass in the pancreas of old, glucose-intolerant rats. Endocrinol 2000;141:4600-4605

[105] Stoffers DA, Kieffer TJ, Hussain MA, *et al.* Insulinotropic glucagon-like peptide 1 agonists stimulate expression of homeodomain protein IDX-1 and increase islet size in mouse pancreas. Diabetes 2000;49:741-748

[106] Toft-Nielsen MB, Damholt MB, Madsbas S, *et al.* Determinants of the impaired secretion of glucagon-like peptide-1 in type 2 diabetes. J Clin Endocrinol Metab 2001;86:3717-3723

[107] Holst JJ. Glucagon-like peptide-1, a gastrointestinal hormone with a pharmaceutical potential. Curr Med Chem 1999;6:1005-1017

[108] Gallwitz B. New therapeutic strategies for the treatment of type 2 diabetes mellitus based on incretins. Rev Diab Studies 2005;2,2:61-69

[109] Bosi E, Lucotti P, Setola E, Monti L, Piatti PM. Incretin-based therapies in type 2 diabetes: A review of clinical results. Diabetes Res Clin Pract 2008;82,Suppl.2:S102-S107

[110] Pratley RE, Gilbert M. Targeting incretins in type 2 diabetes: role of GLP-1 receptor agonists and DPP-4 inhibitors. Rev Diab Studies 2008;5,2:73-94

[111] Eng J, Kleinman WA, Singh G, Raufman JP. Isolation and characterization of exendin-4 an exendin-3 analogue, from Heloderma suspectum venom. Further evidence for an exendin receptor on dispersed acini from guinea pig pancreas. J Biol Chem 1992;267:7402-7405

[112] Nielsen LL, Baron AD. Pharmacology of exenatide (synthetic exendin-4) for the treatment of type 2 diabetes. Curr Opin Invest Drugs 2003;4:401-405

[113] Göke R, Fehmann HC, Linn T, *et al.* Exendin-4 is a high potency agonist and truncated exendin-(9–39)-amide an antagonist at the glucagon-like peptide 1-(7–36)-amide receptor of insulin-secreting beta cells. J Biol Chem 1993;268:19650-19655

[114] Thorens B, Porret A, Bühler L, Deng SP, Morel P, Widmann C. Cloning and functional expression of the human islet GLP-1 receptor. Demonstration that exendin-4 is an agonist and exendin-9(9–39) an antagonist of the receptor. Diabetes 1993;42:1678-1682

[115] Kolterman OG, Kim DD, Shen L, *et al.* Pharmacokinetics, pharmacodynamics, and safety of exenatide in patients with type 2 diabetes mellitus. Am J Health Syst Pharm 2005;62:173-181

[116] Parkes D, Jodka C, Smith P, *et al.* Pharmacokinetic actions of exendin-4 in the rat: comparison with glucagon-like peptide-1. Drug Dev Res 2001;53:260-267

[117] Iltz JL, Baker DE, Setter SM, Campbell RK. Exenatide: An incretin mimetic for the treatment of type 2 diabetes mellitus. Clin Therap 2006;28,5:652-665

[118] Degn KB, Brock B, Juhl CB, *et al.* Effect of intravenous infusion of exenatide (synthetic exendin-4) on glucose-dependent insulin secretion and counterregulation during hypoglycaemia. Diabetes 2004;53:2397-2403

[119] Egan JM, Clocquet AR, Elahi D. The insulinotropic effect of acute exendin-4 administered to humans: Comparison of nondiabetic state to type 2 diabetes. J Clin Endocrinol Metab 2002;87:1281-1290

[120] Buse JB, Henry RR, Han J, Kim DD, Fineman MS, Baron AD. Effects of exenatide (exendin-4) on glycemic control over 30 weeks in sulfonylurea-treated patients with type 2 diabetes. Diabetes Care 2004;27:2628-2635

[121] DeFronzo RA, Ratner RE, Han J, Kim DD, Fineman MS, Baron AD. Effects of exenatide (exendin-4) on glycemic control and weight over 30 weeks in metformin-treated patients with type 2 diabetes. Diabetes Care 2005;28:1092-1100

[122] Kendall DM, Riddle MC, Rosenstock J, *et al.* Effects of exenatide (exendin-4) on glycemic control over 30 weeks in patients with type 2 diabetes treated with metformin and a sulfonylurea. Diabetes Care 2005,28:1083-1091

[123] Schnabel CA, Wintle M, Kolterman O. Metabolic effects of the incretin mimetic exenatide in the treatment of type 2 diabetes. Vasc Health Risk Manag 2006;2,1:69-77

[124] Heine RJ, Van Gaal LF, Johns D, Mihm MJ, Widel MH, Brodows RG. Exenatide versus insulin glargine in patients with suboptimally controlled type 2 diabetes: a randomized trial. Ann Intern Med 2005;143:559-569

[125] Nauck MA, Duran S, Kim D, *et al.* A comparison of twice-daily exenatide and biphasic insulin aspart in patients with type 2 diabetes who were suboptimally controlled with sulfonylurea and metformin: a non-inferiority study. Diabetologia 2007;50:259-267

[126] Knudsen LB, Nielsen PF, Huusfeldt PO, *et al.* Potent derivatives of glucagon-like peptide-1 with pharmacokinetic properties suitable for once daily administration. J Med Chem 2000;43:1664-1669

[127] Madsbad S, Schmitz O, Ranstam J, *et al.* Improved glycemic control with no weight increase in patients with type 2 diabetes after once-daily treatment with the long acting glucagon-like peptide 1 analogue liraglutide (NN2211). Diabetes Care 2004;27:1335-1342

[128] Bregenholt S, Moldrup A, Blume N, *et al.* The long-acting glucagon-like peptide-1 analogue, liraglutide, inhibits beta-cell apoptosis in vitro. Biochem Biophys Res Commun 2005;330:577-584

[129] Nauck MA, Hompesch M, Filipczak R, Le TD, Zdravkovic M, Glumprecht J. Five weeks of treatment with the GLP-1 analogue liraglutide improves glycemic control and lowers weight in subjects with type 2 diabetes. Exp Clin Endocrinol Diabetes 2006;114:417-423

[130] Vilsbøll T, Zdravkovic M, Le-Thi T, *et al.* Liraglutide significantly improves glycemic control, and lowers body weight without risk of either major or minor hypoglycemic episodes in subjects with type 2 diabetes. Diabetes 2006;55,Suppl.1:27-28

[131] Vilsbøll T, Zdravkovic M, Le Thi T, *et al.* Liraglutide, a long-acting human glucagon-like peptide-1 analog, given as monotherapy significantly improves glycemic control and lowers body weight without risk of hypoglycemia in patients with type 2 diabetes. Diabetes Care 2007;30:1608-1610

[132] Deacon CF. Therapeutic strategies based on glucagon-like peptide 1. Diabetes 2004;53:2181-2189

[133] Villhauer EB, Brinkman JA, Naderi GB. 1-3[(3-hydroxy-1adamantyl)amino]acetyl]-2-cyano-(S)-pyrrolidine: a potent, selective, and orally bioavailable dipeptidyl peptidase IV inhibitor with antyhyperglycemic properties. J Med Chem 2003;46:2774-2789

[134] Deacon CF, Holst JJ. Dipeptidyl peptidase IV inhibition as an approach to the treatment and prevention of the type 2 diabetes. A historical perspective. Biochem Biophys Res Commun 2002;294:1-4

[135] Åhren B, Landin-Olsson M, Jansson PA, Svensson M, Holmes D, Schweizer A. Inhibition of dipeptidyl peptidase-4 reduces glycemia, sustains insulin levels, and reduces glucagon levels in type 2 diabetes. J Clin Endocrinol Metab 2004;89:2078-2084

[136] Herman GA, Stevens C, Van Dyck K. Pharmacokinetics and pharmacodynamics of sitagliptin, an inhibitor of dipeptidyl peptidase IV, in healthy subjects: results from two randomized double-blind, placebo-controlled studies with single oral doses. Clin Pharmacol Ther 2005;78:675-688

[137] Vilsbøll T, Agerso H, Krarup T, Holst JJ. Similar elimination rates of glucagon-like peptide-1 in obese type 2 diabetic patients and healthy subjects. J Clin Endocrinol Metab 2003;88:220-224

[138] Xu G, Stoffers DA, Habener JF, Bonner-Weir S. Exendin-4 stimulates both beta-cell replication and neogenesis, resulting in increased beta-cell mass and improved glucose tolerance in diabetic rats. Diabetes 1999;48:2270-2276

[139] He YL, Serra D, Wang Y, et al. Pharmacokinetics and pharmacodynamics of vildagliptin in patients with type 2 diabetes mellitus. Clin Pharmacokinet 2007;46:577-588

[140] He YL, Sadler BM, Sabo R, et al. The absolute oral bioavailability and population-based pharmacokinetic modelling of a novel dipeptidylpeptidase-IV inhibitor, vildagliptin, in healthy volunteers. Clin Pharmacokinet 2007;46:787-802

[141] Sunkara G, Sabo R, Wang Y, et al. Dose proportionality and the effect of food on vildagliptin, a novel dipeptidyl peptidase IV inhibitor, in healthy volunteers. J Clin Pharmacol 2007;47:1152-1158

[142] Pratley RE, Jauffret-Kamel S, Galbreath E, Holmes D. Twelve-week monotherapy with the DPP-4 inhibitor vildagliptin improves glycemic control in subjects with type 2 diabetes. Horm Metab Res 2006;38:423-428

[143] de Valk HW. DPP-4 inhibitors and combined treatment in type 2 diabetes: Re-evaluation of clinical success and safety. Rev Diabet Stud 2007;4:126-133

[144] Åhren B, Gomis R, Stundl E, Mills D, Schweizer A. Twelve- and 52-week efficacy of the dipeptidyl peptidase IV inhibitor LAF237 in metformin-treated patients with type 2 diabetes. Diabetes Care 2004;27:2874-2880

[145] Hayat AS, Shaikh N, Ali P, Shaikh TZ, Khan AH. Clinical efficacy of gliptins for glycemic control in type 2 diabetes mellitus. World Appl Sci J 2009;7,1:1-6

[146] Pi-Sunyer FX, Schweizer A, Mills D, et al. Efficacy and tolerability of vildagliptin monotherapy in drug-naïve patients with type 2 diabetes. Diabetes Res Clin Pract 2007;76:132-138

[147] Fonseca V, Schweizer A, Albrecht D, Baron MA, Chang I, Dejager S. Addition of vildagliptin to insulin improves glycemic control in type 2 diabetes. Diabetologia 2007;50:1148-1155

[148] Garber AJ, Schweizer A, Baron MA, et al. Vildagliptin in combination with pioglitazone improves glycemic control in patients with type 2 diabetes failing thiazolidinedione monotherapy: a randomized, placebo-controlled study. Diabetes Obes Metab 2007;9:166-174

[149] Herman GA, Stevens C, Van Dyck, et al. Pharmacokinetics and pharmacodynamics of sitagliptin, an inhibitor of dipeptidyl peptidase IV, in healthy subjects: results from two randomized double-blind, placebo controlled studies with single oral doses. Clin Pharmacol Ther 2005;78:675-688

[150] Xu L, Stein P, Brazg R, Sanchez M, Dalla Man C, Cobelli C. Sitagliptin, a novel dipeptidyl peptidase-4 inhibitor, improved B-cell function in patients with type 2 diabetes when added to metformin monotherapy. JDF 2006, Abstract 868

[151] Aschner P, Kipnes MS, Lunceford JK, et al. Effect of the dipeptidyl peptidase-4 inhibitor sitagliptin as monotherapy on glycemic control in patients with type 2 diabetes. Diabetes Care 2006;29:2632-2637

[152] Triplitt C, McGill JB, Porte D Jr, Conner CS. The changing landscape of type 2 diabetes: the role of incretin-based therapies and managed care outcomes. J Manag Care Pharm 2007;13:S2-S16

[153] Raz I, Hanefeld M, Xu L, et al. Efficacy and safety of the dipeptidyl peptidase-4 inhibitor sitagliptin as monotherapy in patients with type 2 diabetes mellitus. Diabetologia 2006;49:2564-2571

[154] Charbonnel B, Karasik A, Liu J, et al. Efficacy and safety of the dipeptidyl peptidase-4 inhibitor sitagliptin added to ongoing metformin therapy in patients with type 2 diabetes inadequately controlled with metformin alone. Diabetes Care 2006;29:2638-2643

[155] Rosenstock J, Brazg R, Andryuk PJ, et al. Efficacy and safety of the dipeptidyl peptidase-4 inhibitor sitagliptin added to ongoing pioglitazone therapy in patients with type 2 diabetes: a 24-week, multicenter, randomized, double-blinded, placebo-controlled, parallel-group study. Clin Ther 2006;28:1556-1568

[156] DeFronzo RA, Bonadonna RC, Ferannini E. Pathogenesis of NIDDM: a balanced overview. Diabetes Care 1992;15:318-368

[157] Moller DE. New drug targets for type 2 diabetes and the metabolic syndrome. Nature 2001;414,6865:821-827

[158] Bailey CJ, Turner RC. Metformin. N Engl J Med 1996;334:574-579

[159] Wollen N, Bailey CJ. Inhibition of hepatic gluconeogenesis by metformin. Synergism with insulin. Biochem Pharmacol 1988;37:4353-4358

[160] Stumvoll N, Nurjhan N, Perriello G, Dailey G, Gerich JE. Metabolic effects of metformin in non-insulin-dependent diabetes mellitus. N Engl J Med 1995;333:550-554

[161] Johnson AB, Webster JM, Sum CF, *et al.* The impact of metformin therapy on hepatic glucose production and skeletal muscle synthase activity in overweight type II diabetic patients. Metabol 1993;42:1217-1222

[162] Zangeneh F, Kudva YC, Basu A. Insulin sensitizers. Mayo Clin Proc 2003;78:471-479

[163] Radziuk J, Zhang Z, Wiernsperger N, Pye S. Effects of metformin on lactate uptake and gluconeogenesis in the perfused rat liver. Diabetes 1997;46:1406-1413

[164] He L, Sabet A, Djedjos S, *et al.* Metformin and insulin suppress hepatic gluconeogenesis by inhibiting cAMP signaling through phosphorylation of CREB binding protein (CBP). Cell 2009;137,4:635-646

[165] Argaud D, Roth H, Wiernsperger N, Leverve XM. Metformin decreases gluconeogenesis by enhancing the pyruvate kinase flux in isolated rat hepatocytes. Eur J Biochem 1993;213:1341-1348

[166] Large V, Beylot M. Modifications of citric acid cycle activity and gluconeogenesis in streptozotocin-induced diabetes and effects of metformin. Diabetes 1999;48:1251-1257

[167] Gunton JE, Delhanty PJD, Takahashi S-J, Baxter RC. Metformin rapidly increases insulin receptor activation in human liver and signals preferentially through insulin-receptor substrate-2. J Clin Endocrinol Metab 2003;88,3:1323-1332

[168] Hundal RS, Krssak M, Dufour S, *et al.* Mechanism by which metformin reduces glucose production in type 2 diabetes. Diabetes 2000;49:2063-2069

[169] Luna V, Casauban L, Sajan MP. Metformin improves atypical protein kinase C activation by insulin and phosphatidylinositol-3,4,5-(PO$_4$)$_3$ in muscle of diabetic subjects. Diabetologia 2006;49:375-382

[170] Mahvash Z, Dowling R, Fantus G, Sonenberg N, Pollak M. Metformin is an AMP kinase-dependent growth inhibitor for breast cancer cells. Obstet Gynecol Surv. 2007;62,3:182-183

[171] Rossetti L, DeFronzo RA, Gherzi R, *et al.* Effect of metformin treatment on insulin action in diabetic rats: *in vivo* and *in vitro* correlations. Metabol 1990;39:425-435

[172] Klip A, Leiter RA. Cellular mechanism of action of metformin. Diabetes Care 1990;13:696-704

[173] Zhou G, Meyers R, Li Y, *et al.* Role of AMP-activated protein kinase in mechanism of metformin action. J Clin Invest 2001;108:1167-1174

[174] Kim YB, Ciaraldi TP, Kong A, *et al.* Troglitazone but not metformin restores insulin-stimulated phosphoinositide 3-kinase activity and increases p110 beta protein levels in skeletal muscle of type 2 diabetic subjects. Diabetes 2002;51:443-448

[175] Matthaei S, Reibold JP, Hamann A, *et al. In vivo* metformin treatment ameliorates insulin resistance: evidence for potential of insulin-induced translocation and increased functional activity of glucose transporters in obese (*fa/fa*) Zucker rat adipocytes. Endocrinol 1993;133:304-311

[176] DeFronzo RA, Goodman AM. Efficacy of metformin in patients with non-insulin-dependent diabetes mellitus. The Multicenter Metformin Study Group. N Engl J Med 1995;333:541-549

[177] Poelje PD, Dang Q, Erion MD. Fructose-1,6-bisphosphatase as a therapeutic target for type 2 diabetes. Drug Disc Today Ther Strat 2007;4,2:103-109

[178] Clissold SP, Edwards C. Acarbose. A preliminary review of the pharmacodynamic and pharmacokinetic properties and therapeutic potential. Drugs 1988;35:214-243

[179] Lebovitz HE. A new oral therapy for diabetes management: alfa-glucosidase inhibition with acarbose. Clinical Diabetes 1995;13:99-103

[180] Hillebrand I, Boehme K, Frank G, Fink H, Berchtold P. The effect of the α-glucosidase inhibitor BAY g 5421 (Acarbose) on meal-stimulated elevations of circulating glucose, insulin, and triglyceride levels in man. Res Exp Med (Berl) 1979;179:81-86

[181] Bayraktar M, Van Thiel DH, Adalar N. A comparison of acarbose versus metformin as an adjuvant therapy in sulfonylurea-treated NIDDM patients. Diabetes Care 1996;19:252-254

[182] Van de Laar FA, Lucassen PLBJ, Akkermans RP, Ven de Lisdonk EH, Rutten GEHM, Van Weel C. Alpha-glucosidase inhibitors for type 2 diabetes mellitus. Cochrane Database Syst Rev 2005;2 Art. No.: CD003639, doi:10.1002/14651858.CD003639.pub.2

[183] Lebovitz HE, Banerji MA. Insulin resistance and its treatment by thiazolidinediones. Recent Progr Horm Res 2001;56:265-294

[184] Yu JG, Kruszynska YT, Mulford MI, Olefsky JM. A comparison of troglitazone and metformin on insulin requirements in euglycemic intensively insulin-treated type 2 diabetic patients. Diabetes 1999;48:2414-2421

[185] Cavaghan MK, Ehrmann DA, Byrne MM, Polonsky KS. Treatment with the oral antidiabetic agent troglitazone improves beta cell responses to glucose in subjects with impaired glucose tolerance. J Clin Invest 1997;100:530-537

[186] Buchanan TA, Xiang AH, Peters RK, *et al.* Response of pancreatic beta-cells to improved insulin sensitivity in women at high risk for type 2 diabetes. Diabetes 2000;49:782-788

[187] Joshi P. Oral hypoglycaemic drugs and newer agents use in Type 2 diabetes mellitus. SA Fam Pract 2009;51,1:10-16

[188] Luna B, Feinglos NN. Oral agents in the management of type 2 diabetes. Am Fam Physician 2001;63:1747-1756

[189] Mudaliar S, Henry RR. New oral therapies for type diabetes mellitus: The glitazones or insulin sensitizers. Ann Rev Med 2001;52:239-257

[190] MacIsaac RJ, Jerums G. Clinical indications for thiazolidinediones. Aust Prescr 2004;27:70-74

[191] Granberry MC, Hawkins JB, Franks AM. Thiazolidinediones in patients with type 2 diabetes and heart failure. Am J Health Syst Pharm 2007;64:931-936

[192] Ruder K. Type 2 drug up risk of fractures. Diabetes Forecast 2007;60:29-30

[193] Davis SN. Insulin, hypoglycaemic agents, and the pharmacology of the endocrine pancreas. In: Brunton LL, Parker KL, et al, eds.: Goodman & Gilman's The Pharmacological Basis of Therapeutics, 11th ed. McGraw Hill, New York, NY. 2006:1613-1646

[194] van den Heuvel LP, Assiak K, Willemsen M, Monnens L. Autosomal recessive renal glucosuria attributable to a mutation in the sodium glucose cotransporter (SGLT2) Hum Genet 2002;111:544-547

[195] Calado J, Soto K, Clemente C, Correia P, Rueff J. Novel compound heterozygous mutations in *SLC5A2* are responsible for autosomal recessive renal glucosuria. Hum Genet 2004;114:314-316

[196] Turk E, Zabel B, Mundlos S, Dyer J, Wright EM. Glucose/galactose malabsorption caused by a defect in the Na^+/glucose cotransporter. Nature (Lond) 1991;350:354-356

[197] Martin MG, Turk E, Lostao MP, Kerner C, Wright EM. Defects in Na^+/glucose cotransporter (SGLT1) trafficking and function cause glucose-galactose malabsorption. Nat Genet 1996;12:216-220

[198] Katsumo K, Fujimori Y, Takemura Y, *et al.* Sergliflozin, a novel selective inhibitor of low-affinity sodium glucose cotransporter (SGLT2), validates a critical role of SGLT2 in renal glucose reabsorption and modulates plasma glucose level. J Pharmacol Exp Ther 2007;320,1:323-330

[199] Han S, Hagan DL, Taylor JR, *et al.* Dapagliflozin, a selective SGLT2 inhibitor, improves glucose homeostasis in normal and diabetic rats. Diabetes 2008;57:1723-1729

[200] Peraldi P, Xu M, Spiegelman BM. Thiazolidinediones block tumor necrosis factor-alpha-induced inhibition of insulin signaling. J Clin Invest 1997;100,7:1863-1869

[201] Stuart CA, Howell MEA, Yin D. Overexpression of GLUT5 in diabetic muscle is reversed by pioglitazone. Diabetes Care 2007;30,4:925-931

[202] DeFronzo RA, Jacot E, Jequier F, Maeder E, Wahren J, Felber JP. The effect of insulin on the disposal of intravenous glucose. Results from indirect colorimetry and hepatic and femoral venous catheterization. Diabetes 1981;30:1000-1007

[203] Tuomilehto J, Lindstrom J, Eriksson JG, *et al.* Prevention of Type 2 diabetes mellitus by changes in lifestyle among subjects with impaired glucose tolerance. N Engl J Med 2001;344:1343-1350

[204] Jessen N, Goodyear LJ. Contraction signaling to glucose transport in skeletal muscle. J Appl Physiol 2005;99:330-337

[205] Sato Y, Nagasaki M, Nakai N, Fushimi T. Physical exercise improves glucose metabolism in lifestyle-related diseases. Exp Biol Med 2003;228:1208-1212

[206] Borghouts LB, Keizer HA. Exercise and insulin sensitivity: a review. Int J Sports Med 2000;21:1-12

[207] Oshida Y, Ohsawa I, Sato J, *et al.* Effects of different types of physical training on insulin action in human peripheral tissues – use of the euglycemic clamp technic. Jap J Physical Fit Sports Med 1991;40:315-320

[208] Minuk H, Vranic M, Marliss E, Hanno A, Albisser A, Zinman B. Glucoregulatory and metabolic response to exercise in obese noninsulin-dependent diabetes. Am J Physiol 1981;240:E458-E464

[209] Giacca A, Groenewoud Y, Tsui E, McClean P, Zinman B. Glucose production, utilization, and cycling in response to moderate exercise in obese subjects with type 2 diabetes and mild hyperglycemia. Diabetes 1998;47:1763-1770

[210] McGee SL, Hargreaves M. Exercise and skeletal muscle glucose transporter 4 expression: molecular mechanisms. Clin Exp Pharmacol Physiol 2006;33:395-399

[211] Devlin JT, Hirshman M, Horton ED, Horton ES. Enhanced peripheral and splenchnic insulin sensitivity in NIDDM men after single bout of exercise. Diabetes 1987;36:434-439

[212] Winnick JJ, Sherman WM, Habash DL, *et al.* Short-term aerobic exercise training in obese humans with type 2 diabetes mellitus improves whole-body insulin sensitivity through gains in peripheral not hepatic insulin sensitivity. J Clin Endocrinol Metab 2008;93:771-778

[213]   Henriksen EJ. Effects of acute exercise and exercise training on insulin resistance. J Appl Physiol 2002;93:788-796

[214]   Nesher R, Karl IE, Kipnis DM. Dissociation of effects of insulin and contraction on glucose transport in rat epitrochlearis muscle. Am J Physiol Cell Physiol 1985;249:C226-C232

[215]   Holloszy JO, Narahara HT. Studies of tissue permeability. X changes in permeability to 3-methylglucose associated with contraction of frog muscle. J Biol Chem 1965;240:3493-3500

[216]   Suarez E, Bach D, Cadefau J, Palacin M, Zorzano A, Guma A. A novel role of neuregulin in skeletal muscle. Neuregulin stimulates glucose uptake, glucose transporter translocation, and transporter expression in muscle cells. J Biol Chem 2001;276:18257-18264

[217]   Sakamoto K, Goodyear LJ. Intracellular signaling in contracting skeletal muscle. J Appl Physiol 2002;93:369-383

[218]   Holten MK, Zacho M, Gaster M, Juel C, Wojtaszewski JF, Dela F. Strength training increases insulin-mediated glucose uptake, GLUT4 content, and insulin signaling in skeletal muscle in patients with type 2 diabetes. Diabetes 2004;53,2:294-305

[219]   Daugaard JR, Nielsen JN, Kristiansen S, Andersen JL, Hargreaves M, Richter EA. Fiber type-specific expression of GLUT4 in human skeletal muscle: influence of exercise training. Diabetes 2000;49,7:1092-1095

[220]   Ivy JL, Kuo C-H. Regulation of GLUT4 protein and glycogen synthase during muscle glycogen synthesis after exercise. Acta Physiol Scand 1998;162:295-304

[221]   Gulve EA, Spina RJ. Effect of 7-10 days of cycle ergometer exercise on skeletal muscle GLUT-4 protein content. J Appl Physiol 1995;79:1562-1566

[222]   Houmard JA, Hickey MS, Tyndall GL, Gavigan GL, Dohm GL. Seven days of exercise increase GLUT-4 protein content in human skeletal muscle. J Appl Physiol 1995;79:1936-1938

[223]   Philips SM, Han XX, Green HJ, Bonen A. Increments in skeletal muscle GLUT-1 and GLUT-4 after endurance training in humans. Am J Physiol 1996;270:E456-E462

[224]   Neufer PD, Dohm GL. Exercise induces a transient increase in transcription of the GLUT-4 gene in skeletal muscle. Am J Physiol 1993;265:C1597-C1603

[225]   Kraniou Y, Cameron-Smith D, Misso M, Collier G, Hargreaves M. Effects of exercise on GLUT-4 and glycogenin gene expression in human skeletal muscle. J Appl Physiol 2000;88:794-796

[226]   Kraniou GN, Cameron-Smith D, Hargreaves M. Effect of short-term training on GLUT-4 mRNA and protein expression in human skeletal muscle. Exp Physiol 2004;89,5:559-563

[227]   Chang L, Chiang SH, Saltiel AR. TC10 alpha is required for insulin-stimulated glucose uptake in adipocytes. Endocrinol 2007;148,1:27-33

[228]   Ojuka EO, Jones TE, Nolte LA, *et al.* Regulation of GLUT-4 biogenesis in muscle: evidence for involvement of AMPK and Ca^{2+}. Am J Physiol Endocrinol Metab 2002;282:E1008-E1013

[229]   Kuo CH, Rowning KS, Ivy JL. Regulation of GLUT4 protein expression and glycogen storage after prolonged exercise. Acta Physiol Scand 1999;165:193-201

[230]   Thai MV, Guruswamy S, Cao KT, Pessin JE, Olson AL. Myocyte enhancer factor 2 (MEF2)-binding site is required for GLUT4 gene expression in transgenic mice. Regulation of MEF2 DNA binding activity in insulin-deficient diabetes. J Biol Chem 1998;273:14285-14292

[231]   Oshel K, Knight J, Cao K, Thai M, Olson A. Identification of a 30-base pair regulatory element and novel DNA binding protein that regulates the human GLUT4 promoter in transgenic mice. J Biol Chem 2000;275:2366-23673

[232]   Knight JB, Eyster CA, Grisel BA, Olson AL. Regulation of the human GLUT4 gene promoter: Interaction between a transcriptional activator and myocyte enhancer factor 2A. Proc Natl Acad Sci USA 2003;100:14725-14730

[233]   Moreno H, Serrano AI, Santalucia T, *et al.* Differential regulation of the muscle-specific GLUT4 enhancer in regenerating and adult skeletal muscle. J Biol Chem 2003;278:40557-40564

[234]   McKinsey TA, Zhang CL, Olson EN. MEF2: A calcium-dependent regulator of cell division, differentiation and death. Trends Biochem Sci 2002;27:40-47

[235]   McGee SL, Hargreaves M. Exercise and myocyte enhancer factor 2 regulation in human skeletal muscle. Diabetes 2004;53:1208-1214

[236]   Lund S, Holman GD, Schmitz O, Pedersen O. Contraction stimulates translocation of glucose transporter GLUT4 in skeletal muscle through a mechanism distinct from that of insulin. Proc Natl Acad Sci USA 1995;92:5817-5821

[237]   Kirwan JP, del Aguila LF. Insulin signalling, exercise and cellular integrity. Biochem Soc Trans 2003;31,(Pt6):1281-1285

[238]   Richter EA, Mikines KJ, Galbo H, Kiens B. Effect of exercise on insulin action in human skeletal muscle. J Appl Physiol 1989;66:876-885

[239]   Holloszy JO, Constable SH, Young DA. Activation of glucose transport in muscle by exercise. Diabetes Metab Rev 1986;1:409-423

[240] Perrini S, Henrikson J, Zierath ZR, Widegren U. Exercise-induced protein kinase C isoform-specific activation in human skeletal muscle. Diabetes 2004;53:21-24

[241] Nielsen JN, Frosig C, Sajan MP, *et al.* Increased atypical PKC activity in endurance-trained human skeletal muscle. Biochem Biophys Res Commun 2003;312:1147-1153

[242] Kannel WB. Role of diabetes in cardiac disease: conclusions from population studies. In: Diabetes and the Heart, Zonaraich S ed., Springfield IL. 1978:97-112

[243] Sprafka JM, Burke GL, Folsom AR, McGovern PG, Hahn LP. Trends in prevalence of diabetes mellitus in patients with myocardial infarction and effect of diabetic survival: the Minnesota Heart Survey. Diabetes Care 1991;14:537-543

[244] Stanley WC, Hall JL, Smith KR, Cartee GD, Hacker TA, Wisneski JA. Myocardial glucose transporters and glycolytic metabolism during ischemia in hyperglycemic diabetes swine. Metabolism 1994;43:61-69

[245] Nadeau A, Rousseau-Migneron S, Tancrede G. Exercise training improves early survival rate in diabetic rats submitted to acute coronary artery ligation. Diabetes Care 1988;9:37-40

[246] Kainulainen H, Virtanen P, Ruskoaho H, Takala TES. Training increases cardiac glucose uptake during rest and exercise in rats. Am J Physiol 1989;257 (Heart Circ Physiol. 26): H839-H845

[247] Paulson DJ, Mathews R, Bowman J, Zhao J. Metabolic effects of treadmill exercise training in the diabetic heart. J Appl Physiol 1992;73:265-271

[248] Hall JL, Sexton WL, Stanley WC. Exercise training attenuates the reduction in myocardial GLUT-4 in diabetic rats. J Appl Physiol 1995;78:76-81

[249] Osborn BA, Daar JT, Laddaga RA, Romano FD, Paulson DJ. Exercise training increases sarcolemmal GLUT-4 protein and mRNA content in diabetic heart. J Appl Physiol 1997;82,3:828-834

[250] Folli F, Saad MJA, Backer JM, Kahn CR, Saad MJ. Insulin stimulation of phosphatidylinositol 3-kinase activity and association with insulin receptor substrate 1 in liver and muscle of the intact rat. J Biol Chem 1992;267:22171-22177

[251] Goodyear LJ, Giorgino F, Balon TW, Condorelli G, Smith RJ. Effects of contractile activity on tyrosine phosphoproteins and phosphatidylinositol 3-kinase activity in rat skeletal muscle. Am J Physiol Endocrinol Metab 1995;268:E987-995

[252] Kemp BE, Mitchelhill KJ, Stapleton D, Michell BJ, Chen ZP, Witters LA. Dealing with energy demand: the AMP-activated protein kinase. Trends Biochem Sci 1999;24:22-25

[253] Rasmussen BB, Hancock CR, Winder WW. Postexercise recovery of skeletal muscle malonyl-CoA, acetyl-CoA carboxylase, and AMP-activated protein kinase. J Appl Physiol 1998;85:1629-1634

[254] Goodyear LJ, Chang PY, Sherwood DJ, Dufresne SD, Moller DE. Effects of exercise and insulin on mitogen-activated protein kinase signaling pathways in rat skeletal muscle. Am J Physiol Endocrinol Metab 1996;271:E403-E408

[255] Fujii N, Hayashi T, Hirshman MF, *et al.* Exercise induces isoform-specific increase in 5'AMP-activated protein kinase activity in human skeletal muscle. Biochem Biophys Res Commun 2000;273:1150-1155

[256] Chen ZP, McConell GK, Michell BJ, Snow RJ, Canny BJ, Kemp BE. AMPK signaling in contracting human skeletal muscle: acetyl-CoA carboxylase and NO synthase phosphorylation. Am J Physiol Endocrinol Metab 2000;279:E1202-E1206

[257] Hayashi T, Hirshman MF, Dufresne SD, Goodyear LJ. Skeletal muscle contractile activity *in vitro* stimulates mitogen-activated protein kinase signaling. Am J Physiol Cell Physiol 1999;277:C701-C707

[258] Ryder JW, Fahlman R, Wellberg-Henriksson H, Alessi DR, Krook A, Zierath JR. Effect of contraction on mitogen-activated protein kinase signal transduction in skeletal muscle. J Biol Chem 2000;275:1457-1462

[259] Martineau LC, Gardiner PF. Insight mechanotransduction: MAPK activation is quantitavely related to tension. J Appl Physiol 2001;91:693-702

[260] Nader GA, Esser KA. Intracellular signaling specificity in skeletal muscle in response to different modes of exercise. J Appl Physiol 2001;90:1936-1942

[261] Boppart MD, Hirshman MF, Sakamoto K, Fielding RA, Goodyear LJ. Static stretch increases c-Jun NH_2-terminal kinase activity and p38 phosphorylation in rat skeletal muscle. Am J Physiol Cell Physiol 2001;280:C352-C358

[262] Dufresne SD, Bjorbaek C, El Haschimi K, *et al.* Altered extracellular signal-regulated kinase signaling and glycogen metabolism in skeletal muscle from p90 ribosomal S6 kinase 2 knockout mice. Mol Cell Biol 2001;21:81-87

[263] Aronson D, Violan MA, Dufresne SD, Zangen D, Fielding RA. Foodyear LJ. Exercise stimulates the mitogen-activated protein kinase pathway in human skeletal muscle. J Clin Invest 1997;99:1251-1257

[264] Aronson D, Dufresne SD, Goodyear LJ. Contractile activity stimulates the c-Jun NH_2-terminal kinase pathway in rat skeletal muscle. J Biol Chem 1997;272:25636-25640

[265] Aronson D, Boppart MD, Dufresne SD, Fielding RA, Goodyear LJ. Exercise stimulates c-Jun NH_2-terminal kinase activity and c-Jun transcriptional activity in human skeletal muscle. Biochem Biophys Res Commun 1998;251:106-110

[266] Boppart MD, Asp S, Wojtaszewski JF, Fielding RA, Mohr T, Goodyear LJ. Marathon running transiently increases c-Jun NH_2-terminal kinase and p38 activities in human skeletal muscle. J Physiol 2000;526:663-669

[267] Somwar R, Perreault M, Kapur S, *et al.* Activation of p38 mitogen-activated protein kinase α and β by insulin and contraction in rat skeletal muscle: potential role in the stimulation of glucose transport. Diabetes 2000;49:1794-1800

[268] Wretman C, Lionikas A, Widegren U, Lannergren J, Westerblad H, Henriksson J. Effects of concentric and eccentric contractions on phosphorylation of $MAPK^{erk1/2}$ and $MAPK^{p38}$ in isolated rat skeletal muscle. J Physiol 2001;535:155-164

[269] Widegren U, Jiang XJ, Krook A, *et al.* Divergent effects of exercise on metabolic and mitogenic signaling pathways in human skeletal muscle. FASEB J 1998;12:1379-1389

[270] Merall NW, Plevin RJ, Stokoe D, Cohen P, Nebreda AR, Gould GW. Mitogen-activated protein kinase (MAP kinase), MAP kinase kinase and c-Mos stimulate glucose transport in Xenopus oocytes. Biochem J 1993;295:351-355

[271] Hayashi T, Hirshman MF, Kurth EJ, Winder WW, Goodyear LJ. Evidence for 5' AMP-activated protein kinase mediation of the effect of muscle contraction on glucose transport. Diabetes 1998;47:1369-1373

[272] Banks EA, Brozinick JT Jr, Yaspelkis BB III, Kang HY, Ivy JL. Muscle glucose transport, GLUT-4 content, and degree of exercise in obese Zucker rats. Am J Physiol Endocrinol Metab 1992;263:E1010-E1015

[273] Brozinick JT Jr, Etgen GJ, Yaspelkis BB III, Kang HY, Ivy JL. Effects of exercise training on muscle GLUT-4 protein content and translocation in obese Zucker rats. Am J Physiol Endocrinol Metab 1993;265:E419-E427

[274] Etgen GJ, Jensen J, Wilson CM, Hunt DG, Cushman SW, Ivy JL. Exercise training reverses insulin resistance in muscle by enhanced recruitment of GLUT-4 to the cell surface. Am J Physiol Endocrinol Metab 1997;272:E864-E869

[275] Holoszy JO, Constable SH, Young DA. Activation of glucose transport in muscle by exercise. Diabetes Metab Rev 1986;1:409-424

[276] Holoszy JO, Hansen PA. Regulation of glucose transport into skeletal muscle. Rev Physiol Biochem Pharmacol 1996;128:99-193

[277] Krogh A, Lindhard J. The relative value of fat and carbohydrate as sources of muscular energy. Biochem J 1920;14:290-363

[278] Laurent D, Hundal RS, Dresner A, *et al.* Mechanism of muscle glycogen autoregulation in humans. Am J Physiol Endocrinol Metab 2000;278,4:E663-E668

[279] Coyle EF, Jeukendrup AF, Oseto MC, Hodgkinson B, Zderic TW. Low-diet alters intramuscular substrates and reduces lipolysis and fat oxidation during exercise. Am J Physiol Endocrinol Metab 2001;280,3:E391-E398

[280] Kiens B, Helge JW. Effect of high-fat diets on exercise performance. Proc Nutr Soc 1998;57,1:73-75

[281] Jeukendrup AE. Modulation of carbohydrate and fat utilization by diet, exercise and environment. Biochem Soc Trans 2003;31,6:1270-1273

[282] Kahn BB. Dietary regulation of glucose transporter gene expression: tissue specific effects in adipose cells and muscle. J Nutr 1994;124:1289S-1295S

[283] Kraegen EW, James DE, Storlien LH, Burleigh KM, Chisholm DJ. *In vivo* insulin resistance in individual peripheral tissues of the high fat fed rats: assessment by euglycemic clamp plus deoxyglucose administration. Diabetologia 1986:29;192-198

[284] Penicaud L, Kande J, Le Magnen J, Girand JR. Insulin action during fasting and refeeding in rat determined by euglycemic clamp. Am J Physiol 1985;249:E514-E518

[285] Kahn BB, Pedersen O. Suppression of GLUT4 expression in skeletal muscle of rats which are obese from high fat feeding but not from high carbohydrate feeding or genetic obesity. Endocrinol 1993;132:13-22

[286] Kahn BB, Cushman SW, Flier JS. Regulation of glucose transporter specific mRNA levels in rat adipose cells with fasting and refeeding: Implications for *in vivo* control of glucose transporter number. J Clin Invest 1989;33:199-204

[287] American Diabetes Association. Standards of medical care in diabetes. Diabetes Care 2008;31:S12-S54

[288] American Diabetes Association. Nutrition recommendations and interventions for diabetes: a position statement of the American Diabetes Association. Diabetes Care 2008;31:S61-S78

[289] Carey VJ, Walters EE, Colditz GA, *et al.* Body fat distribution and risk of non-insulin-dependent diabetes mellitus in women. Am J Epidemiol 1997;145:614-619

[290] Lyen KR. The insulin receptor. Ann Acad Med Singapore 1985;14:364-371

[291] Olefsky JM, Koltermann OG, Scarlett JA. Insulin action and resistance in obesity and non-insulin-dependent type II diabetes mellitus. Am J Physiol 1982;243:E15-E30

[292] Beck-Nielson H, Pederson O, Lindkov HO. Normalization of insulin sensitivity and the cellular insulin binding during treatment of diabetics for one year. Acta Endocrinol (Copenh) 1979;90:103-112

[293] Pedersen O, Hjollund E, Sorensen NS. Insulin receptor binding and insulin action in human fat cells, effects of obesity and fasting. Metabol 1982;31:884-895

[294] Anderson JW, Kendall CWC, Jenkins DJA. Importance of weight management in type 2 diabetes: review with meta-analysis of clinical studies. J Am Coll Nutr 2003;22,5:331-339

[295] Colditz GA, Willett WC, Stampfer MJ, *et al.* Weight as a risk factor for clinical diabetes in women. Am J Epidemiol 1990;132:501-513

[296] Nielsen JV, Joensson E. Low-carbohydrate diet in type 2 diabetes stable improvement of bodyweight and glycemic control during 22 months follow-up. Nutr Metabol 2006;3:22, doi:10.1186/1743-7075-3-22

[297] Hu FB, Manson JE, Stampfer MJ, *et al.* Diet, lifestyle, and the risk of type 2 diabetes mellitus in women. N Engl J Med 2001;345,11:790-797

[298] Zierath JR, Houseknecht KL, Gnudi L, Kahn BB. High-fat feeding impairs insulin-stimulated GLUT4 recruitment via an early insulin-signaling defect. Diabetes 1997;46:215-223

[299] Cerf ME. High fat diet modulation of glucose sensing in the beta-cell. Med Sci Monit 2007;13,1:RA12-17

[300] Kahn SE, Hull RL, Utzschneider KM. Mechanisms linking obesity to insulin resistance and type 2 diabetes. Nature 2006;444:840-846

[301] Kahn BB, Flier JS. Obesity and insulin resistance. J Clin Invest 2000;106,4:473-481

[302] Hu G, Lindström J, Valle TT, *et al.* Physical activity, body mass index, and risk of type 2 diabetes in patients with normal and impaired glucose regulation. Arch Int Med 2004;164,8:892-896

[303] Zorzano A, Palacín M, Gumà A. Mechanisms regulating GLUT4 glucose transporter expression and glucose transport in skeletal muscle. Acta Physiol Scand 2005;183:43-58

Index

Printed in Poland
by Amazon Fulfillment
Poland Sp. z o.o., Wrocław